Prevention, Diagnosis and Treatments of Early-Stage NSCLC: New Advances and Future Prospective

Prevention, Diagnosis and Treatments of Early-Stage NSCLC: New Advances and Future Prospective

Guest Editor

Monica Casiraghi

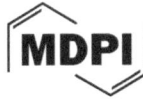

Basel • Beijing • Wuhan • Barcelona • Belgrade • Novi Sad • Cluj • Manchester

Guest Editor
Monica Casiraghi
Department of Thoracic Surgery
European Institute of Oncology-IEO
Milan
Italy

Editorial Office
MDPI AG
Grosspeteranlage 5
4052 Basel, Switzerland

This is a reprint of the Special Issue, published open access by the journal *Journal of Clinical Medicine* (ISSN 2077-0383), freely accessible at: https://www.mdpi.com/journal/jcm/special_issues/17359Y35JL.

For citation purposes, cite each article independently as indicated on the article page online and as indicated below:

Lastname, A.A.; Lastname, B.B. Article Title. *Journal Name* **Year**, *Volume Number*, Page Range.

ISBN 978-3-7258-3419-8 (Hbk)
ISBN 978-3-7258-3420-4 (PDF)
https://doi.org/10.3390/books978-3-7258-3420-4

© 2025 by the authors. Articles in this book are Open Access and distributed under the Creative Commons Attribution (CC BY) license. The book as a whole is distributed by MDPI under the terms and conditions of the Creative Commons Attribution-NonCommercial-NoDerivs (CC BY-NC-ND) license (https://creativecommons.org/licenses/by-nc-nd/4.0/).

Contents

About the Editor vii

Ian Diebels, Marc Dubois and Paul E. Y. Van Schil
Sublobar Resection for Early-Stage Lung Cancer: An Oncologically Valid Procedure?
Reprinted from: *J. Clin. Med.* **2023**, 12, 2674, https://doi.org/10.3390/jcm12072674 1

Monica Casiraghi, Francesco Petrella, Claudia Bardoni, Shehab Mohamed, Giulia Sedda, Juliana Guarize, et al.
Surgically Treated pT2aN0M0 (Stage IB) Non-Small Cell Lung Cancer: A 20-Year Sin-Gle-Center Retrospective Study
Reprinted from: *J. Clin. Med.* **2023**, 12, 2081, https://doi.org/10.3390/jcm12052081 5

Filippo Lococo, Dania Nachira, Marco Chiappetta, Isabella Sperduti, Maria Teresa Congedo, Elisa Meacci, et al.
Rate and Predictors of Unforeseen PN1/PN2-Disease in Surgically Treated cN0 NSCLC-Patients with Primary Tumor > 3 cm: Nationwide Results from Italian VATS-Group Database
Reprinted from: *J. Clin. Med.* **2023**, 12, 2345, https://doi.org/10.3390/jcm12062345 15

Beatrice Trabalza Marinucci, Cecilia Menna, Paolo Scanagatta, Silvia Fiorelli, Matteo Tiracorrendo, Giuseppe Naldi, et al.
Do More with Less? Lobectomy vs. Segmentectomy for Patients with Congenital Pulmonary Malformations
Reprinted from: *J. Clin. Med.* **2023**, 12, 5237, https://doi.org/10.3390/jcm12165237 26

Lisa Jungblut, Harry Etienne, Caroline Zellweger, Alessandra Matter, Miriam Patella, Thomas Frauenfelder and Isabelle Opitz
Swiss Pilot Low-Dose CT Lung Cancer Screening Study: First Baseline Screening Results
Reprinted from: *J. Clin. Med.* **2023**, 12, 5771, https://doi.org/10.3390/jcm12185771 37

Nicole Asemota, Alessandro Maraschi, Savvas Lampridis, John Pilling, Juliet King, Corinne Le Reun and Andrea Bille
Comparison of Quality of Life after Robotic, Video-Assisted, and Open Surgery for Lung Cancer
Reprinted from: *J. Clin. Med.* **2023**, 12, 6230, https://doi.org/10.3390/jcm12196230 47

Giulia Fabbri, Federico Femia, Savvas Lampridis, Eleonora Farinelli, Alessandro Maraschi, Tom Routledge and Andrea Bille
Long-Term Oncologic Outcomes in Robot-Assisted and Video-Assisted Lobectomies for Non-Small Cell Lung Cancer
Reprinted from: *J. Clin. Med.* **2023**, 12, 6609, https://doi.org/10.3390/jcm12206609 62

Jolanta Smok-Kalwat, Paulina Mertowska, Izabela Korona-Głowniak, Sebastian Mertowski, Paulina Niedźwiedzka-Rystwej, Dominika Bębnowska, et al.
Enhancing Immune Response in Non-Small-Cell Lung Cancer Patients: Impact of the 13-Valent Pneumococcal Conjugate Vaccine
Reprinted from: *J. Clin. Med.* **2024**, 13, 1520, https://doi.org/10.3390/jcm13051520 75

Jolanta Smok-Kalwat, Paulina Mertowska, Sebastian Mertowski, Stanisław Góźdź, Izabela Korona-Głowniak, Wojciech Kwaśniewski and Ewelina Grywalska
Analysis of Selected Toll-like Receptors in the Pathogenesis and Advancement of Non-Small-Cell Lung Cancer
Reprinted from: *J. Clin. Med.* **2024**, 13, 2793, https://doi.org/10.3390/jcm13102793 97

Jibran Ahmad Khan, Ibrahem Albalkhi, Sarah Garatli and Marcello Migliore
Recent Advancements in Minimally Invasive Surgery for Early Stage Non-Small Cell Lung Cancer: A Narrative Review
Reprinted from: *J. Clin. Med.* **2024**, *13*, 3354, https://doi.org/10.3390/jcm13113354 . . . . **122**

Ilaria Attili, Riccardo Asnaghi, Davide Vacirca, Riccardo Adorisio, Alessandra Rappa, Alberto Ranghiero, et al.
Co-Occurring Driver Genomic Alterations in Advanced Non-Small-Cell Lung Cancer (NSCLC): A Retrospective Analysis
Reprinted from: *J. Clin. Med.* **2024**, *13*, 4476, https://doi.org/10.3390/jcm13154476 . . . . **135**

Beatrice Trabalza Marinucci, Alessandra Siciliani, Claudio Andreetti, Matteo Tiracorrendo, Fabiana Messa, Giorgia Piccioni, et al.
Mini-Invasive Thoracic Surgery for Early-Stage Lung Cancer: Which Is the Surgeon's Best Approach for Video-Assisted Thoracic Surgery?
Reprinted from: *J. Clin. Med.* **2024**, *13*, 6447, https://doi.org/10.3390/jcm13216447 . . . . **148**

Luis Gerardo García-Herreros, Enid Ximena Rico-Rivera and Olga Milena García Morales
Two-Year Experience of a Center of Excellence for the Comprehensive Management of Non-Small Cell Lung Cancer at a Fourth-Level Hospital in Bogota, Colombia: Observational Case Series Study and Retrospective Analysis
Reprinted from: *J. Clin. Med.* **2024**, *13*, 6820, https://doi.org/10.3390/jcm13226820 . . . . **159**

About the Editor

Monica Casiraghi

Dr. Monica Casiraghi is the Deputy Director of the Division of Thoracic Surgery at the European Institute of Oncology in Milan and Assistant Professor of the Department of Oncology and Hemato-Oncology at the University of Milan, Italy. Since 2008, she has worked at the European Institute of Oncology in Milan where she became an expert in minimally invasive techniques such as robotic surgery. She obtained her Ph.D. at Alma Mater Studiorum—University of Bologna in March 2021. Dr. Casiraghi serves as the editor and reviewer of a number of international journals. She is a board member of the Thoracic Domain, chair of the Surgical Oncology task force of the EACTS, and a member of the ESTS Robotic Working Group and Women in General Thoracic Surgery.

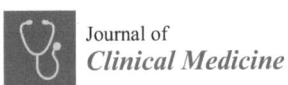

Editorial

Sublobar Resection for Early-Stage Lung Cancer: An Oncologically Valid Procedure?

Ian Diebels [1], Marc Dubois [1] and Paul E. Y. Van Schil [2,*]

[1] Department of Thoracic and Vascular Surgery, Heilig Hart Ziekenhuis, 2500 Lier, Belgium
[2] Department of Thoracic and Vascular Surgery, Antwerp University Hospital, 2650 Edegem, Belgium
* Correspondence: paul.van.schil@uza.be

Keywords: non-small-cell lung cancer (NSCLC); minimally invasive surgery; sublobar resection; segmentectomy; wedge excision; lobectomy

In the era of minimally invasive surgery, the role of sublobar resection comprising anatomical segmentectomy and wide wedge excision remains controversial. Its precise role from an oncological point of view still has to be exactly defined. Theoretically, a less invasive resection should lead to overall better post-operative respiratory function. However, until recently, hard evidence of survival equality or benefit over lobectomy was still lacking. Thus, lobectomy has been the preferred treatment of choice for most non-small cell lung cancer (NSCLC). Recently, two milestone trials have investigated the role of sublobar resection in the treatment of NSCLC.

The surgical goal of oncologic resections is achieving a microscopically complete resection (R0), which can be defined by free resection margins as per the latest, eighth edition of the tumour, node, metastasis (TNM) classification [1]. Correct staging is crucial as it determines treatment modalities and prognostic relevance [2]. Hence, it is concerning that local or regional recurrences still occur in R0 resected patients. Therefore, according to published guidelines, standard tumour resection and lymph node (LN) dissection are necessary to ensure true complete resection and correct evaluation in clinical trials. For this reason, the 2005 Complete Resection Subcommittee of the International Association for the Study of Lung Cancer (IASLC) proposed adding an additional stratification term, 'uncertain resection R(un)' [3]. R(un) is defined as a resection of a lung cancer with margins free of microscopic disease, but one of the following is present: incomplete LN dissection according to the standard systematic or lobe-specific criteria, metastasis in the highest resected mediastinal LN, carcinoma in situ confirmed at the bronchial resection margin, or positive cytology obtained during intraoperative pleural lavage [3]. The clinical significance of R(un) was confirmed by a re-analysis of 14,712 patients from the IASLC database, based on the previously mentioned criteria, whereby 57% of the R0 resections had to be reclassified to R(un). The R descriptor has an important impact on prognosis. In the conventional resection (R) status analysis, the 5-year overall survival (OS) was 73% for R0, which decreased to 36% for R1- and 28% for R2 resections. However, when the R0 dataset was reanalysed, now including R(un) with a positive highest resected LN, the 5-year OS for R0 resection was 55% while for R(un), it was only 45% [4]. The prognostic significance of the R factor is further analysed in other trials.

The first sublobar, landmark prospective randomised trial by Ginsberg et al., published in 1995, showed the inferiority of sublobar resection. The study included patients with a peripheral cT1N0 (<3 cm) lung cancer who were intraoperatively randomised between sublobar resections (n = 122, of which 82 were segmentectomies) and lobectomy (n = 125) [5]. Interestingly, 50% of NSCLC patients were excluded intraoperatively due to tumour size >3 cm, tumour location or configuration, or positive mediastinal LNs. A sublobar resection demonstrated a three-fold increase in the local recurrence rate (*p* = 0.008). A 30% increase in

Citation: Diebels, I.; Dubois, M.; Van Schil, P.E.Y. Sublobar Resection for Early-Stage Lung Cancer: An Oncologically Valid Procedure? *J. Clin. Med.* **2023**, *12*, 2674. https://doi.org/10.3390/jcm12072674

Received: 22 February 2023
Revised: 18 March 2023
Accepted: 20 March 2023
Published: 3 April 2023

Copyright: © 2023 by the authors. Licensee MDPI, Basel, Switzerland. This article is an open access article distributed under the terms and conditions of the Creative Commons Attribution (CC BY) license (https://creativecommons.org/licenses/by/4.0/).

overall death rate (p = 0.08) and 50% increase in death with cancer rate were found during long-term follow-up in the lesser resection arm. Because of missing data in the original publication, a re-analysis was performed showing that overall survival was not statistically significantly different between both treatment arms, but this correction was published only one year later [6].

In the years that followed, several retrospective studies reported outcomes comparing lobectomy with sublobar resection. Kraeve et al. reported the 10-year outcomes of patients in the Surveillance, Epidemiology and End-Results (SEER) database, and found that patients undergoing lobectomy had significantly better survival rates when compared to segmentectomy in tumours <3 cm (cT1N0, stage IA) [7]. However, Kaplan–Meier survival curves remained similar in the first 3 years of follow-up. The general advice remained that lobectomy was the preferred treatment of choice for NSCLC, but a role might be present for sublobar resections in smaller, stage IA NSCLC patients. Other retrospective studies have demonstrated similar survival rates and local recurrence rates in favour of lobectomy [8–15]. A problem is that these studies frequently lacked adjustment for preoperative risk factors; thus, given the retrospective nature of these studies, it is possible that a selection bias was present, i.e., fitter patients would receive a lobectomy whilst sublobar resections were reserved for patients in poor overall health, resulting in lower OS. This was also confirmed in the systematic review by De Zoysa et al., concluding that lobectomy should be performed for early-stage NSCLC in younger patients with acceptable cardiopulmonary reserve [16]. The advantage of a decreased complication rate does not outweigh the increased locoregional recurrence rate. On the other hand, in elderly patients, a sublobar resection may yield comparable survival rates to lobectomy.

A meta-analysis by Ijsseldijk et al. compared lobar resection with parenchymal sparing resections for pT1a NSCLC [17]. Five-year OS and disease-free survival (DFS) after segmentectomy were similar to lobectomy with a relative risk (RR) = 1.08 (95% CI: 0.99–1.18). In most comparisons, wedge resections were similar to segmentectomy or lobectomy. Thus, for T1a NSCLC, parenchymal-sparing surgery has similar outcomes to lobectomy; however, an important concern is the risk of nodal upstaging. Two randomised trials were initiated to obtain more evidence: JCOG0802/WJOG4607L in Japan, and CALBG 140503 in North America.

In the Cancer and Lymphoma Group B (CALBG 140503) trial, patients with a suspected or confirmed cT1aN0 peripheral NASCLC $\leq$ 2 cm were included. After confirmation of diagnosis and negative hilar and mediastinal LNs, patients were intraoperatively randomised to lobectomy or to sublobar resection, comprising segmentectomy and wedge resection [18,19]. Pure ground-glass opacities (GGO) were excluded. The primary endpoint was DFS with the following secondary endpoints: OS, pulmonary function and recurrence rates. In total, 357 patients were included in the lobectomy group and 340 patients in the sublobar group, of which 58.8% were wedge resections. There was no significant difference in 5-year DFS between 63.6% (sublobar resection) and 64.1% (lobar resection). For OS, non-inferiority of sublobar resection was confirmed with a one-sided p = 0.014. There was no significant difference in lung- and non-lung related deaths or disease recurrence in both arms. When comparing pulmonary functions at 6 months to the baseline function, there was a significant difference in median forced expiratory volume in one second (FEV1) change from baseline for lobectomy and sublobar resection (p = 0.0006). Change in forced vital capacity (FVC)% approached significance, but remained at p = 0.0712 in favour of sublobar resection.

Sublobar resection was not inferior to lobectomy for the primary endpoint of DFS or the secondary endpoint of OS. Disease recurrence at 30% was also similar in both study arms. Even though differences in respiratory functions were observed, in favour of sublobar resection, the clinical significance is questionable. This trial confirms the non-inferiority of sublobar resection which still entails a 30% recurrence rate.

In the Japan Clinical Oncology Group and the West Japan Oncology Group trial (JCOG 0802/WJOG4607L), patients were included with a cT1a peripheral NSCLC or suspected nodule, a maximum tumour diameter of ≤2 cm and in the case of GGO, a consolidation-to-tumour ratio (CTR) >0.5 [20]. Patients were then randomised to lobectomy or segmentectomy (wedge excisions were not allowed). The primary endpoint of 5-year OS demonstrated a better outcome for segmentectomy of 94.3% vs. 91.1% (HR 0.663 (95% CI: 0.474–0.927) p = 0.0082) for superiority. Secondary endpoints however, showed similar 5-year relapse-free survival with segmentectomy at 88.0% and lobectomy at 87.9% (HR 0.998 (95% CI: 0.753–1.323) p = 0.9889). The recurrence pattern demonstrated a significantly higher proportion of local recurrences of 10.5% in the segmentectomy arm and 5.4% in the lobectomy group (p = 0.0018). However, the total number of lung cancer deaths were similar at 4.7% for segmentectomy versus 4.1% for lobectomy. The overall mortality was higher in the lobectomy group at 14.9% vs. 10.5%. However, this was primarily due to other deaths such as other malignancies at 5.6% (lobectomy) and 2.2% (segmentectomy) and non-malignant disease at 3.8% (lobectomy) vs. 2.7% (segmentectomy). This remains to be further explored.

NCT02011997 is an ongoing Chinese randomised control trial comparing complete Video-Assisted Thoracoscopic Surgery (cVATS) lobectomy to cVATS segmentectomy. An estimated 500 patients will be included involving a stage IA NSCLC with adenocarcinoma in situ or with microinvasion. A 5-year postoperative follow-up will be performed and recurrence-free survival has been chosen as the primary endpoint. The secondary endpoints are: 5-year survival rate, pulmonary function at 6 months follow-up, postoperative complications, and quality of life assessment. Patient enrolment commenced in December 2013; however, no results have been published yet.

With the new evidence provided, sublobar resection should be the new standard treatment modality in patients with peripheral small stage IA NSCLC tumours (≤2 cm) without lymph node metastases. There might be a place for tumours up to 3 cm in the outer third of the lung parenchyma; however, compelling evidence is lacking. Further subgroup analysis with the merging of data from recent randomised trials might contribute to outcome differences in the type of sublobar resection (wide wedge excision and anatomical segmentectomy), NSCLC histology, secondary cancers, and comorbidity.

Author Contributions: Writing—original draft preparation, I.D.; writing—review and editing, M.D.; writing—review and editing, P.E.Y.V.S.; supervision, P.E.Y.V.S. All authors have read and agreed to the published version of the manuscript.

Conflicts of Interest: P.E.Y.V.S. reports external expert and/or honoraries for lectures of AstraZeneca, Roche, BMS, MSD and Janssen. P.E.Y.V.S. is also unpaid Treasurer of Belgian Association for Cardiothoracic Surgery and unpaid President-elect of International Association for the Study of Lung Cancer. The other authors have no conflicts of interest to declare.

References

1. Brierley, J.D.; Gospodarowicz, M.K.; Wittekind, C.; Union International Cancer Control. *TNM Classification of Malignant Tumours*, 8th ed.; John Wiley & Sons: Hoboken, NJ, USA, 2017; pp. 1–272.
2. Smeltzer, M.P.; Lin, C.C.; Kong (Spring), F.M.; Jemal, A.; Osarogiagbon, R.U. Survival impact of postoperative therapy modalities according to margin status in non-small cell lung cancer patients in the United States. *J. Thorac. Cardiovasc. Surg.* **2017**, *154*, 661–672. [CrossRef] [PubMed]
3. Rami-Porta, R.; Wittekind, C.; Goldstraw, P. Complete resection in lung cancer surgery: Proposed definition. *Lung Cancer* **2005**, *49*, 25–33. [CrossRef] [PubMed]
4. Edwards, J.G.; Chansky, K.; Van Schil, P.; Nicholson, A.G.; Boubia, S.; Brambilla, E.; Donington, J.; Galateau-Sallé, F.; Hoffmann, H.; Infante, M.; et al. The IASLC Lung Cancer Staging Project: Analysis of Resection Margin Status and Proposals for Residual Tumor Descriptors for Non-Small Cell Lung Cancer. *J. Thorac. Oncol.* **2020**, *15*, 344–359. [CrossRef] [PubMed]
5. Ginsberg, R.J.; Rubinstein, L.V. Randomized trial of lobectomy versus limited resection for T1 N0 non-small cell lung cancer. *Ann. Thorac. Surg.* **1995**, *60*, 615–623. [CrossRef] [PubMed]
6. Rubinstein, L.V.; Ginsberg, R.J. Lobectomy versus limited resection in T1N0 lung cancer. *Ann. Thorac. Surg.* **1996**, *62*, 1249–1250.
7. Kraev, A.; Rassias, D.; Vetto, J.; Torosoff, M.; Ravichandran, P.; Clement, C.; Kadri, A.; Ilves, R. Wedge resection vs lobectomy: 10-year survival in stage I primary lung cancer. *Chest* **2007**, *131*, 136–140. [CrossRef] [PubMed]

8. Landreneau, R.J.; Sugarbaker, D.J.; Mack, M.J.; Hazelrigg, S.R.; Luketich, J.D.; Fetterman, L.; Liptay, M.J.; Bartley, S.; Boley, T.M.; Keenan, R.J.; et al. Wedge resection versus lobectomy for stage I (T1 N0 M0) non-small-cell lung cancer. *J. Thorac. Cardiovasc. Surg.* **1997**, *113*, 691–700. [CrossRef] [PubMed]
9. Koike, T.; Yamato, Y.; Yoshiya, K.; Shimoyama, T.; Suzuki, R. Intentional limited pulmonary resection for peripheral T1 N0 M0 small-sized lung cancer. *J. Thorac. Cardiovasc. Surg.* **2003**, *125*, 924–928. [CrossRef] [PubMed]
10. Okada, M.; Koike, T.; Higashiyama, M.; Yamato, Y.; Kodama, K.; Tsubota, N. Radical sublobar resection for small-sized non-small cell lung cancer: A multicenter study. *J. Thorac. Cardiovasc. Surg.* **2006**, *132*, 769–775. [CrossRef] [PubMed]
11. Fernando, H.C.; Santos, R.S.; Benfield, J.R.; Grannis, F.W.; Keenan, R.J.; Luketich, J.D.; Close, J.M.; Landreneau, R.J. Lobar and sublobar resection with and without brachytherapy for small stage IA non-small cell lung cancer. *J. Thorac. Cardiovasc. Surg.* **2005**, *129*, 261–267. [CrossRef] [PubMed]
12. Okada, M.; Nishio, W.; Sakamoto, T.; Uchino, K.; Yuki, T.; Nakagawa, A.; Tsubota, N. Effect of tumor size on prognosis in patients with non-small cell lung cancer: The role of segmentectomy as a type of lesser resection. *J. Thorac. Cardiovasc. Surg.* **2005**, *129*, 87–93. [CrossRef] [PubMed]
13. Schuchert, M.J.; Kilic, A.; Pennathur, A.; Nason, K.S.; Wilson, D.O.; Luketich, J.D.; Landreneau, R.J. Oncologic outcomes after surgical resection of subcentimeter non-small cell lung cancer. *Ann. Thorac. Surg.* **2011**, *91*, 1681–1688. [CrossRef] [PubMed]
14. Schuchert, M.J.; Abbas, G.; Awais, O.; Pennathur, A.; Nason, K.S.; Wilson, D.O.; Siegfried, J.M.; Luketich, J.D.; Landreneau, R.J. Anatomic segmentectomy for the solitary pulmonary nodule and early-stage lung cancer. *Ann. Thorac. Surg.* **2012**, *93*, 1780–1787. [CrossRef] [PubMed]
15. Donahue, J.M.; Morse, C.R.; Wigle, D.A.; Allen, M.S.; Nichols, F.C.; Shen, K.R.; Deschamps, C.; Cassivi, S.D. Oncologic efficacy of anatomic segmentectomy in stage IA lung cancer patients with T1a tumors. *Ann. Thorac. Surg.* **2012**, *93*, 381–388. [CrossRef] [PubMed]
16. De Zoysa, M.K.; Hamed, D.; Routledge, T.; Scarci, M. Is limited pulmonary resection equivalent to lobectomy for surgical management of stage I non-small-cell lung cancer? *Interact. Cardiovasc. Thorac. Surg.* **2012**, *14*, 816–820. [CrossRef] [PubMed]
17. Ijsseldijk, M.A.; Shoni, M.; Siegert, C.; Seegers, J.; van Engelenburg, A.K.C.; Tsai, T.C.; Lebenthal, A.; ten Broek, R.P.G. Oncological Outcomes of Lobar Resection, Segmentectomy, and Wedge Resection for T1a Non-Small-Cell Lung Carcinoma: A Systematic Review and Meta-Analysis. *Semin. Thorac. Cardiovasc. Surg.* **2020**, *32*, 582–590. [CrossRef] [PubMed]
18. Altorki, N.K.; Wang, X.; Kozono, D.; Watt, C.; Landreneau, R.; Wigle, D.; Port, J.; Jones, D.R.; Conti, M.; Ashrafi, A.S.; et al. PL03.06 Lobar or Sub-lobar Resection for Peripheral Clinical Stage IA = 2 cm Non-small Cell Lung Cancer (NSCLC): Results From an International Randomized Phase III Trial (CALGB 140503 [Alliance]). *J. Thorac. Oncol.* **2022**, *17*, S1–S2. [CrossRef]
19. Altorki, N.K.; Wang, X.; Wigle, D.; Gu, L.; Darling, G.; Ashrafi, A.S.; Landrenau, R.; Miller, D.; Liberman, M.; Jones, D.R.; et al. Perioperative mortality and morbidity after sublobar versus lobar resection for early-stage non-small-cell lung cancer: Post-hoc analysis of an international, randomised, phase 3 trial (CALGB/Alliance 140503). *Lancet Respir. Med.* **2018**, *6*, 915–924. [CrossRef] [PubMed]
20. Saji, H.; Okada, M.; Tsuboi, M.; Nakajima, R.; Suzuki, K.; Aokage, K.; Aoki, T.; Okami, J.; Yoshino, I.; Ito, H.; et al. Segmentectomy versus lobectomy in small-sized peripheral non-small-cell lung cancer (JCOG0802/WJOG4607L): A multicentre, open-label, phase 3, randomised, controlled, non-inferiority trial. *Lancet* **2022**, *399*, 1607–1617. [CrossRef] [PubMed]

Disclaimer/Publisher's Note: The statements, opinions and data contained in all publications are solely those of the individual author(s) and contributor(s) and not of MDPI and/or the editor(s). MDPI and/or the editor(s) disclaim responsibility for any injury to people or property resulting from any ideas, methods, instructions or products referred to in the content.

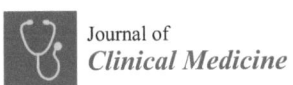

Article

Surgically Treated pT2aN0M0 (Stage IB) Non-Small Cell Lung Cancer: A 20-Year Single-Center Retrospective Study

Monica Casiraghi [1,2,*], Francesco Petrella [1,2], Claudia Bardoni [1], Shehab Mohamed [1], Giulia Sedda [1], Juliana Guarize [1], Antonio Passaro [3], Filippo De Marinis [3], Patrick Maisonneuve [4] and Lorenzo Spaggiari [1,2]

1. Department of Thoracic Surgery, IEO, European Institute of Oncology IRCCS, 20141 Milan, Italy
2. Department of Oncology and Hemato-Oncology, University of Milan, 20141 Milan, Italy
3. Division of Oncology, IEO, European Institute of Oncology IRCCS, 20141 Milan, Italy
4. Division of Epidemiology and Biostatistics, IEO, European Institute of Oncology IRCCS, 20141 Milan, Italy
* Correspondence: monica.casiraghi@ieo.it; Tel.: +39-0257489667

Abstract: Introduction The suitability of adjuvant therapy (AT) in patients with stage IB non-small cell lung cancer (NSCLC) is still under debate considering the cost–benefit ratio between improvement in survival and side effects. We retrospectively evaluated survival and incidence of recurrence in radically resected stage IB NSCLC, to determine whether AT could significantly improve prognosis. **Methods** Between 1998 and 2020, 4692 consecutive patients underwent lobectomy and systematic lymphadenectomy for NSCLC. Two hundred nineteen patients were pathological T2aN0M0 (>3 and ≤4 cm) NSCLC 8th TNM. None received preoperative or AT. Overall survival (OS), cancer specific survival (CSS) and the cumulative incidence of relapse were plotted and log-rank or Gray's tests were used to assess the difference in outcome between groups. **Results** The most frequent histology was adenocarcinoma (66.7%). Median OS was 146 months. The 5-, 10-, and 15-year OS rates were 79%, 60%, and 47%, whereas the 5-, 10-, and 15-year CSS were 88%, 85%, and 83%, respectively. OS was significantly related to age ($p < 0.001$) and cardiovascular comorbidities ($p = 0.04$), whereas number of LNs removed was an independent prognostic factor of CSS ($p = 0.02$). Cumulative incidence of relapse at 5-, 10-, and 15-year were 23%, 31%, and 32%, respectively, and significantly related to the number of LNs removed ($p = 0.01$). Patients with more than 20 LNs removed and clinical stage I had a significantly lower relapse ($p = 0.02$). **Conclusions** Excellent CSS, up to 83% at 15-year, and relatively low risk of recurrence for stage IB NSCLC (8th TNM) patients suggested that AT for those patients could be reserved only for very selected high-risk cases.

Keywords: stage IB; non-small cell lung cancer; T2aN0M0; surgery

1. Introduction

Lung cancer is still one of the leading causes of death worldwide, being the second most commonly diagnosed cancer after female breast cancer. In the last decades, owing to the wide diffusion of lung cancer screening programs, the vast majority of early-stage NSCLC cases, in particular of the adenocarcinoma type, were readily detected [1,2]. Nevertheless, the 5-year overall survival (OS) of patients with radically resected stage I NSCLC is still considerably heterogeneous, varying from 90% for stage IA1 to 73% for stage IB [3], with a relatively high propensity for recurrence.

Whereas it is widely recognized that NSCLC patients with lymph node involvement have poor prognosis and that their survival could improve with adjuvant treatment (AT) [4,5], the appropriateness of administering AT to stage IB patients (T3-4cmN0M0, T2CentrN0M0, and T2ViscPlN0M0) is still under debate as the cost–benefit ratio between survival rate improvement and side effects are being evaluated.

Retrospective, single-center studies on the topic have given controversial and inconclusive results [6–13], and raised many doubts suggesting discordant recommendations [14–16], mostly related to the changes made to the definition of stage IB and IIA

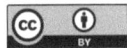

NSCLC in the 8th edition of the tumor, node, metastasis (TNM) staging system. Indeed, in the 8th TNM staging system, T2 has been split into T2a (<3–4 cm), the real stage IB, and T2b (>4–5 cm), with T2bN0M0 classed as IIA. This has had an unprecedented effect on the population eligible to receive AT, and has created confusion in interpreting data from studies, which still consider lesions greater than 4 cm as stage IB.

The only multicenter randomized clinical trial (CALGB 9633) specifically designed for stage IB NSCLC patients showed that AT had failed to improve survival except in patients with tumors larger than 4 cm [17]. Thus, the current National Comprehensive Cancer Network (NCCN) guidelines recommend postoperative chemotherapy only for T2bN0M0 NSCLC patients with a tumor $\geq$4 cm in size (stage IIA according to the 8th TNM), while currently T2aN0M0 patients (stage IB based on the 8th TNM) are usually tailored-treated following the oncologist's recommendations, unless in case of a high-risk of recurrence.

The aim of this study is to retrospectively analyze radically resected T2aN0M0 (stage IB) NSCLC patients to evaluate their survival and the incidence of recurrence, and to determine whether AT could improve their prognosis.

2. Materials and Methods

The study was conducted according to the guidelines of the Declaration of Helsinki; the Ethics Committee of our Institution waived the need for ethics approval and the need to obtain consent for the collection, analysis, and publication of the retrospectively obtained and anonymized data for this non-interventional study. Written informed consent was obtained from all patients at the time of surgery. All data underlying this article are available in the article and in its online Supplementary Materials. This study was reported based on the Strengthening the Reporting of Observational Studies in Epidemiology (STROBE) checklist for cross-sectional studies.

We selected patients who, according to the 8th TNM edition, were affected by pathological T2a NSCLC (tumor size >3 and $\leq$4 cm) and that showed no pathological lymph node involvement. We excluded from the study all patients with one or more of the following characteristics: prior treatments or history of cancer within the previous 5 years, histology other than NSCLC, incomplete preoperative staging, incomplete lymphadenectomy, anatomical resection other than lobectomy, incomplete resection (R1 or R2 resection), preoperative or adjuvant treatments such as chemotherapy, biological therapy, immunotherapy, or radiotherapy.

For all patients, preoperative staging was based on total body computed tomography scan (CT-scan), positron emission tomography (PET) with fluorodeoxyglucose (FDG), cardiological examination, and pulmonary function test followed by anesthesia evaluation. Whenever possible, suspected mediastinal lymph node involvement was verified with either endobronchial ultrasound-guided transbronchial needle aspiration (EBUS-TBNA) or mediastinoscopy [18]. Staging and functional exams were always performed in the 5 weeks before surgery. During the multidisciplinary meetings, thoracic surgeons and oncologists confirmed patient resectability and medical treatment plans.

All patients underwent pulmonary lobectomy and radical lymphadenectomy. In all patients, systematic lymph node dissection was performed according to the classification of the American Thoracic Society by removing all lymphatic tissue from stations 2R, 4R, 7, and 10R for right-sided tumors and from stations 5, 6, 7, and 10 L for left-sided tumors. A complete pathologically resection was defined R0, microscopic residual disease at pathology was defined R1, whereas a macroscopically incomplete resection was defined R2. Postoperative complications were defined according to the Clavien–Dindo classification [19].

Patients received a physical follow-up, chest X-ray, and blood tests at 1 month after surgery; then, they received a physical examination plus a chest and upper abdomen CT-scan every 4 months for the first 2 years, every 6 months for the following 3 years, and annually after 5 years from surgery.

Recurrence at the site of surgery (hilar/mediastinal region or lung parenchyma close to the previous resection), in the chest cavity (ipsilateral and contralateral such as new pulmonary nodules or pleural diffusion) and distant metastasis were recorded and classified as local, regional, and distant, respectively. We did not consider recurrence but a second primary tumor when a distinct pulmonary malignancy displayed different histology or different morphology by comprehensive histologic assessment, and/or it was diagnosed 2 or more years after the first primary lung cancer, in the absence of nodal or systemic metastases. In the case of adenocarcinoma histology, considering the retrospective nature of the study and the impossibility to have a molecular mutational analysis performed on any paired primary tumor and suspected recurrent tumor to distinguish true recurrence from second primary tumor, the second event was considered recurrence.

Statistical Analysis

Overall survival (OS) and cancer-specific survival (CSS) were calculated using the date of surgery and the date of either last contact or death. Relapse was defined from the date of surgery to the date of any relapse (local, regional, or distant), last contact, or death. OS and CSS were plotted using the Kaplan–Meier method, and the log-rank test was used to assess outcome differences between groups. For time to recurrence, we considered death as competing risk and use cumulative incidence plots with the Fine and Gray test. Analyses were performed with SAS software version 9.4 (SAS Institute, Cary, NC, USA). All P values were two-sided; $p < 0.05$ was considered statistically significant.

3. Results

We retrospectively evaluated 4692 consecutive patients who, between January 1998 and December 2020, underwent lobectomy and systematic lymphadenectomy for NSCLC at the European Institute of Oncology (IEO) in Milan, Italy. Among them, 219 were pathological T2aN0M0 (stage IB) NSCLC patients whose characteristics and tumor details are shown in Table 1: they were mostly men (68.9%); aged 41–89 years; with at least one comorbidity (88.1%); 8 patients out of 219 were clinical stage IA1 (3.6%), 35 IA2 (16%), 59 IA3 (26.9%), 71 IB (32.4%), 40 IIA (18.3%), and 6 IIB (2.7%).

Table 1. Characteristics of 219 patients with stage IB (pT2aN0M0) NSCLC operated at the IEO during 1998–2020, who did not receive neoadjuvant or adjuvant therapy for primary cancer.

Patients' Characteristics	N (%)	Surgical Characteristics	N (%)	Tumor Characteristics	N (%)
Age, years, Median [range]	67 [40–88]	Surgical approach		Histology	
<60	36 (16.4)	Open lobectomy	149 (68.0)	Adenocarcinoma	146 (66.7)
60–69	100 (45.7)	RATS	56 (25.6)	Squamous	61 (27.9)
70+	83 (37.9)	VATS	14 (6.4)	Adeno-squamous	10 (4.6)
Sex		Conversion	3 (1.4)	NSCLC	2 (0.9)
Men	151 (68.9)	Sleeve	7 (3.2)	Tumor size	
Women	68 (31.1)	Nodule site		30–35mm	142 (64.8)
Comorbidities		Upper lobe	146 (66.7)	36–40mm	77 (35.2)
Other Cardiac	125 (57.1)	Middle lobe	6 (2.7)	Tumor grade	
Ischemic heart disease	21 (9.6)	Lower lobe	67 (30.6)	G1	18 (8.2)
Hypertension	87 (39.7)	Nodule side		G2	78 (35.6)
Pulmonary	33 (15.1)	Left	132 (60.3)	G3	115 (52.5)
COPD	25 (11.4)	Right	87 (39.7)	Missing	8 (3.7)
Other	176 (80.4)	Lymph nodes removed		Visceral pleura infiltration	
Clinical Stage		Total, median [range]	16 [4–40]	Absent	141 (64.4)
I	173 (79.0)	N1, median [range]	6 [1–28]	Present	78 (35.6)
II	46 (21.0)	N2, median [range]	8 [0–25]		

COPD: chronic obstructive pulmonary disease; RATS: robotic-assisted thoracic surgery; VATS: video-assisted thoracic surgery; NSCLC: non-small cell lung cancer; VP: visceral pleura.

Open surgery was performed in 156 patients (71.2%), whereas 56 (25.6%) were surgically approached in RATS, and 14 (6.4%) in VATS. Three patients were converted to open surgery from either VATS (n = 2) or RATS (n = 1), due to adhesions.

All patients underwent lobectomy and systematic lymphadenectomy; 7 patients out of 219 (3.2%) underwent sleeve resection (6 bronchial and 1 bronchial and vascular). All 219 patients had a pathological radical resection (R0).

The pathological size of the primary tumor was 30–35 mm in 142 patients (64.8%), and 36–40 mm in 77 (35.2%).

Adenocarcinoma was the most frequently found histologic type (n = 146; 66.7%), followed by squamous carcinoma (n = 61; 27.9%), and adeno-squamous carcinoma (n = 10; 4.6%). The median total number of lymph nodes removed was 16 (range 4–40). Visceral pleural infiltration was evident in 78 cases (35.6%).

Postoperative complications and outcomes are listed in Supplementary Table S1. Major complications (Clavien–Dindo 3 and 4) were observed in 9 patients (4.1%): 1 hemothorax and 1 chylothorax, both requiring surgical intervention; 1 bronchopleural fistula, treated with a completion pneumonectomy; 1 acute cholecystitis, requiring cholecystectomy; 1 empyema treated with chest tube and antibiotic therapy; 2 bronchial toilettes, and 2 acute respiratory distress syndrome (ARDS) requiring intensive care unit (ICU). Minor complications (Clavien–Dindo 1 and 2) occurred in 58 patients (26.48%), mostly atrial fibrillation (n = 27; 12.32%) and pleural air leak (n = 17; 7.76%).

The mean hospital stay for all patients was 6 days (range, 3–44 days). No intraoperative mortality was observed.

The median OS was 146 months, with 5-, 10-, and 15-year OS rates of 79%, 60%, and 47%, whereas the CSS at 5-, 10-, and 15-year were 88%, 85%, and 83%, respectively (Figure 1).

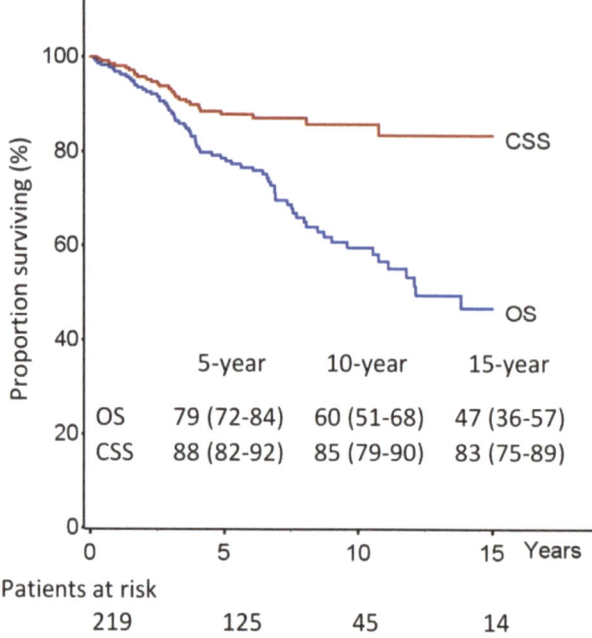

Figure 1. Overall survival (OS) and lung cancer specific survival (CSS).

Whereas OS was significantly related to age ($p < 0.001$) and to cardiovascular comorbidities ($p = 0.04$), the number of lymph nodes removed was an independent prognostic factor of CSS ($p = 0.02$) (Figure 2 and Table 2).

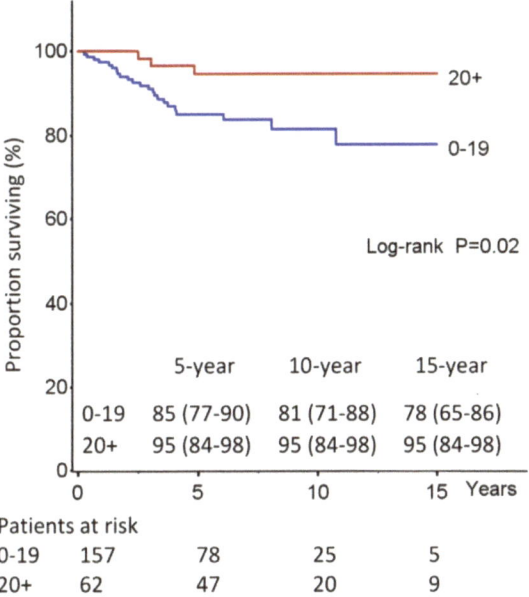

Figure 2. Lung cancer specific survival (CSS) by number of LN removed.

Table 2. Factors associated with tumor relapse, cancer specific survival (CSS), and overall survival (OS).

Characteristics			Tumor Relapse			Cancer Specific Survival (CSS)			Overall Survival (OS)		
	N (%)	Events	HR (95% CI)	Gray's Test	Deaths	HR (95% CI)	Log-Rank	Deaths	HR (95% CI)	Log-Rank
Total		219	55						75		
Age											
<60	36 (16.4)	6	1.00		3	1.00		5	1.00	
60–69	100 (45.7)	26	1.63 (0.68–3.90)		11	1.44 (0.40–4.16)		30	2.67 (1.03–6.91)	
70+	83 (37.9)	23	1.80 (0.74–4.38)	0.41	12	2.04 (0.57–7.31)	0.47	40	5.99 (2.33–15.4)	<0.0001
Sex											
Men	151 (68.9)	37	1.00		15	1.00		54	1.00	
Women	68 (31.1)	18	1.10 (0.63–1.93)	0.73	11	1.65 (0.76–3.60)	0.20	21	0.83 (0.50–1.40)	0.49
Comorbidities											
Cardiac	125 (57.1)	32	1.15 (0.68–1.94)	0.60	15	1.20 (0.55–2.63)	0.65	45	1.64 (1.02–2.63)	0.04
Myocardial infarction	21 (9.6)	6	1.06 (0.47–2.37)	0.90	2	0.80 (0.19–3.39)	0.76	11	1.85 (0.97–3.52)	0.06
Hypertension	87 (39.7)	22	1.07 (0.63–1.84)	0.77	9	0.93 (0.41–2.09)	0.86	28	1.27 (0.79–2.04)	0.32
Pulmonary	33 (15.1)	7	0.80 (0.37–1.76)	0.59	4	1.00 (0.34–2.99)	0.99	12	1.12 (0.60–2.07)	0.73
COPD	25 (11.4)	7	1.07 (0.49–2.37)	0.86	4	1.30 (0.45–3.77)	0.63	11	1.26 (0.66–2.39)	0.48
Other	176 (80.4)	50	3.06 (1.2–7.67)	0.01	21	1.24 (0.46–3.33)	0.67	56	1.27 (0.74–2.19)	0.39
Clinical Stage											
I	173 (79.0)	40	1.00		21	1.00		60	1.00	
II	46 (21.0)	15	1.68 (0.92–3.09)	0.08	5	1.00 (0.38–2.65)	0.99	15	1.14 (0.64–2.01)	0.66
Surgical approach											
Open lobectomy	149 (68.0)	39	1.00		21	1.00		61	1.00	
RATS	56 (25.6)	13	1.09 (0.58–2.05)		4	0.45 (0.23–1.94)	0.62	10	0.80 (0.40–1.57)	
VATS	14 (6.4)	3	0.78 (0.27–2.29)	0.86	1	0.50 (0.07–3.76)		4	0.85 (0.31–2.36)	0.78
Conversion	3 (1.4)	0	-	0.30	0	-	0.50	2	1.43 (0.35–5.87)	0.61
Sleeve	7 (3.2)	1	0.47 (0.06–3.56)	0.43	1	0.99 (0.14–7.38)	0.99	3	0.79 (0.25–2.51)	0.68
Nodule site											
Upper lobe	146 (66.7)	34	1.00		17	1.00		49	1.00	
Middle lobe	6 (2.7)	1	1.30 (0.75–2.24)		0	-		1	1.13 (0.69–1.83)	
Lower lobe	67 (30.6)	20	0.70 (0.10–4.78)	0.58	9	1.13 (0.51–2.54)	0.65	25	0.42 (0.06–3.06)	0.58
Nodule side											
Left	132 (60.3)	20	1.00		13	1.00		30	1.00	
Right	87 (39.7)	35	1.13 (0.65–1.96)	0.66	13	0.65 (0.30–1.40)	0.26	45	1.06 (0.67–1.70)	0.80
Lymph nodes removed											
≥20	62 (28.3)	10	1.00		3	1.00		24	1.00	
<20	157 (71.7)	45	2.27 (1.17–4.39)	0.01	23	3.79 (1.13–12.6)	0.02	51	1.25 (0.77–2.05)	0.37
Histology											
Adenocarcinoma	146 (66.7)	40	1.00		16	1.00		39	1.00	
Squamous	61 (27.9)	12	0.64 (0.33–1.24)		7	0.96 (0.40–2.34)		31	1.48 (0.91–2.38)	
Adeno-squamous	10 (4.6)	3	1.12 (0.34–3.63)		3	2.87 (0.83–9.88)		4	1.51 (0.54–4.24)	
NSCLC	2 (0.9)	0	-	0.43	0	-	0.32	1	2.29 (0.31–16.8)	0.36
Tumor size											
30–35 mm	142 (64.8)	39	1.00		15	1.00		48	1.00	
36–40 mm	77 (35.2)	16	0.76 (0.42–1.36)	0.35	11	1.41 (0.65–3.07)	0.39	27	1.12 (0.70–1.81)	0.63
Tumor grade											
G1	18 (8.2)	3	1.00		2	1.00		5	1.00	
G2	78 (35.6)	22	2.12 (0.68–6.58)		9	1.33 (0.29–6.15)		26	1.78 (0.68–4.66)	
G3	115 (52.5)	28	1.69 (0.55–5.21)	0.39	14	1.30 (0.30–5.72)	0.93	42	1.77 (0.70–4.48)	0.46
Missing	8 (3.7)	2	-		1					
Visceral pleura infiltration											
Absent	141 (64,4)	34	1.00		19	1.00		53	1.00	
Present	78 (35.6)	21	1.11 (0.65–1.89)	0.71	7	0.66 (0.29–1.57)	0.34	22	0.80 (0.48–1.31)	0.37

CSS: cancer specific survival; OS: overall survival; COPD: chronic obstructive pulmonary disease; RATS: robotic-assisted thoracic surgery; VATS: video-assisted thoracic surgery; NSCLC: non-small cell lung cancer. Bold text indicates a statistically significant difference with a *p*-value less than 0.05.

A total of 55 (25.1%) patients developed recurrences of the disease (Table S1 and Figure 1): 15 (6.8%) had local relapse, 18 (8.2%) regional recurrences, and 26 (11.9%) distant metastases (2 patients had simultaneous local and distant relapse and 1 patient simultaneous local, regional and distant relapse).

Of the 55 patients with recurrences, 38 (73.1%) developed adenocarcinoma, with 3 of them (5.7%) harboring EGFR mutations. The recurrences were mostly treated with radiotherapy alone (n = 21, 40.4%), followed by platinum-based chemotherapy (n = 18, 34.6%). The three patients with EGFR mutations were treated with Osimertinib. Combined treatments (platinum-based chemotherapy with either radiotherapy or immunotherapy) were indicated in eight patients (15.4%) who developed distant metastasis. Instead, one patient who developed a single metastasis in the contralateral lung underwent surgical metastasectomy.

The cumulative incidence of relapse at 5-, 10-, and 15-year was 23%, 31%, and 32%, respectively (Figure 3), and related to clinical stage (p = 0.08) and number of LNs removed (p = 0.01) (Figure 4 and Table 2); patients with more than 20 LNs removed and clinical stage I had a significantly lower probability of relapse than patients with less than 20 LNs removed or clinical stage II (p = 0.02) (Figure S1), whereas the CSS was significantly related only to the number of LNs removed (p = 0.02).

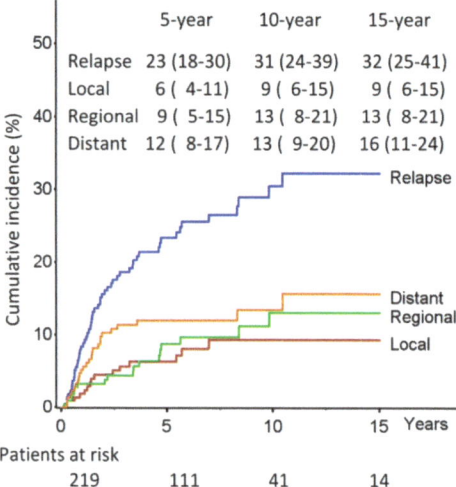

Figure 3. Lung cancer recurrence.

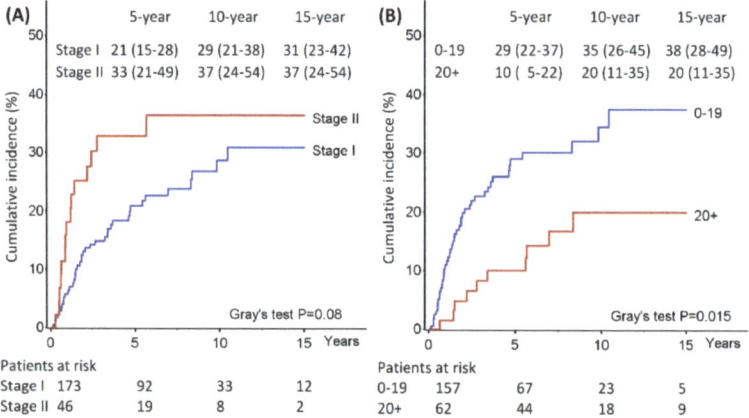

Figure 4. Cumulative incidence of relapse by clinical stage (**A**) or number of resected nodes (**B**).

4. Discussion

When taking as reference the 8th edition of the TNM staging system, the 5-year OS rate for NSCLC patients is about 73% for stage IB cases and 80–90% for stage IA cases. Thus, in the last decade, oncologists and surgeons have often discussed the opportunity to propose to stage IB patients a postoperative treatment aimed to improve survival and to reduce recurrences. The latest guidelines include recommendations for postoperative treatment in resected stage II–IIIA and in selected stage IB NSCLC patients, usually associated with poor prognosis and disease recurrence [15,16]. However, mostly due to the incorrect staging of these patients and the confusion in interpreting data that still consider lesions larger than 4 cm as stage IB, based on the 7th edition of the TNM staging system, there are still many doubts on the benefits of postoperative treatment on the survival of these patients. Furthermore, rates of relapse after surgery still remain highly dependent on disease stages (45% for stage IB disease; 62% for stage II disease; 76% for stage III disease), notwithstanding the use of adjuvant chemotherapy [20].

The Cancer and Leukemia Group B 9633 study showed that adjuvant chemotherapy improved survival in patients with tumors larger than 4 cm in size, but not in those with tumors smaller than 4 cm (HR, 1.12; 90% CI, 0.75 to 1.07; $p = 0.32$) [21]. However, when reanalyzing the patient population based on the 8th TNM edition, only a few stage IB NSCLC patients were included without considering possible high-risk factors. Even the ANITA trial, which showed the benefits of adjuvant chemotherapy mainly in patients with lymph node metastasis, unfortunately considered only stage IB cases as defined in the 7th TNM edition.

In 2021, Wang [22] performed the largest and most recent systematic review and meta-analysis (including 12 eligible studies for a total of 15,678 patients) and showed that AT might provide survival benefits in patients with stage IB NSCLC, independently from histology or regimens. This study also addressed the issue of whether AT should be administered in the case of malignancies <4 cm: only 7 out of the 12 studies taken into consideration showed better OS and gave support to the routine use of AT for stage IB NSCLC patients. This number decreased to only two in the case of adenocarcinoma histology [22].

In our study, we analyzed selected T2aN0M0 (size 3–4 cm, stage IB in the 8th TNM edition) NSCLC patients surgically treated without AT and found that the 5-year OS was 79%, and the 5-year CSS was 88%, staying at up to 83% for as long as 15 years. In comparison to the available literature, we showed a higher survival rate and the importance of correct staging and data interpretation. Real stage IB cases, as defined in the 8th TNM, are indeed smaller than 4 cm in size and have better survival outcomes than those similarly staged in the previous edition of the staging system. Therefore, AT should not be prescribed a priori to improve survival in patients with an already good prognosis, and used only in carefully selected high-risk cases.

Several are the factors that are considered to be high-risk, among them poor tumor differentiation, vascular invasion, wedge resection, visceral pleural involvement, and incomplete lymph node dissection [14], but a clear, clinically applicable risk-stratification model for the identification of stage IB NSCLC is not yet available. It is unknown whether there is a risk difference between them and the efficacy of adjuvant chemotherapy in those high-risk patients, creating confusion in clinical practice, as the use of adjuvant chemotherapy relies on the clinician's judgment [23,24].

In a recent study, Zhai et al. proposed a clinical risk score (CRS) based on the patients' detailed risk factors, predicted the prognosis of patients with stage IB-IIA NSCLC, and found a significant association between adjuvant chemotherapy and the prognosis of patients with stage IB-IIA NSCLC, particularly those with a high clinical risk score and non-squamous cell histology. Unfortunately, they did not manage to make a clear distinction between stage IB and IIA cases [25].

In 2022, Choi et al. published a retrospective multicenter study including 285 stage IB NSCLC patients with high-risk factors as defined by the 8th TNM edition. They showed that adjuvant chemotherapy was beneficial in this cohort of patients and that it significantly reduced their risk of recurrence and mortality. In the multivariate analysis, the adjuvant chemotherapy group had a significantly lower recurrence rate and risk of mortality than the control group, in particular in patients with high-risk factors such as visceral pleural involvement or vascular invasion [26].

In the phase 3 ADAURA study (NCT02511106) [27], Osimertinib was found to have a clinically meaningful effect on disease-free survival in patients with resected stages IB to IIIA EGFR-mutated (EGFRm) NSCLC, irrespective of whether patients had previously received chemotherapy or not. However, only 26% of patients with stage IB disease received adjuvant chemotherapy compared to 76% of II to IIIA stage cases. Moreover, also in the ADAURA study, stage IB cases were classified as such according to the 7th TNM edition, and were therefore actual stage IIA cases.

In our study, the incidence of relapse rates at 5-, 10-, and 15-year were 23%, 31%, and 32%, respectively, and significantly associated with the number of lymph nodes removed ($p = 0.01$); moreover, in a subgroup analysis, patients with more than 20 lymph nodes removed and clinical stage I had a probability of relapse significantly lower than patients with less than 20 lymph nodes removed or clinical stage II ($p = 0.02$) (Figure 4). Additionally, the number of lymph nodes removed was also an independent prognostic factor of CSS ($p = 0.02$), making it the only high-risk factor related to survival, unlike size and visceral pleura which, on the other hand, did not correlate with either survival or risk of recurrence.

This was an important finding as the high survival rate we observed in our study could be explained with a proper postoperative staging resulting from the radical and systematic lymphadenectomy we routinely performed. The lower survival rates found by others could be due to cases being wrongly staged as IB following incomplete removal of lymph nodes.

Our study presents a few limitations. Firstly, its retrospective nature placed limits and introduced biases on all the variables included in the analysis. Secondly, it did not include a control group undergoing AT, as we do not routinely administer AT to stage IB NSCLC, except for a highly selected cohort of high-risk patients. As the use of Osimertinib was allowed only recently in cases carrying EGFR mutations, only three patients were included in this study, too few to make any considerations. The main strength of our study is in relying on data from a single center, with uniform indications and patients' selection over the years. In addition, the data presented herein were collected by a high-volume referral center for more than twenty years, so that noteworthy conclusions can be drawn from them.

5. Conclusions

Based on the excellent CSS (up to 86% at 15-year, with a relatively low risk of recurrence) observed for the stage IB (8th TNM) patients in our study, AT could be prescribed only to selected high-risk factors cases.

Supplementary Materials: The following supporting information can be downloaded at: https://www.mdpi.com/article/10.3390/jcm12052081/s1, Table S1: Patients' outcomes; Figure S1: Relapse according to clinical stage and number of lymph nodes removed.

Author Contributions: Conceptualization, M.C.; methodology, M.C.; software, P.M.; validation, F.P., J.G., and A.P.; formal analysis, G.S.; investigation, C.B.; resources, S.M.; data curation, C.B. and S.M.; writing—original draft preparation, M.C.; writing—review and editing, M.C. and F.P.; visualization, A.P.; supervision, L.S. and F.D.M. All authors have read and agreed to the published version of the manuscript.

Funding: The study was supported partially by the Italian Ministry of Health with Ricerca Corrente and 5×1000 funds.

Institutional Review Board Statement: The study was conducted according to the guidelines of the Declaration of Helsinki; the Ethics Committee of our Institution waived the need for ethics approval and the need to obtain consent for the collection, analysis, and publication of the retrospectively obtained and anonymized data for this non-interventional study.

Informed Consent Statement: Informed consent was obtained from all subjects involved in the study.

Data Availability Statement: Available upon request.

Acknowledgments: This article was revised by Claudia Crovace. The abstract has been submitted to the 103rd AATS Annual Meeting, Saturday, 6 May 2023–Tuesday, 9 May 2023, Los Angeles, CA, USA.

Conflicts of Interest: The authors declare no conflict of interest.

References

1. Arenberg, D. Update on screening for lung cancer. *Transl. Lung Cancer Res.* **2019**, *8*, S77–S87. [CrossRef] [PubMed]
2. National Lung Screening Trial Research Team. Reduced lung-cancer mortality with low-dose computed tomographic screening. *N. Engl. J. Med.* **2011**, *365*, 395–409. [CrossRef] [PubMed]
3. Siegel, R.L.; Miller, K.D.; Fuchs, H.E.; Jemal, A. Cancer Statistics, 2021. *CA Cancer J. Clin.* **2021**, *71*, 7–33. [CrossRef]
4. Douillard, J.Y.; Rosell, R.; De Lena, M.; Carpagnano, F.; Ramlau, R.; Gonzales-Larriba, J.L.; Grodzki, T.; Pereira, J.R.; Groumellec, A.L.; Lorusso, P.V.; et al. Adjuvant vinorelbine plus cisplatin versus observation in patients with completely resected stage IB-IIIA non-small-cell lung cancer (Adjuvant Navelbine International Trialist Association [ANITA]): A randomised controlled trial. *Lancet Oncol.* **2006**, *7*, 719e27. [CrossRef]
5. Winton, T.; Livingston, R.; Johnson, D.; Rigas, J.; Johnston, M.; Butts, C.; Cormier, Y.; Goss, G.; Inculet, R.; Vallieres, E.; et al. Vinorelbine plus cisplatin vs. observation in resected non-small-cell lung cancer. *N. Engl. J. Med.* **2005**, *352*, 2589e97. [CrossRef]
6. Qian, F.; Yang, W.; Wang, R.; Xu, J.; Wang, S.; Zhang, Y.; Jin, B.; Yu, K.; Han, B. Prognostic significance and adjuvant chemotherapy survival benefits of a solid or micropapillary pattern in patients with resected stage IB lung adenocarcinoma. *J. Thorac. Cardiovasc. Surg.* **2018**, *155*, 1227–1235.e2. [CrossRef]
7. Xu, J.; Wang, S.; Zhong, H.; Zhang, B.; Qian, J.; Yang, W.; Qian, F.; Qiao, R.; Teng, J.; Lou, Y.; et al. Adjuvant Chemotherapy Improves Survival in Surgically Resected Stage IB Squamous Lung Cancer. *Ann. Thorac. Surg.* **2019**, *107*, 1683–1689. [CrossRef]
8. Chen, D.; Wang, X.; Zhang, F.; Han, R.; Ding, Q.; Xu, X.; Shu, J.; Ye, F.; Shi, L.; Mao, Y.; et al. Could tumor spread through air spaces benefit from adjuvant chemotherapy in stage I lung adenocarcinoma? A multi-institutional study. *Ther. Adv. Med. Oncol.* **2020**, *12*, 1758835920978147. [CrossRef]
9. Jang, H.J.; Cho, S.; Kim, K.; Jheon, S.; Yang, H.C.; Kim, D.K. Effect of Adjuvant Chemotherapy after Complete Resection for Pathologic Stage IB Lung Adenocarcinoma in High-Risk Patients as Defined by a New Recurrence Risk Scoring Model. *Cancer Res. Treat.* **2017**, *49*, 898–905. [CrossRef] [PubMed]
10. Ito, H.; Nakayama, H.; Nagashima, T.; Samejima, J.; Inafuku, K.; Eriguchi, D.; Yamada, K.; Suzuki, M.; Yokose, T. The adjuvant chemotherapy can be omitted for lepidic predominant lung adenocarcinoma in stage IB of the 8th TNM staging system. *Res. Sq.* **2020**. [CrossRef]
11. Cao, S.; Teng, J.; Xu, J.; Han, B.; Zhong, H. Value of adjuvant chemotherapy in patients with resected stage IB solid predominant and solid non-predominant lung adenocarcinoma. *Thorac. Cancer* **2019**, *10*, 249–255. [CrossRef] [PubMed]
12. Chen, T.; Luo, J.; Gu, H.; Gu, Y.; Huang, Q.; Wang, Y.; Zheng, J.; Yang, Y.; Chen, H. Impact of Solid Minor Histologic Subtype in Postsurgical Prognosis of Stage I Lung Adenocarcinoma. *Ann. Thorac. Surg.* **2018**, *105*, 302–308. [CrossRef] [PubMed]
13. Wang, J.; Wu, N.; Lv, C.; Yan, S.; Yang, Y. Should patients with stage IB non-small cell lung cancer receive adjuvant chemotherapy? A comparison of survival between the 8th and 7th editions of the AJCC TNM staging system for stage IB patients. *J. Cancer Res. Clin. Oncol.* **2019**, *145*, 463–469. [CrossRef] [PubMed]
14. National Comprehensive Cancer Network, Non-Small Cell Lung Cancer (Version 2022). Available online: https://www.nccn.org/patientresources/patient-resources/guidelines-forpatients/guidelines-for-patients-details?patientGuidelineId=11 (accessed on 1 November 2022).
15. Postmus, P.E.; Kerr, K.M.; Oudkerk, M.; Senan, S.; Waller, D.A.; Vansteenkiste, J.; Escriu, C.; Peters, S. Early and locally advance non-small cell lung cancer (NSCLC): ESMO clinical practice guidelines for diagnosis, treatment and follow-up. *Ann. Oncol.* **2017**, *28* (Suppl. 4), iv1–iv21. [CrossRef]
16. Kris, M.G.; Gaspar, L.E.; Chaft, J.E.; Kennedy, E.B.; Azzoli, C.G.; Ellis, P.M.; Lin, S.H.; Pass, H.I.; Seth, R.; Shepherd, F.A.; et al. Adjuvant systemic therapy and adjuvant radiation therapy for stage I to IIIA completely resected non-small-cell lung cancers: American Society of Clinical Oncology/Cancer Care Ontario clinical practice guideline update. *J. Clin. Oncol.* **2017**, *35*, 2960–2974. [CrossRef]
17. Wakelee, H.A.; Schiller, J.H.; Gandara, D.R. Current status of adjuvant chemotherapy for stage IB non-small-cell lung cancer: Implications for the New Intergroup Trial. *Clin. Lung Cancer* **2006**, *8*, 18–21. [CrossRef] [PubMed]
18. Guarize, J.; Casiraghi, M.; Donghi, S.; Diotti, C.; Vanoni, N.; Romano, R.; Casadio, C.; Brambilla, D.; Maisonneuve, P.; Petrella, F.; et al. Endobronchial Ultrasound Transbronchial Needle Aspiration in Thoracic Diseases: Much More than Mediastinal Staging. *Can. Respir. J.* **2018**, *2018*, 4269798. [CrossRef]
19. Dindo, D.; Demartines, N.; Clavien, P.-A. Classification of Surgical Complications. *Ann. Surg.* **2004**, *240*, 205–213. [CrossRef]
20. Pignon, J.-P.; Tribodet, H.; Scagliotti, G.V.; Douillard, J.-Y.; Shepherd, F.A.; Stephens, R.J.; Dunant, A.; Torri, V.; Rosell, R.; Seymour, L.; et al. Lung adjuvant cisplatin evaluation: A pooled analysis by the LACE Collaborative Group. *J. Clin. Oncol.* **2008**, *26*, 3552–3559. [CrossRef]

21. Strauss, G.M.; Herndon, J.E., 2nd; Maddaus, M.A.; Johnstone, D.W.; Johnson, E.A.; Harpole, D.H.; Gillenwater, H.H.; Watson, D.M.; Sugarbaker, D.J.; Schilsky, R.L.; et al. Adjuvant paclitaxel plus carboplatin compared with observation in stage IB non-small-cell lung cancer: CALGB 9633 with the Cancer and Leukemia Group B, Radiation Therapy Oncology Group, and North Central Cancer Treatment Group Study Groups. *J. Clin. Oncol.* **2008**, *26*, 5043–5051. [CrossRef]
22. Wang, X.; Chen, D.; Wen, J.; Mao, Y.; Zhu, X.; Fan, M.; Chen, Y. Benefit of adjuvant chemotherapy for patients with stage IB non-small cell lung cancer: A systematic review and meta-analysis. *Ann. Transl. Med.* **2021**, *9*, 1430. [CrossRef] [PubMed]
23. Nentwich, M.F.; Bohn, B.A.; Uzunoglu, F.G.; Reeh, M.; Quaas, A.; Grob, T.J.; Perez, D.; Kutup, A.; Bockhorn, M.; Izbicki, J.R.; et al. Lymphatic invasion predicts survival in patients with early node-negative non-small cell lung cancer. *J. Thorac. Cardiovasc. Surg.* **2013**, *146*, 781e7. [CrossRef] [PubMed]
24. Mizuno, T.; Ishii, G.; Nagai, K.; Yoshida, J.; Nishimura, M.; Mochizuki, T.; Kawai, O.; Hasebe, T.; Ochiai, A. Identification of a low-risk subgroup of stage IB lung adenocarcinoma patient. *Lung Cancer* **2008**, *62*, 302e8. [CrossRef] [PubMed]
25. Zhai, W.; Duan, F.; Li, D.; Yan, Q.; Dai, S.; Zhang, B.; Wang, J. Risk stratification and adjuvant chemotherapy after radical resection based on the clinical risk scores of patients with stage IB-IIA non-small cell lung cancer. *Eur. J. Surg. Oncol.* **2022**, *48*, 752–760. [CrossRef] [PubMed]
26. Choi, J.; Oh, J.Y.; Lee, Y.S.; Min, K.H.; Shim, J.J.; Choi, S.I.; Park, D.W.; Park, C.K.; Kang, E.J.; Yong, H.S.; et al. Clinical efficacy of adjuvant chemotherapy in stage IB (<4 cm) non-small cell lung cancer patients with high-risk factors. *Korean J. Intern. Med.* **2022**, *37*, 127–136.
27. Wu, Y.L.; John, T.; Grohe, C.; Majem, M.; Goldman, J.W.; Kim, S.W.; Kato, T.; Laktionov, K.; Vu, H.V.; Wang, Z.; et al. Postoperative Chemotherapy Use and Outcomes From ADAURA: Osimertinib as Adjuvant Therapy for Resected EGFR-Mutated NSCLC. *J. Thorac. Oncol.* **2022**, *17*, 423–433. [CrossRef]

Disclaimer/Publisher's Note: The statements, opinions and data contained in all publications are solely those of the individual author(s) and contributor(s) and not of MDPI and/or the editor(s). MDPI and/or the editor(s) disclaim responsibility for any injury to people or property resulting from any ideas, methods, instructions or products referred to in the content.

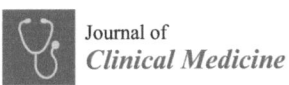

Journal of
Clinical Medicine

Article

Rate and Predictors of Unforeseen PN1/PN2-Disease in Surgically Treated cN0 NSCLC-Patients with Primary Tumor > 3 cm: Nationwide Results from Italian VATS-Group Database

Filippo Lococo [1,2,†], Dania Nachira [1,2,†], Marco Chiappetta [1,2,*], Isabella Sperduti [3], Maria Teresa Congedo [1,2], Elisa Meacci [1,2], Fausto Leoncini [1,4], Rocco Trisolini [1,4], Roberto Crisci [5], Carlo Curcio [6], Monica Casiraghi [7,8], Stefano Margaritora [1,2] and on the behalf of the Italian VATS Group [‡]

1. Università Cattolica del Sacro Cuore, 00168 Rome, Italy
2. Thoracic Surgery, Fondazione Policlinico Universitario A. Gemelli IRCCS, 00168 Rome, Italy
3. Biostatistics, IRCCS Regina Elena National Cancer Institute, 00144 Rome, Italy
4. Interventional Pulmonology Unit, Fondazione Policlinico Universitario A. Gemelli IRCCS, 00168 Rome, Italy
5. Thoracic Surgery, University of L'Aquila, 67100 L'Aquila, Italy
6. Division of Thoracic Surgery, Monaldi Hospital, 80100 Naples, Italy
7. Department of Thoracic Surgery, IEO-European Institute of Oncology IRCCS, 20141 Milan, Italy
8. Department of Oncology and Hemato-Oncology, University of Milan, 20141 Milan, Italy
* Correspondence: marcokiaps@hotmail.it or marco.chiappetta@policlinicogemelli.it; Tel.: +39-3282224738
† These authors contributed equally to this work.
‡ Collaborators of the Italian VATS Group is provided in the Acknowledgments.

Abstract: Background. Since no robust data are available on the real rate of unforeseen N1-N2 disease (uN) and the relative predictive factors in clinical-N0 NSCLC with peripheral tumours > 3 cm, the usefulness of performing a (mini)invasive mediastinal staging in this setting is debated. Herein, we investigated these issues in a nationwide database. **Methods.** From 01/2014 to 06/2020, 15,784 thoracoscopic major lung resections were prospectively recorded in the "Italian VATS-Group" database. Among them, 1982 clinical-N0 peripheral solid-type NSCLC > 3 cm were identified, and information was retrospectively reviewed. A mean comparison of more than two groups was made by ANOVA (Bonferroni correction for multiple comparisons), while associations between the categorical variables were estimated with a Chi-square test. The multivariate logistic regression model and Kaplan–Meyer method were used to identify the independent predictors of nodal upstaging and survival results, respectively. **Results.** At pathological staging, 229 patients had N1-involvement (11.6%), and 169 had uN2 disease (8.5%). Independent predictors of uN1 were SUVmax (OR: 1.98; CI 95: 1.44–2.73, $p = 0.0001$) and tumour-size (OR: 1.52; CI: 1.11–2.10, $p = 0.01$), while independent predictors of uN2 were age (OR: 0.98; CI 95: 0.96–0.99, $p = 0.039$), histology (OR: 0.48; CI 95: 0.30–0.78, $p = 0.003$), SUVmax (OR: 2.07; CI 95: 1.15–3.72, $p = 0.015$), and the number of resected lymph nodes (OR: 1.03; CI 95: 1.01–1.05, $p = 0.002$). **Conclusions.** The unforeseen N1-N2 disease in cN0/NSCLCs > 3 cm undergoing VATS resection is observable in between 12 and 8% of all cases. We have identified predictors that could guide physicians in selecting the best candidate for (mini)invasive mediastinal staging.

Keywords: NSCLC; surgery; nodal upstaging; staging; VATS; VATS-Group

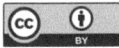

1. Introduction

The treatment plan in non-small cell lung cancer (NSCLC) is substantially based on the tumour stage and general clinical condition of the patient. Basically, while surgery remains the best treatment in clinical N0/N1 disease, multimodal combined treatment (including surgery) is preferable in N2 disease. Therefore, the clinical stage (performed by imaging and (mini)invasive procedures) should be as accurate as possible in order to reduce, at minimum, the number of unforeseen node diseases (pN1-N2) at pathological staging after surgery [1].

Indeed, pathological nodal involvement is one of the most important prognostic factors in NSCLC to evaluate any possible adjuvant therapy and is a good parameter for the effectiveness of the lymphadenectomy and, therefore, of the surgical approach employed [2].

Since no robust data are available on the real rate of unforeseen N1-N2 disease (uN), its prognostic impact, and the relative predictive factors in clinical-N0 NSCLC with peripheral tumours > 3 cm, means that the usefulness of performing a (mini)invasive mediastinal staging in this setting is debated.

In particular, the role of (mini)invasive mediastinal procedures for patients with no detectable lymph node metastases on imaging studies is unclear, and it is questionable whether aggressive invasive lymph node staging affects the prognosis of patients with clinical stage I disease on imaging.

The primary endpoint of this work is to investigate the rate and (secondary endpoint) predictors of unforeseen pN1/pN2-disease in surgically treated cN0-NSCLC patients with a primary tumour > 3 cm in a nationwide database.

2. Materials and Methods

2.1. Patients

All the data used in this analysis were retrospectively extracted from the Italian VATS Group Registry. This database was created in January 2014 to prospectively collect data on VATS lobectomies performed by 56 Italian-certified thoracic surgery centres. Among 15784 cases, 1982 met the inclusion criteria for our study (diagnosis of NSCLC, clinical N0, solid-type tumour measuring > 3 cm).

We excluded from our population study those patients who did not undergo a PET/CT scan before surgery and those with suspected Hilo-mediastinal lymph nodes at CT and/or PET, even if investigated by the (mini) invasive staging of the mediastinum [3]. Moreover, we excluded NSCLC patients who were converted to thoracotomy, those who underwent neoadjuvant treatments, and those with a pathological diagnosis that was different from NSCLC (see the consort diagram reported in Figure 1). We also did not consider patients with sub-solid/non-solid NSCLC, synchronous lung cancer, or multiple nodules.

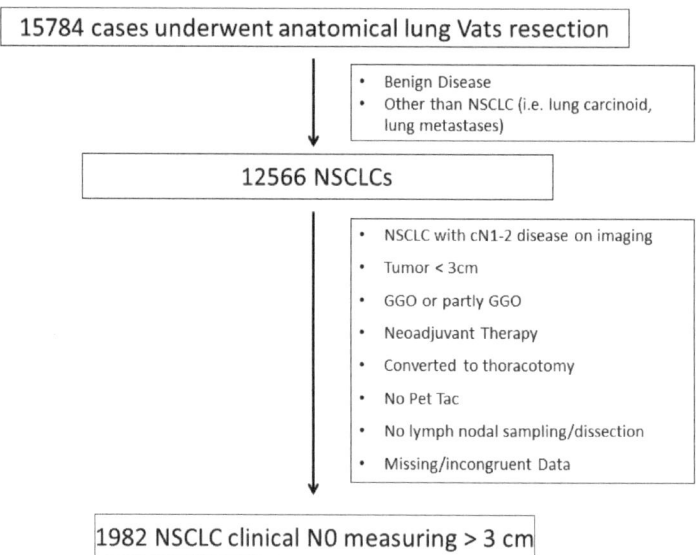

Figure 1. Consort diagram.

For each patient, we recorded the preoperative characteristics such as the age, sex, clinical (c) TNM, intraoperative details, pathological (p) TNM, and the final pathology report, excluding cases where these variables were incomplete or data incongruent.

Despite unavoidable differences between centres, the principles at the basis of surgical lymph node dissection were those described by ESTS [4]. As well, the definitions of systematic nodal dissection, systematic nodal sampling, and nodal sampling followed the ESTS standardized tassonomy defined in 2004 [4].

The rate of nodal upstaging was defined by comparing cTNM to pTNM based on the eighth edition of TNM classification [5]. Nodal micrometastases are defined as clusters of cells measuring between 0.2 and 2 mm in their greatest diameter, usually with mitoses and vascular or lymphatic invasion, and when identified, are considered similar to other nodal metastases with consequent tumour upstaging [6].

2.2. Statistical Methods

Descriptive statistics were used to summarize the pertinent study information. Associations between categorical variables were analysed according to the Pearson chi-square test or Fisher exact test when indicated.

Survival curves were calculated by the Kaplan–Meier method from the date of surgery until relapse or death. The log-rank test was used to assess differences between the subgroups. Significance was defined at the $p \leq 0.05$ level.

The odds ratio (OR) and the 95% confidence intervals (95% CI) were estimated using the logistic regression model.

Factors considered for the univariable analysis of uN1 and uN2 occurrence were: age (continuous), sex, side, type of surgery, histology, lymphadenectomy, primary tumour SUVmax, tumour size, tumour location, the number of resected nodes, type of surgical approach.

Multivariate logistic regression was developed using stepwise regression (forward selection, enter with a limit or a removed limit, $p = 0.10$ and $p = 0.15$, respectively) to identify independent predictors of outcome.

The SPSS (version 21.0; SPSS, Inc., Chicago, IL, USA) and MedCalc (version 14.2.1; MedCalc Software, Ostend, Belgium) licensed statistical programs were used for all analyses.

All of the patients included in this national registry gave their written informed consent, and this database project was approved by the Institutional Research Review Board (IRRB) of each participating centre.

3. Results

From 01/2014 to 06/2020, 15784 thoracoscopic major lung resections were prospectively recorded in the "Italian VATS-Group" database. Among them, the data of 1982 patients who underwent VATS lobectomy from

January 2014 to April 2017 and met the inclusion criteria were extracted from the database (Figure 1) and retrospectively analysed.

Among those, 1315 (67%) were males, 667 (33%) were females, and the median age was 69.7 ± 8.9 years. The main clinical and surgical features are summarized in Table 1.

In particular, the tumour size distribution was: 3–5 cm in 76.9% of cases, 5–7 cm in 18.8%, and >7 cm in 4.1%. The main histology was adenocarcinoma (more than 70% of all tumours), while the median uptake SUVmax value was 8.7 ± 6.4. The surgery consisted of an anatomical resection, in all cases, with only 1.6% of sublobar resection. The main surgical approach was triportal (78%; mainly anterior by "Copenhagen"), followed by biportal (11.9%) and uniportal (10.1%). Two-thirds of the patients underwent systematic lymph nodal dissection, with a mean number of dissected lymph nodes at 13.7 ± 8.3. Finally, no marked differences in terms of the nodal stations and the number of lymph nodes harvested were observed between the different approaches used.

Table 1. Clinical and pathological characteristics.

Variables	
Gender	
M	1315 (66.3%)
F	667 (33.6%)
Age of Diagnosis	
Mean ± SD	69.7 ± 8.9
<70 years	952 (48.0%)
≥70 years	1030 (51.9%)
Side	
Left	828 (41.7%)
Right	1154 (58.2%)
Tumour Location	
Upper	785 (39.6%)
Middle	77 (3.8%)
Lower	1120 (56.5%)
Primary tumour PET SUVmax	
Mean ± SD	8.7 ± 6.4
SUVmax < 2.5	267 (13.4%)
SUVmax ≥ 2.5	1563 (78.8%)
Histology	
Adenocarcinoma	1418 (71.5%)
Squamous cell carcinoma	456 (23.0%)
Others	108 (5.4%)
Tumour-size	
3–5 cm	1526 (76.9%)
5–7 cm	373 (18.8%)
>7 cm	83 (4.1%)
Surgery	
(Bi)Lobar Resection	1949 (98.3%)
Sublobar Resection	33 (1.6 %)
Type of surgical approach	
Triportal	1546 (78.0%)
Biportal	236 (11.9%)
Uniportal	200 (10.1%)
Lymph Node Assessment	
Radical Dissection	1341 (67.6%)
Systematic Sampling or Sampling	641 (32.3%)
Number of LFN dissected (Mean ± SD)	13.7 ± 8.3
All	1982

3.1. Clinico-Pathological Characteristics in N0, uN1 and uN2 Disease

At pathological staging, 229 patients had N1-involvement (11.6%), and 169 had uN2 disease (8.5%). Among pN1 patients, the main number of positive lymph nodes and the rate of micrometastases were 2.0 ± 1.3 and 17.5% (40 patients), respectively, while in pN2 patients, they were 3.0 ± 1.4 and 17.7% (30 patients), respectively.

The distribution of the p-N status according to clinic-pathological variables is reported in Table 2.

Table 2. The distribution of p-N status according to clinic-pathological variables. In this table we describe the clinico-pathological characteristics in the different groups according to N-status.

Variables	pN0 (n, %)	uN1 (n, %)	uN2 (n, %)
Population	1584 (79.9%)	229 (11.6%)	169 (8.5%)
Gender			
M	1064 (80.9%)	145 (11.0%)	106 (8.1%)
F	520 (78.0%)	84 (12.6%)	63 (9.4%)
Age of Diagnosis			
Mean ± SD	70.3 ± 5.4	69 ± 8.5	68 ± 11.0
<70 years	744 (78.2%)	119 (12.5%)	89 (9.3%)
≥70 years	840 (81.5%)	110 (10.7%)	80 (7.8%)
Side			
Left	642 (77.6%)	109 (13.2%)	77 (9.3%)
Right	942 (81.6%)	120 (10.4%)	92 (8.0%)
Tumour Location			
Upper	610 (77.7%)	103 (13.1%)	72 (9.2%)
Middle	63 (81.8%)	7 (9.1%)	7 (9.1%)
Lower	1001 (89.4%)	119 (10.6%)	90 (8.0%)
Primary tumour PET SUVmax			
Mean ± SD	7.8 ± 5.9	10.1 ± 6.1	8.8 ± 5.5
SUVmax < 2.5	235 (88.0%)	19 (7.1%)	13 (4.9%)
SUVmax ≥ 2.5	1226 (78.5%)	191 (12.2%)	146 (9.3%)
Histology			
Adenocarcinoma	1109 (78.2%)	170 (11.9%)	139 (9.8%)
Squamous cell carcinoma	386 (84.7%)	49 (10.7%)	21 (4.6%)
Others	89 (82.4%)	10 (9.3%)	9 (8.3%)
Tumour-size			
3–5 cm	1238 (81.1%)	157 (10.2%)	131 (8.7%)
5–7 cm	284 (76.1%)	58 (15.5%)	31 (8.3%)
>7 cm	62 (74.7%)	14 (16.9%)	7 (8.4%)
Surgery			
(Bi)Lobar Resection	1553 (79.7%)	228 (11.7%)	168 (8.6%)
Sublobar Resection	31 (94.0%)	1 (3.0%)	1 (3.0%)
Lymph Node Assessment			
Radical Dissection	1061 (79.1%)	163 (12.2%)	117 (8.7%)
Sampling	523 (81.6%)	66 (10.3%)	52 (8.1%)
Number of nodes dissected (Mean ± SD)	12.4 ± 6.6	15.7 ± 9.8	15.7 ± 8.6

A significant difference ($p = 0.001$) was observed for the uN1/uN2 rate compared to tumours with a low FDG uptake and high FDG uptake, and in addition, higher SUVmax values were associated in patients with uN1/uN2 disease compared with N0 disease. Similarly, the rate of N2 disease was higher in adenocarcinoma (9.8% vs. 4.6%, $p = 0.008$) compared to squamous cell carcinoma, while the rate of uN1 disease was substantially similar. Interestingly, the larger the tumour size, the higher the rate of uN1 disease was ($p = 0.003$), while the rate of uN2 disease was similar in all subgroups. Finally, the mean number of dissected lymph nodes was significantly ($p < 0.001$) higher in uN1/uN2 disease (both 15.7%) compared to that observed in N0-disease (12.4%).

3.2. Predictive Factors for uN1 and uN2

Using a multivariate logistic regression model, independent predictors of uN1 were SUVmax (OR: 1.98; CI95%: 1.44–2.73, $p = 0.0001$), and a tumour-size >5 cm (OR: 1.52; CI95%: 1.11–2.10, $p = 0.01$), while independent predictors of uN2 were age (OR: 0.98; CI95%: 0.96–0.99, $p = 0.039$), adenocarcinoma histology (OR: 0.48; CI95%: 0.30–0.78, $p = 0.003$), SUVmax > 6 (OR: 1.807; CI95%: 1.27–2.58, $p = 0.001$), lymph node resected > 6 (OR: 2.37; CI95%: 1.26–4.45, $p = 0.007$) (Table 3).

Table 3. Multivariable analysis for unforeseen pN1 and pN2.

Variable	N1 Upstaging OR (CI95%)	p Value
SUVmax ≥ 6	1.98 (1.44–2.73)	<0.0001
Tumour-size ≥ 5 cm	1.52 (1.11–2.10)	0.01
Variable	N2 Upstaging OR (CI95%)	p Value
Age	0.98 (0.96–0.99)	0.039
Histology (Ref:SCC)	0.48 (0.30–0.78)	0.003
SUVmax ≥ 6	1.807 (1.27–2.58)	0.001
Resected-LN ≥ 6	2.37 (1.26–4.45)	0.007

3.3. Survival Results According to N-Status

The five-year overall survival (Figure 2) was 73.1% in pN0 patients vs. 35.3% and 31.1% in pN1 and pN2 patients, respectively ($p < 0.0001$), while five-year cancer-specific survival was 81.1% in pN0 vs. 40.0% and 37.8% in pN1 and pN2, respectively ($p < 0.0001$).

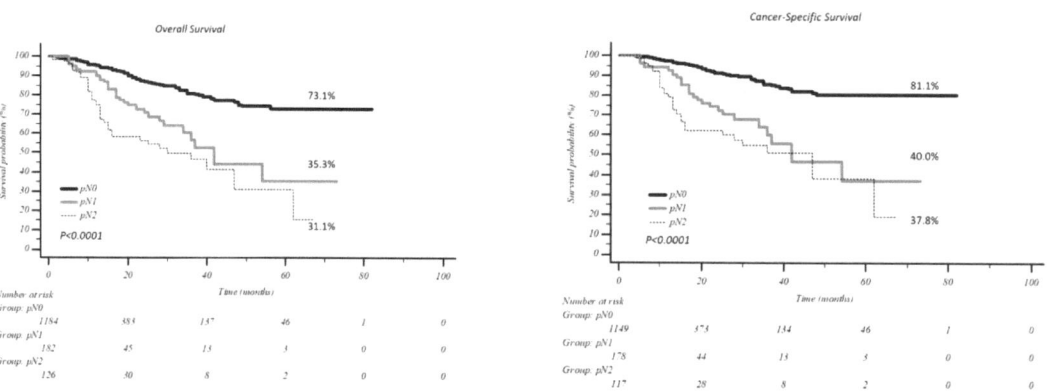

Figure 2. Overall and cancer specific survival according to nodal involvement.

According to tumour dimension, no difference in survival was present in patients with pN0 and pN1 and a tumour >5 cm vs. <5 cm, 5years overall survival was 74.7% vs. 72.8% ($p = 0.612$) in pN0 patients and 36.0% vs. 36.7% in pN1 patients ($p = 0.338$, Figure 3). Conversely, in uN2 patients, the difference in survival was statistically significant: five-year overall survival of 35.1% was recorded in tumours <5 cm vs. 25.5% in tumours >5 cm ($p = 0.031$, Figure 3).

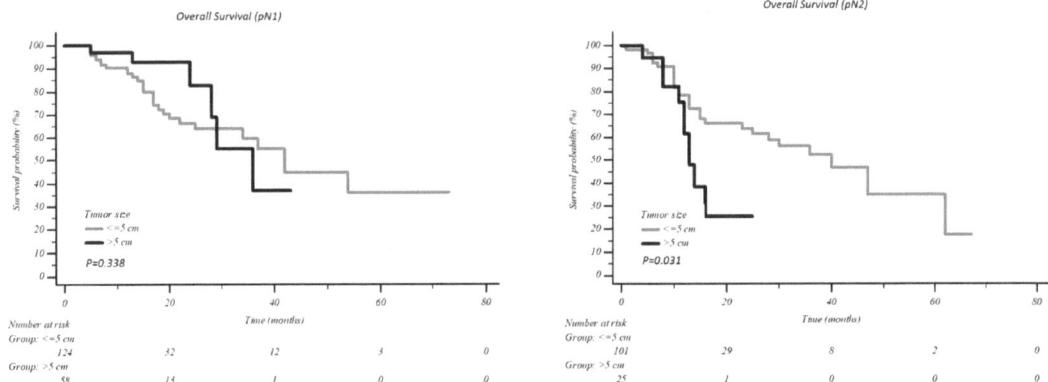

Figure 3. Overall survival according to the tumour dimension in patients with pN1 and pN2.

4. Discussion

The American College of Chest Physicians (ACCP) guidelines [7] and the ESTS guidelines [4] suggest performing mediastinal staging by mediastinoscopy or video-assisted mediastinoscopy (VAM) in some specific subsets of patients with negative lymph nodes at preoperative CT and/or PET-CT. In the case of central tumours, tumours greater than 3 cm or cN1, or with adenocarcinoma histology, the ACCP indicates endoscopic staging by EBUS/EUS with FNA as a first step (level of evidence 2B), while the ESTS concludes that the choice between mediastinoscopy/pre-surgical lymphadenectomy (VAMLA or TEMLA) and EBUS/EUS must rely on local expertise (level of evidence V). The reported sensitivity of EBUS was 0.17–0.41 in cN0 patients and 0.38–0.53 in cN1 ones for early-stage NSCLC, and 0.86–0.88 in N2/N3 NSCLC; the sensitivity of combined EUS/EBUS was 0.83 (95% CI 0.77–0.8). Negative EUS/EBUS results in patients at risk were confirmed by mediastinoscopy, which, to date, remains the gold standard in the staging process, with a sensitivity ranging from 0.78 to 0.97 and a negative predictive value of 0.83–0.99 [3,8].

Nevertheless, not all thoracic centres perform mediastinoscopy as a confirmation in patients with suspicious nodal enlargement or large tumours but with negative PET-CT after a negative EBUS [9]. A retrospective study on Italian VATS-Group data concluded that only 3.5% of patients (22.1% cT2 and 1.8% cT3) underwent an invasive mediastinal staging with an incidence of pN2-upstaging of 6.5% [9].

The main risk factors involved in nodal upstaging in early-stage lung cancer are still debated, and several works also investigated the topic in relation to different surgical approaches, including open, VATS, or both. Indeed, while some authors have been concerned about the safety and effectiveness of VATS in performing an oncological radical lymphadenectomy compared to open or RATS surgery, Toker et al. [2] believed that VATS lymphadenectomy could have some limits only in the hands of novice surgeons. In fact, while RATS surgery gives the possibility to everyone to replicate open dissection, thanks to the high technological instrumentations in assisting movements, VATS requires certain expertise. Therefore, after overcoming the learning curve, a surgical approach should not influence nodal upstaging.

In recent years, several—manly retrospective—studies (Table 4) were identified as predictive risk factors for post-operative nodal upstaging: T stage, tumour size, number of dissected nodes, type of surgical approach, lower lobes, SUVmax, adenocarcinoma histology [1,10–14], etc.

Table 4. An overview of studies on the nodal upstaging.

Study	Patients	Inclusion Criteria	pN1/N2-Upstaging (%)	Upstaging Risk Factors	Survival pN0	Survival u-pN1	Survival u-pN2
Rocha, 2004 [10] (prospective; thoracotomy)	109	c-stage: I/II (cN0, cN1) NSCLC	upN1: 5.5% upN2: 8.3%	-lower lobe location ($p < 0.006$)	NA	NA	NA
Lee, 2007 [14] (retrospective; thoracotomy)	224	c-stage: I NSCLC	upN1: 9.8% upN2: 6.5% (T1)-8.7% (T2)	-central tumours ($p < 0.001$) -larger cT size ($p < 0.001$) -adeno-carcinoma histology (p: 0.082) -higher tumour PET-SUV$_{max}$ (p: 0.017)	NA	NA	NA
Licht, 2013 [1] (retrospective on a National registry; Thoracotomy vs. VATS)	1513	c-stage: I NSCLC	upN1: 13.1% vs. 8.1% ($p < 0.001$) upN2: 11.5 vs. 3.8% ($p < 0.001$)	-cT stage ($p = 0.01$) -invasive mediastinal staging ($p < 0.001$) -number of nodal stations dissected ($p = 0.02$) -surgical approach ($p < 0.001$) -lower lobe ($p = 0.045$).	HR: 1	HR: 1.84	HR: 2.79 ($p < 0.001$)
Marulli, 2018 [12] (retrospective; VATS)	231	cT1-T3N0, I-IIB NSCLC	upN1: 9.1% upN2: 7.4%	-T size (p: 0.027) -adenocarcinoma histology (p: 0.0382)	NA	NA	NA
Ismail, 2018 [15] (retrospective; VATS)	136	c-stage: I-IIB	upN1: 7.4% upN2: 5.2%	-positive nodes in stations 2–4 (0.009) and 5–6 (0.027)	NA	NA	NA
Moon, 2018 [11] (retrospective; Thoracotomy)	486	Peripheral cT1N0	upN1: 4.7% upN2: 3.9%	-tumour diameter (p: 0.039) -consolidation/tumour ratio ($p = 0.001$)	NA	NA	NA
Marulli, 2019 [13] (retrospective on a National registry; VATS)	3276	cT1-T3N0, I-IIB NSCLC	upN1: 6.2% upN2: 2.4%	-adenocarcinoma histology ($p < 0.001$) -higher tumour grade ($p < 0.001$) -higher pathologicT status ($p < 0.001$) -tumour size > 3 cm ($p < 0.001$) -upper lobe tumours ($p = 0.049$) ->12 nodes resected ($p < 0.001$)	NA	NA	NA
Present series 2021 (retrospective on a National registry; VATS)	1982	cN0 peripheral solid-type NSCLC > 3 cm	upN1: 11.6% upN2: 8.5%	uN1: -SUVmax (OR: 1.98; CI95: 1.44–2.73, $p = 0.0001$), -tumour-size (OR: 1.52; CI: 1.11–2.10, $p = 0.01$); uN2: -age, $p = 0.039$), -histology ($p = 0.003$), -SUVmax ($p = 0.015$), -number of resected nodes ($p = 0.002$).	5 y: 73%	5 y: 35%	5 y: 31% ($p < 0.0001$)

In our series of 1982 patients with cN0 peripheral solid-type NSCLC > 3 cm, both the N1- and N-2 involvements were higher (11.6% vs. 6.2% and 8.5% vs. 2.4%) compared to cT1-T3N0 patients of Marulli's series [13] from the same national database. This could be explained by the presence of only larger tumours (>3 cm) in our dataset. Indeed, a previous retrospective analysis on 160 cN0 NSCLC patients [16] who underwent an open or Uniportal VATS approach identified the main risk factor for pN1 upstaging only in central/larger (>3 cm) tumours (p: 0.0004).

Our analysis confirmed most of the results of previous studies [13,14], identifying, in particular, SUVmax > 6 ($p = 0.0001$) and the tumour size >5 cm ($p = 0.01$) as predictor factors for pN1 nodal upstaging, while age ($p = 0.039$), adenocarcinoma histology ($p = 0.003$), SUVmax > 6 ($p = 0.001$), and more than six lymph nodes resected ($p = 0.007$) as predictors for pN2. In particular, we confirmed the role of histology in predicting N2 upstaging, as other authors reported previously [12–14]. The number of retrieved nodes predictive of pathological upstaging is also an argument of debate among the authors. Ismail and colleagues [15] concluded that the resection of 18 nodes could be the best predictor of general nodal upstaging (13.3%) in a single-centre VATS series of 136 patients and suggested the removal of at least seven nodes from hilar stations and eleven from mediastinal ones to enhance the possibilities of detecting an unforeseen nodal disease.

On the other hand, in our study, tumour dimension resulted as a predictive factor for N1 upstaging and not for N2, but this result could explain considering the kind of N1 involvement. Indeed, despite N2, metastases are only due to lymphatic spreading, and N1 involvement may be related to lymphatic dissemination or direct nodal invasion. Unfortunately, in the database, it was not possible to know if N1 positive nodes were related to direct infiltration, but the rate of these cases may explain this difference considering the tumour dimension on this topic.

Interestingly, age resulted in an independent prognostic factor for N2 upstaging, which is, to our knowledge, the first report of this risk factor. However, even if we found a correlation between age and N2 upstaging, it was hard to understand the possible correlation. One possibility was the presence of more aggressive tumours in younger patients [17], but further studies are needed to validate this hypothesis.

Accurate identification of the predictive factors of upstaging is pivotal for selecting the best candidates for a (mini)invasive mediastinal staging. From a theoretical point of view, we could reserve the staging (mini-invasive) procedures only for cN0-NSCLC patients with a higher risk of N+ disease with several practical implications: (i) to optimize resources and reducing costs; (ii) to avoid complications from unnecessary procedures; (iii) to reduce an interval in surgery. Obviously, these results should be confirmed on the prospective clinical cohort of patients, and clear recommendations should guide physicians in the diagnostic pathway.

Moreover, an accurate definition of N-status before surgery has several potential implications. In particular, a correct staging could help in planning the most appropriate and tailored treatment for patients at risk—not only in terms of adjuvant therapies—but to increase their overall survival. Indeed, limited sub-lobar resections or sampling/limited lobe-specific lymphadenectomy should be avoided in patients with risk factors of nodal upstaging.

While some authors [18–20] believe that nodal involvement in the post-operative period and unexpected pN2 disease could worsen survival, Obiols et al. [21] showed a reasonable survival rate (40% at 5-year follow-up vs. 10–30%) of that reported in the above-mentioned studies [18,19]. The authors explained the results by accurate preoperative staging, which reduced the number of uN2 if conducted according to the ESTS guidelines. Furthermore, they concluded that surgery might be reasonable in pN2 patients if complete resection can be achieved.

Our survival results showed a five-year overall survival of 35.3% and 31.1% in pN1 and pN2 patients, respectively, compared to 73.1% in pN0 patients ($p < 0.0001$). From these results, the importance of accurately defining the N-status before surgery clearly emerged, even if pN2 patients should not be excluded a priori from surgery but discussed in a multidisciplinary setting.

Our large series reflects the real scenario adopted in most parts of Italian Thoracic Centres in the preoperative management and staging procedures of this subset of NSCLC patients. The main biases of this work are the retrospective nature of the study on a prospective collected national database, the selection bias (only VATS procedures), and above all, the no uniform adherence to ESTS guidelines by thoracic surgeons in performing pre-operative staging in the case of large (>3 cm) peripheral cN0. Moreover, since we found that the mean number of dissected lymph nodes was significantly higher in uN1/uN2 disease compared to that observed in N0-disease, the rate of uN1/N2 could be under-estimated in those patients with a few lymph nodes sampled during surgery. Then, the unforeseen postoperative nodal involvement is a mirror for a series of factors, such as the surgeons' expertise in VATS, the intrinsic risk factors related to the tumour, and, above all, the incorrect preoperative management of those patients.

5. Conclusions

The unforeseen N1-N2 disease in cN0/NSCLCs measuring >3 cm and undergoing VATS resection is observed in between 12 and 8% of all cases, respectively, and seems to have a prognostic impact. Considering the importance of identifying predictive factors in this subpopulation of NSCLC patients, we have herein identified different predictors of unforeseen N1 and uN2 on a large cohort of patients who underwent video-assisted surgery.

These findings should be confirmed in prospective studies and, in the near future, could guide physicians to select the best candidate for (mini)invasive mediastinal staging and to adopt a tailored strategy of care.

Author Contributions: Italian VATS group: data source; Conceptualization, F.L. (Filippo Lococo); Data curation, D.N. and F.L. (Fausto Leoncini); Formal analysis, I.S.; Investigation, F.L. (Filippo Lococo) and D.N.; Methodology, F.L. (Filippo Lococo); Project administration, M.C. (Monica Casiraghi); Supervision, E.M., R.C. and C.C.; Validation, D.N.; Visualization, M.T.C. and R.T.; Writing—original draft, F.L. (Filippo Lococo); Writing—review and editing, M.C. (Marco Chiappetta) and S.M. All authors have read and agreed to the published version of the manuscript.

Funding: This research received no external funding.

Institutional Review Board Statement: Ethical review and approval were waived for this study due to the use of a multicentric national database.

Informed Consent Statement: Patient consent was waived due to the use of a multicentric national database.

Data Availability Statement: Data are the property of the Italian VATS group.

Acknowledgments: We would like to thank Franziska M. Lohmeyer, Fondazione Policlinico Universitario A. Gemelli IRCCS, for her support in revising the language of our manuscript. Collaborators on the behalf of the Italian VATS Group: Mancuso Maurizio, Pernazza Fausto, Refai Majed, Stella Franco, Argnani Desideria, Marulli Giuseppe, De Palma Angela, Bortolotti Luigi, Rizzardi Giovanna, Solli Piergiorgio, Dolci Giampiero, Perkmann Reinhold, Zaraca Francesco, Benvenuti Mauro Roberto, Gavezzoli Diego, Cherchi Roberto, Ferrari Paolo Albino, Mucilli Felice, Camplese Pierpaolo, Melloni Giulio, Mazza Federico, Cavallesco Giorgio, Maniscalco Pio, Voltolini Luca, Gonfiotti Alessandro, Sollitto Francesco, Ardò Nicoletta Pia, Pariscenti Gian Luca, Risso Carlo, Surrente Corrado, Lopez Camillo, Droghetti Andrea, Giovanardi Michele, Breda Cristiano, Lo Giudice Fabio, Alloisio Marco, Bottoni Edoardo, Spaggiari Lorenzo, Gasparri Roberto, Torre Massimo, Rinaldo Alessandro, Nosotti Mario, Tosi Davide, Negri Giampiero, Bandiera Alessandro, Baisi Alessandro, Raveglia Federico, Stefani Alessandro, Natali Pamela, Scarci Marco, Pirondini Emanuele, Curcio Carlo, Amore Dario, Rena Ottavio, Nicotra Samuele, Dell' Amore Andrea, Bertani Alessandro, Tancredi Giorgia, Ampollini Luca, Carbognani Paolo, Puma Francesco, Vinci Damiano, Cardillo Giuseppe, Carleo Francesco, Margaritora Stefano, Meacci Elisa, Paladini Piero, Ghisalberti Marco, Crisci Roberto, Divisi Duilio, Fontana Diego, Della Beffa Vittorio, Morelli Angelo, Londero Francesco, Imperatori Andrea, Rotolo Nicola, Alberto, Viti Andrea, Infante Maurizio, Benato Cristiano.

Conflicts of Interest: The authors declare no conflict of interest.

References

1. Licht, P.B.; Jørgensen, O.D.; Ladegaard, L.; Jakobsen, E. A national study of nodal upstaging after thoracoscopic versus open lobectomy for clinical stage I lung cancer. *Ann. Thorac. Surg.* **2013**, *96*, 943–949; discussion 949–950. [CrossRef] [PubMed]
2. Toker, A.; Özyurtkan, M.O.; Kaba, E. Nodal upstaging: Effects of instrumentation and three-dimensional view in clinical stage I lung cancer. *J. Vis. Surg.* **2017**, *3*, 76. [CrossRef]
3. De Leyn, P.; Dooms, C.; Kuzdzal, J.; Lardinois, D.; Passlick, B.; Rami-Porta, R.; Zielinski, M. Revised ESTS guidelines for preoperative mediastinal lymph node staging for non-small-cell lung cancer. *Eur. J. Cardio-Thorac. Surg.* **2014**, *45*, 787–798. [CrossRef] [PubMed]

4. Lardinois, D.; De Leyn, P.; Van Schil, P.; Porta, R.R.; Waller, D.; Passlick, B.; Zielinski, M.; Junker, K.; Rendina, E.A.; Ris, H.-B. ESTS guidelines for intraoperative lymph node staging in nonsmall cell lung cancer. *Eur. J. Cardio-Thorac. Surg.* **2006**, *30*, 787–792. [CrossRef]
5. Asamura, H.; Chansky, K.; Crowley, J.; Goldstraw, P.; Rusch, V.W.; Vansteenkiste, J.F.; Watanabe, H.; Wu, Y.L.; Zielinski, M.; Ball, D.; et al. International Association for the Study of Lung Cancer Staging and Prognostic Factors Committee, Advisory Board Members, and Participating Institutions. The International Association for the Study of Lung Cancer Lung Cancer Staging Project: Proposals for the Revision of the N Descriptors in the Forthcoming 8th Edition of the TNM Classification for Lung Cancer. *J. Thorac. Oncol.* **2015**, *10*, 1675–1684. [CrossRef]
6. Garelli, E.; Renaud, S.; Falcoz, P.E.; Weingertner, N.; Olland, A.; Santelmo, N.; Massard, G. Microscopic N2 disease exhibits a better prognosis in resected non-small-cell lung cancer. *Eur. J. Cardio-Thorac. Surg.* **2016**, *50*, 322–328. [CrossRef]
7. Silvestri, G.A.; Gonzalez, A.V.; Jantz, M.A.; Margolis, M.L.; Gould, M.K.; Tanoue, L.T.; Harris, L.J.; Detterbeck, F.C. Diagnosis and management of lung cancer, 3rd ed: American College of Chest Physicians evidence-based clinical practice guidelines. *Chest* **2013**, *143* (Suppl. 5), e211S–e250S. [CrossRef]
8. Rami-Porta, R.; Call, S.; Dooms, C.; Obiols, C.; Sánchez, M.; Travis, W.D.; Vollmer, I. Lung cancer staging: A concise update. *Eur. Respir. J.* **2018**, *51*, 1800190. [CrossRef]
9. Bertani, A.; Gonfiotti, A.; Nosotti, M.; Ferrari, P.A.; De Monte, L.; Russo, E.; Guerrera, F. Nodal management and upstaging of disease: Initial results from the Italian VATS Lobectomy Registry. *J. Thorac. Dis.* **2017**, *9*, 2061–2070. [CrossRef]
10. Rocha, A.T.; McCormack, M.; Montana, G.; Schreiber, G. Association between lower lobe location and upstaging for early-stage non-small cell lung cancer. *Chest* **2004**, *125*, 1424–1430. [CrossRef] [PubMed]
11. Moon, Y.; Kil Park, J.; Lee, K.Y.; Namkoong, M.; Ahn, S. Consolidation/Tumor Ratio on Chest Computed Tomography as Predictor of Postoperative Nodal Upstaging in Clinical T1N0 Lung Cancer. *World J. Surg.* **2018**, *42*, 2872–2878. [CrossRef]
12. Marulli, G.; Verderi, E.; Comacchio, G.M.; Monaci, N.; Natale, G.; Nicotra, S.; Rea, F. Predictors of unexpected nodal upstaging in patients with cT1-3N0 non-small cell lung cancer (NSCLC) submitted to thoracoscopic lobectomy. *J. Vis. Surg.* **2018**, *4*, 15. [CrossRef]
13. Marulli, G.; Faccioli, E.; Mammana, M.; Nicotra, S.; Comacchio, G.; Verderi, E.; De Palma, A.; Rea, F.; Italian VATS Group. Predictors of nodal upstaging in patients with cT1-3N0 non-small cell lung cancer (NSCLC): Results from the Italian VATS Group Registry. *Surg. Today* **2020**, *50*, 711–718, Erratum in *Surg. Today* **2020**, *50*, 719–720. [CrossRef]
14. Lee, P.C.; Port, J.L.; Korst, R.J.; Liss, Y.; Meherally, D.N.; Altorki, N.K. Risk factors for occult mediastinal metastases in clinical stage I non-small cell lung cancer. *Ann. Thorac. Surg.* **2007**, *84*, 177–181. [CrossRef] [PubMed]
15. Ismail, M.; Nachira, D.; Swierzy, M.; Ferretti, G.M.; Englisch, J.P.; Saidy, R.R.O.; Li, F.; Badakhshi, H.; Rueckert, J.C. Lymph node upstaging for non-small cell lung cancer after uniportal video-assisted thoracoscopy. *J. Thorac. Dis.* **2018**, *10* (Suppl. 31), S3648–S3654. [CrossRef]
16. Nachira, D.; Meacci, E.; Congedo, M.T.; Chiappetta, M.; Petracca Ciavarella, L.; Vita, M.L.; Margaritora, S. Upstaging, centrality and survival in early stage non-small cell lung cancer video-assisted surgery: Lymph nodal upstaging in lung cancer surgery: Is it really a surgical technique problem? *Lung Cancer* **2020**, *144*, 85–86. [CrossRef] [PubMed]
17. Hughes, D.J.; Kapiris, M.; Podvez Nevajda, A.; McGrath, H.; Stavraka, C.; Ahmad, S.; Taylor, B.; Cook, G.J.R.; Ghosh, S.; Josephs, D.; et al. Non-Small Cell Lung Cancer (NSCLC) in Young Adults, Age < 50, Is Associated with Late Stage at Presentation and a Very Poor Prognosis in Patients That Do Not Have a Targeted Therapy Option: A Real-World Study. *Cancers* **2022**, *14*, 6056. [CrossRef] [PubMed]
18. Cerfolio, R.J.; Bryant, A.S. Survival of patients with unsuspected N2 (stage IIIA) nonsmall-cell lung cancer. *Ann. Thorac. Surg.* **2008**, *86*, 362–366; discussion 366–367. [CrossRef]
19. Boada, M.; Sánchez-Lorente, D.; Libreros, A.; Lucena, C.M.; Marrades, R.; Sánchez, M.; Paredes, P.; Serrano, M.; Guirao, A.; Guzmán, R.; et al. Is invasive mediastinal staging necessary in intermediate risk patients with negative PET/CT? *J. Thorac. Dis.* **2020**, *12*, 3976–3986. [CrossRef]
20. Chiappetta, M.; Leuzzi, G.; Sperduti, I.; Bria, E.; Mucilli, F.; Lococo, F.; Filosso, P.L.; Ratto, G.B.; Spaggiari, L.; Facciolo, F. Mediastinal Up-Staging During Surgery in Non-Small-Cell Lung Cancer: Which Mediastinal Lymph Node Metastasis Patterns Better Predict the Outcome? A Multicenter Analysis. *Clin. Lung Cancer* **2020**, *21*, 464–471.e1. [CrossRef]
21. Obiols, C.; Call, S.; Rami-Porta, R.; Trujillo-Reyes, J.C.; Saumench, R.; Iglesias, M.; Serra-Mitjans, M.; Gonzalez-Pont, G.; Belda-Sanchís, J. Survival of patients with unsuspected pN2 non-small cell lung cancer after an accurate preoperative mediastinal staging. *Ann. Thorac. Surg.* **2014**, *97*, 957–964. [CrossRef] [PubMed]

Disclaimer/Publisher's Note: The statements, opinions and data contained in all publications are solely those of the individual author(s) and contributor(s) and not of MDPI and/or the editor(s). MDPI and/or the editor(s) disclaim responsibility for any injury to people or property resulting from any ideas, methods, instructions or products referred to in the content.

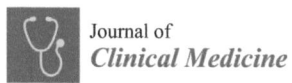
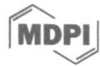

Article

Do More with Less? Lobectomy vs. Segmentectomy for Patients with Congenital Pulmonary Malformations

Beatrice Trabalza Marinucci [1,*], Cecilia Menna [1], Paolo Scanagatta [2], Silvia Fiorelli [3], Matteo Tiracorrendo [1], Giuseppe Naldi [2], Alessandro Inserra [4], Francesco Macchini [5], Erino Angelo Rendina [1] and Mohsen Ibrahim [1]

[1] Thoracic Surgery Sant'Andrea Hospital, La Sapienza University, 00186 Rome, Italy; cecilia.menna@uniroma1.it (C.M.); tiracorrendomatteo@gmail.com (M.T.); erinoangelo.rendina@uniroma1.it (E.A.R.); mohsen.ibrahim@uniroma1.it (M.I.)
[2] Thoracic Surgery—Morelli Hospital, ASST Valtellina e Alto Lario, 23100 Sondalo, Italy; paoscan@hotmail.com (P.S.); giuseppe.naldi@asst-val.it (G.N.)
[3] Anesthesiology and Intensive Care, Sant'Andrea Hospital, La Sapienza University, 00186 Rome, Italy; silvia.fiorelli@uniroma1.it
[4] General and Thoracic Surgery—Bambino Gesù Children's Research Hospital IRCCS, 00165 Rome, Italy; alessandro.inserra@opbg.net
[5] Paediatric Surgery—Niguarda Hospital, ASST Grande Ospedale Niguarda, 20162 Milan, Italy; francesco.macchini@ospedaleniguarda.it
* Correspondence: beatrice.trabalzamarinucci@uniroma1.it; Tel.: +39-3397444709

Abstract: Background: Congenital Pulmonary Malformations (CPMs) are rare benign lesions potentially causing infective complications and/or malignant transformation, requiring surgery even when asymptomatic. CPMs are rare in adulthood but potentially detected at any age. There is not a consensus on the correct extent of resection in both adults and paediatrics. This retrospective multicentric study aims to identify the appropriate surgical resection to prevent the recurrence of the related respiratory symptoms. Methods: Between 2010 and 2020, a total of 96 patients (adults and pediatrics) underwent surgery for CPMs in 4 centers. A 2:1 propensity score matching (considering sex and lesion side) was performed, identifying 2 groups: 50 patients underwent lobectomy (group A) and 25 sub-lobar resections (group B). Clinical and histopathological characteristics, early and late complications, and symptom recurrence were retrospectively analyzed and compared between the two groups by univariate and multivariate analysis. Results: Patients who underwent lobectomy had a statistically significant lower rate of recurrence (4% vs. 24% of group B, $p = 0.014$) and a lower rate of intraoperative complications ($p = 0.014$). Logistic regression identified sub-lobar resection ($p = 0.040$), intra- and post-operative complications ($p = 0.105$ and 0.022), and associated developed neoplasm ($p = 0.062$) as possible risk factors for symptom recurrence after surgery. Conclusions: Pulmonary lobectomy seems to be the most effective surgical treatment for CPMs, guaranteeing the stable remission of symptoms and a lower rate of intra- and postoperative complications. To our knowledge, this is one of the largest studies comparing lobectomy and sub-lobar resections in patients affected by CPMs, considering the low incidence worldwide.

Keywords: Congenital Pulmonary Malformations; thoracic surgery; lobectomy; pulmonary sequestration; congenital cystic adenomatoid malformation

Citation: Marinucci, B.T.; Menna, C.; Scanagatta, P.; Fiorelli, S.; Tiracorrendo, M.; Naldi, G.; Inserra, A.; Macchini, F.; Rendina, E.A.; Ibrahim, M. Do More with Less? Lobectomy vs. Segmentectomy for Patients with Congenital Pulmonary Malformations. *J. Clin. Med.* 2023, 12, 5237. https://doi.org/10.3390/jcm12165237

Academic Editor: David Barnes

Received: 6 July 2023
Revised: 29 July 2023
Accepted: 9 August 2023
Published: 11 August 2023

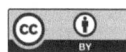

Copyright: © 2023 by the authors. Licensee MDPI, Basel, Switzerland. This article is an open access article distributed under the terms and conditions of the Creative Commons Attribution (CC BY) license (https://creativecommons.org/licenses/by/4.0/).

1. Introduction

CPMs (Congenital Pulmonary Malformations) are a wide spectrum of congenital lung benign lesions such as pulmonary sequestration (PS), congenital cystic adenomatoid malformation (CCAM), congenital lobar emphysema, bronchial atresia, and others intermediary forms.

CCAMs are the most frequent, occurring in 25% of all CPMs [1] and consisting of hamartomatous cystic replacement of the normal lung parenchyma. CCAMs are gland-like cystic lesions of different sizes first classified by Stocker et al. [2] as type 1 (large cysts of 3–10 cm in diameter), type 2 (smaller cysts of <2 cm), and type 3 (minute cysts of <0.3 cm). Later, two other types were added: type 0 (solid malformation often not compatible with life) and type 4 (few peripheral cysts lined by alveolar epithelium).

Pulmonary sequestration (PS) represents 0.15–6.45% of CPMs [3]; it is characterized by a mass of non-functioning lung tissue separated from the normal tracheobronchial tree and receiving vascular supply from a systemic artery (Figure 1). It is classified as intra-lobar PS (IL-PS) when it is incorporated in the parenchyma of a lobe and as extra-lobar PS (EL-PS) when it is separated from the adjacent normal parenchyma by its own pleural envelope.

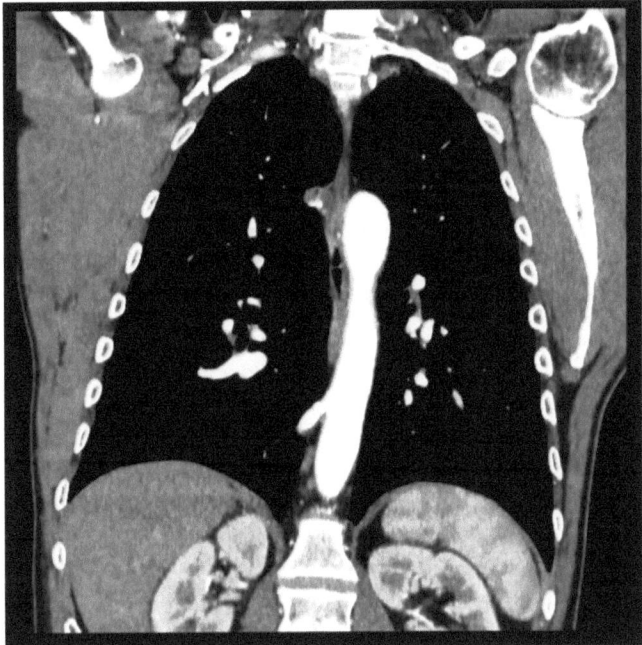

Figure 1. CT evidence of systemic arterial vascularization from descending thoracic aorta.

CPMs represent anomalies occurring because of the abnormal embryonal development of the bronchial tree and they can often be associated with other congenital anomalies or with each other. In fact, CCAM is described in 50% of extra-lobar PS and in 15% of intra-lobar PS [4].

In the past decades, the spread of prenatal ultrasonography has led to a progressive increase in the antenatal detection of CPMs, confirmed by radiological images (chest Rx or CT scan) early after birth.

Most neonates are asymptomatic at birth (>75%). The clinical presentation and severity depend on the extent and on the localization of the lesion [5,6]. CPMs clinically present with respiratory symptoms (such pneumonia, hemoptysis, productive coughing, recurrent wheeze) due to infective complications, occurring most frequently at an average age of 7 months or later during growth. In fact, prenatal diagnosis is sometimes missed, and detection may occur later, either by chance or because of unexplained recurrent or persistent respiratory symptoms or signs, occurring beyond infancy, in adolescence, and/or adulthood. As previously reported in the literature, the most frequent symptoms related to CPMs are pneumonia, recurrent bronchitis, bronchiolitis, severe cough, hemoptysis, dyspnea, and respiratory distress [7,8].

Surgical treatment is mandatory for symptomatic lesions. On the contrary, the management of asymptomatic lesions is rather controversial, as some authors sustain a conservative approach before respiratory symptoms occur. Nevertheless, there is wide concern in literature about the indication of surgical resection even for asymptomatic lesions, to prevent recurrent respiratory symptoms, to ensure a safer surgery before inflammation complicates the anatomy of the lesion and, finally, to avoid the rare but possible malignant transformation [6]. A preliminary study from Rotterdam evaluating pulmonary function in children undergoing pulmonary lobectomy before and after the age of 2 years, showed no differences. Early resection before the development of respiratory complications may also facilitate the thoracoscopic approach of surgical treatment in experienced hands.

Consequently, surgery is indicated early after lesion detection. Moreover, considering that detection is most frequent in neonates and infants, parenchyma-sparing techniques have been proposed depending on the lesion's size and localization. However, the potential lung growth in paediatric patients is described to justify an early lobectomy [7]. To date, there is not a consensus indicating the correct extent of surgical resection between lobectomy and sub-lobar resection for CPMs in adult or paediatric patients.

This retrospective multicentric study aims to identify the appropriate surgical treatment to prevent the recurrence of respiratory symptoms related to the lesions.

2. Materials and Methods

This multi-institutional retrospective observational study included 96 consecutive paediatric and adult patients surgically treated between 2010 and 2020 for CPMs in 4 centres: La Sapienza University of Rome, ASST Valtellina e Alto Lario of Sondrio, Bambino Gesu 'Children's Research Hospital of Rome, and IRCCS Ca' Granda Foundation—Policlinico of Milan.

Lesions were detected radiologically by prenatal ultrasonography of the second pregnancy trimester, then confirmed by computed tomography (CT) scan within the first 3 months after birth, or immediately in symptomatic lesions. Lesions detected prenatally were surgically treated within the first year of age, as previously reported [8]. In all the other cases, lesions were detected incidentally or when symptomatic by CT scan and treated early after the diagnosis.

Preoperative assessment included respiratory functional tests (spirometry and blood gas analysis) and cardiovascular tests (electrocardiography and echocardiography when required). In infants under 5 years old, infant pulmonary function test was used to assess functional capacity [9].

To minimize selection bias, 2:1 propensity score matching was performed based on predetermined confounders and baseline characteristics (sex and lesion side) to identify two homogenous groups of patients: finally, 75 patients with homogenous characteristics were selected and divided into group A (50) treated by lobectomy; group B (25) treated by sub-lobar resections (segmentectomies). Based on the propensity score matching, 21 patients were excluded because they did not match the variables. Videothoracoscopy was performed with a bi-portal access. Thoracotomy was performed with a muscle-sparing technique when VATS was not eligible because of lesion dimensions, localization, and surgical expertise to manage intra-operative complications. The choice to perform lobectomy or sub-lobar resection was made considering radiological and intra-operative characteristics of the lesion (lesions distant < 1 cm from the fissure and/or bigger than 4 cm of maximum diameter at pre-operative CT scan and/or involving two or more pulmonary segments, were considered for lobectomy).

ICU (Intensive Care Unit) admission depended on patient characteristics, comorbidities, intra-operative events, and complications; so surgical team (surgeons and anaesthesiologists) make a decision on its necessity case by case.

An accurate histopathological analysis was conducted. Paediatric patients underwent clinical follow-up once a year up to 18 years and then addressed their general practitioner, who indicated new surgical consulting in case of relapse. Adult patients were followed up for the first year; then, the general practitioner was addressed as well. Demographics characteristics, diagnosis technique, histology, time of surgery, length of hospital stay, length of chest tube permanence, intra-operative and post-operative complications, and symptom recurrence were compared between the two groups.

The study was approved by the institutional review board of Sant'Andrea Hospital (PROT. N. 188 SA/2022) and informed consent was obtained before surgery.

Data were prospectively collected and stored in Excel database (Microsoft Corp, Redmond, WA, USA). Quantitative variables were expressed as mean ± standard deviation and compared using t-test. Nominal variables were expressed binarily (presence—1 or absence—0) and compared by Chi square, after Fisher's exact test was performed. p-values less than 0.05 were considered statistically significant.

A univariate logistic regression analysis was performed to derive crude estimates of association between predictors and outcomes. After univariate analysis, variables with p-values less than 0.05 were included in a multivariate logistic regression model to identify potential independent protective or risk factors for symptom recurrence. The adjusted odd ratios (ORs) and 95% confidence intervals (CI) were calculated to estimate and measure the association using 1000 bootstrapping samples.

Data were analyzed using statistical package SPSS, version 25.0 (SPSS Software, IBM Corp., Armonk, NY, USA).

3. Results

The general characteristics of the patients and postoperative results are shown in Table 1.

Table 1. Descriptive statistical of the population.

	Lobectomy (Group A) (n = 50)	Segmentectomy (Group B) (n = 25)	p (<0.05)
Sex (n; %)			
M	30; 60%	12; 48%	
F	20; 40%	13; 52%	0.338
Symptoms (n; %)			
Yes	17; 34%	6; 24%	
No	33; 66%	19; 76%	0.271
Incidental diagnosis (n; %)			
Yes	1; 2%	6; 24%	
No	49; 98%	19; 76%	0.005
Prenatal diagnosis (n; %)			
Yes	42; 84%	18; 72%	
No	8; 16%	7; 28%	0.178
Histology (n; %) CCAM + SEQ			
Yes	29; 58%	8; 32%	
No	21; 42%	17; 68%	0.030
Histology CCAM (n; %)			
Yes	19; 38%	2; 8%	
No	31; 62%	23; 92%	0.005
Histology SEQ (n; %)			
Yes	2; 4%	15; 60%	
No	48; 96%	10; 40%	0.000
Side (n; %)			
Right	28; 56%	10; 40%	
Left	22; 44%	15; 60%	0.144
Surgical access (n; %)			
VATS	31; 62%	16; 64%	
Minithoracothomy	19; 38%	9; 36%	1.000

Table 1. Cont.

	Lobectomy (Group A) (n = 50)	Segmentectomy (Group B) (n = 25)	p (<0.05)
Lesions dimensions in cm (mean ± SD)	6.6 ± 4	2.5 ± 3	0.005
Intra-operatory complications (n; %)			
Yes	2; 4%	6; 24%	
No	48; 96%	19; 76%	0.014
Post-operatory complications (n; %)			
Yes	5; 10%	3; 12%	
No	45; 90%	22; 88%	0.538
Recurrence (n; %)			
Yes	2; 4%	6; 24%	
No	48; 96%	19; 76%	0.014
Surgery time (n; %)			
<120 min	18; 36%	8; 32%	
>120 min	32; 64%	17; 68%	0.469
Days of hospital stay (n; %)			
<7 days	38; 76%	16; 64%	
>7 days	12; 24%	9; 36%	0.205
Days of chest tube (n; %)			
<7 days	44; 88%	16; 64%	
>7 days	6; 12%	9; 36%	0.018
Neoplasm (n; %)			
Yes	2; 4%	1; 4%	
No	48; 96%	24; 96%	0.710
Age (mean ± SD)	12.70 ± 11.90	4.20 ± 11.60	0.012
Length of in-hospital stay (mean ± SD)	8.80 ± 9.11	8.40 ± 6.63	0.846
Surgery time (mean ± SD)	167.38 ± 62.38	161.48 ± 55.44	0.690
Length of chest tube permanence (mean ± SD)	3.74 ± 4.14	6.64 ± 3.94	0.005

The average age was 12.7 years in group A and 4.2 years in group B, with a statistically significant difference in the *t*-test analysis ($p = 0.012$).

There were 30 (60%) male patients in group A and 12 (48%) in group B.

In group A, 42 (84%) patients had a prenatal diagnosis and 17 (34%) were symptomatic at the diagnosis, while in group B, 18 (72%) patients had a prenatal diagnosis and 6 (24%) were symptomatic.

The lesion was right-sided in 28 (56%) patients in group A and in 10 (40%) patients in group B.

The mean operatory time was 167 min in group A and 161 min in group B, without a statistical significance in the *t*-test analysis.

VATS was performed in 31 (62%) patients in group A and in 16 (64%) in group B, all in the last 10 years. Mini-thoracotomy was performed in 19 (38%) patients in group A and in 9 (36%) in group B.

Histopathological analysis detected 29 (58%) cases of combined lesions (PS and CCAM) in group A and 8 (32%) cases in group B, with a significant statistical difference ($p = 0.030$). Equally, CCAM alone was detected in 19 (38%) of patients in group A and in 2 (8%) in group B, with a significant statistical difference ($p = 0.005$).

Intra-operative complications (pulmonary laceration, hematoma, hemorrhage) were significantly higher in sub-lobar resection group: 6 (24%) in group B vs. 2 (4%) in group A, ($p = 0.014$).

Post-operative complications (persistent air leak, slow re-expansion, bleeding, chest wall hematoma, prolonged liquid leaks) occurred in 5 (10%) of patients in group A vs. 3 (12%) in group B, without a significative difference.

Hospital stay was <7 days for 38 (76%) in group A and for 16 (64%) in group B, without a significant difference. The average hospital stay was 8 days for group B (median of 7 days) and 8.80 days for group A (median of 5 days), without a significant difference in t-test analysis.

The length of chest tube permanence was >7 days for 6 (12%) patients in group A and for 9 (36%) patients in group B, with significant difference ($p = 0.018$). An average of 3.7 days for group A (median of 3 days) and 6.6 days for group B (median of 6 days), with a significant difference in t-test analysis ($p = 0.005$).

Finally, the recurrence of respiratory symptoms related to the lesion was higher in the sub-lobar group (6; 24% in group B vs. 2; 4% in group A; $p = 0.002$) as it is shown in Table 2, which reports differences among patients who experienced symptom recurrence and patients who did not.

Table 2. Statistical description of symptom recurrence.

	Recurrence ($n = 8$)	No Recurrence ($n = 67$)	p (<0.05)
Sex (n; %)			
M	5; 62.5%	37; 55.223%	
F	3; 37.5%	30; 44.776%	0.499
Pre-operatory symptoms (n; %)			
Yes	2; 25%	21; 31.343%	
No	6; 75%	46; 68.656%	0.532
Incidental diagnosis (n; %)			
Yes	1; 12.5%	6; 8.955%	
No	7; 87.5%	61; 91.044%	0.562
Prenatal diagnosis (n; %)			
Yes	7; 87.5%	53; 79.104%	
No	1; 12.5%	14; 20.895%	0.495
Histology CCAM + SEQ (n; %)			
Yes	2; 25%	35; 52.238%	
No	6; 75%	32; 47.761%	0.140
Histology CCAM (n; %)			
Yes	0; 0%	21; 31.343%	
No	8; 100%	46; 68.656%	0.062
Histology (n; %)			
Yes	6; 75%	11; 16.417%	
No	2; 25%	56; 83.582%	0.001
Side (n; %)			
Right	6; 75%	32; 47.761%	
Left	2; 25%	35; 52.238%	0.140
Intra-operatory complications (n; %)			
Yes	3; 37.5%	5; 7.462%	
No	5; 62.5%	62; 92.537%	0.035
Post-operatory complications (n; %)			
Yes	3; 37.5%	5; 7.462%	
No	5; 62.5%	62; 92.537%	0.035
Surgery time (n; %)			
<120 min	2; 25%	24; 35.82%	
>120 min	6; 75%	43; 64.179%	0.428

Table 2. Cont.

	Recurrence (n = 8)	No Recurrence (n = 67)	p (<0.05)
Days of hospital stay (n; %)			
<7 days	6; 75%	48; 71.641%	
>7 days	2; 25%	19; 28.358%	0.604
Days of chest tube (n; %)			
<7 days	7; 87.5%	53; 79.104%	
>7 days	1; 12.5%	14; 20.895%	0.495
Neoplasm (n; %)			
Yes	2; 25%	1; 1.492%	
No	6; 75%	66; 98.507%	0.029
Surgery (n; %)			
Lobectomy	2; 25%	48; 71.641%	
Segmentectomy	6; 75%	19; 28.358%	0.014

The average follow-up period was 10.5 years.

Univariate analysis identified the following risk factors for symptom recurrence after surgical treatment: pulmonary sequestration (p = 0.002), sub-lobar resection (p = 0.019), intra-operative (p = 0.020) and post-operative (p = 0.020) complications, and associated neoplasm (p = 0.017). Multivariate logistic regression confirmed the following risk factors for symptoms recurrence after surgical treatment: sub-lobar resection (p = 0.040), post-operative complications (p = 0.022), and associated developed neoplasm (at the edge of statistical significance) (Table 3).

Table 3. Univariate and multivariate logistic regression.

	p	OR (95% CI)	p	OR (95% CI)
Sequestration	0.002	15.273 (2719–85.797)		
Segmentectomy	0.019	7579 (1404–40.917)	0.040	10.412 (0.958–113.096)
Intraop Compl	0.020	7440 (1364–40.595)	0.105	6629 (0.674–65.180)
Postop Compl	0.020	7440 (1364–40.595)	0.022	14.279 (1472–138.461)
Neoplasm	0.017	22.000 (1732–279.449)	0.062	33.298 (0.842–1316.492)

4. Discussion

CPMs are rare benign lesions involving 30–42 cases per 100.00 inhabitants per year [9–11] with an increased risk of infective complications. In the last decades, the extensive use of prenatal ultrasonography has led to a progressive increase in the antenatal detection of CPMs. For this reason, the highest incidence of the pathology occurs in pediatric patients, but the diagnosis may be missed until later in life, even in adulthood. Surgery is mandatory for symptomatic lesions to solve respiratory symptoms, to prevent infective complications, and to avoid the rare risk of malignant transformation. Nevertheless, there is a wide concern in the literature on surgical indication, even for asymptomatic lesions, to prevent late infections and/or malignancies, to guarantee more time for alveolar compensatory growth, and to reduce the risk for emergency surgery. The incidence of post-operative complications is assumed to be lower after early elective operation for CPMs than after an urgent intervention for CPMs when infective complications occurred [10].

Surgery for CPMs is indicated early after lesion detection and many studies in literature discuss surgical treatment options (thoracotomy vs. VATS) [12–15]; however, there is no standardized consensus on the extension of surgical resection between lobectomy and sub-lobar resections. A study by Baird et al. [12] recommends lobectomy (recommendation: weakly agree) as the procedure of choice, especially when the lesion is confined to a single lobe. There are no guidelines in the literature on the correct extension of surgical resection but considering the best practice, formal lobectomy is superior to segmentectomy. The present study investigates the possibility of identifying a consensus among surgeons who approach these pathologies.

In our series, the patients who underwent sub-lobar resections had an average age of 4.2 years vs. 12.7 years in the lobectomy group. Theoretically, it is possible to speculate that parenchyma-saving resection is the optimal choice for children for preserving total lung capacity. Nevertheless, it should be noted that parenchyma-saving resection can be complicated by prolonged air leak in the early postoperative period; moreover, in patients with residual lesion, malignant transformation as well as recurrent infections could develop during the follow-up period, even requiring the surgery to be repeated. However, it is demonstrated that neonates and infant patients have the potential for lung growth within the first years of life [16]. Infants and children tolerate lobectomy well, so that the total lung volume and gas exchange capacity return toward normal during somatic maturation [7]. For these reasons, the ideal extent of resection is still debated [17].

Both video-thoracoscopy (VATS) and thoracotomy were described for the treatment of CPMs. VATS is the procedure of choice; it is demonstrated to be safe and effective, and it is recommended to reduce morbidity related to thoracotomy, guaranteeing cosmetic benefit, and reducing pain [18]. Thoracotomy allows easy access to hilar structures using different intercostal spaces, making the management of anomalous vascularization and the variable size of the lesions easier than VATS. Moreover, dense adhesions due to recurrent infections of the lesion can make VATS dissection more difficult and thoracotomy is sometimes required to better manage an eventual vessel injury when the aberrant or varicose bronchial arteries are not well defined by preoperative imaging (Figure 2); therefore, it is mandatory to consider conversion whenever necessary. In our series, VATS was performed in 31 (62%) patients in group A and 16 (64%) patients in group B in the last 10 years, reflecting the increasing surgical expertise in mini-invasive surgery over the years. Conversion was required only for two patients to manage intra-operative complications (anomalous vessel laceration; tough adhesions). No differences in outcome were found in comparison with the open access approach in the present series.

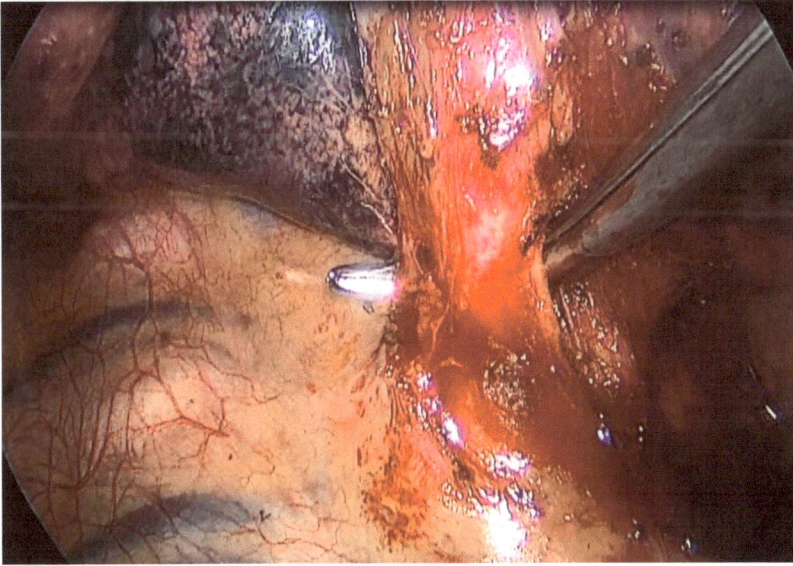

Figure 2. Intraoperative isolation of an extralobar pulmonary sequestration's arterial branch derived from thoracic aorta.

The results reported are in line with previous smaller published studies (Kim et al., Stanton et al.) [16,17] reporting the superiority of lobectomy for the stable remission of symptom recurrence.

Our comparative analysis showed that symptom recurrence after surgical treatment for CPMs was lower in the lobectomy group compared to the sub-lobar group, with statistical significative difference ($p = 0.014$). Even intra-operative complications (pulmonary laceration, hematoma, hemorrhage) were more frequent in sub-lobar resections (24% vs. 4%, $p = 0.014$), probably because these kinds of lesions rarely are limited to an anatomic pulmonary segment. This result probably explains the longer period of chest tube permanence in group B than in group A, with a statistically significant difference. There was not a significant difference in post-operative complications, surgical time, or hospital stay in the two groups, although there was a difference in chest tube drainage permanence, which was longer in the sub-lobar group, probably due to the more frequent intra-operative complications registered in the abovementioned group; nevertheless, the prognosis of post-operative complications was good and patients that experienced post-operative complications had a good recovery at the mean follow-up time.

The comparison of histopathological samples showed an increased frequency of CCAM (isolated lesion or associated with sequestration) in the lobectomy group than in the sub-lobar resection group. Histopathological analysis represents the definitive diagnosis [19] because radiological definition is not always conclusive. In fact, contrast chest CT is considered the most accurate examination, but hyperlucent lesions presuppose an overlapping spectrum and consensus and cooperation between radiologists and histopathologists are of paramount importance for the definitive diagnosis [20]. Therefore, prenatal imaging is not predictive of post-natal histology and surgical resection is also recommended to obtain a final diagnosis of the lesion, to distinguish isolated lesions from associated CPMs, generally related to a higher risk of infective complications and/or malignant transformation [21].

Analyzing the causes of symptom recurrence (present in 8 patients, 11% of the entire population), the presence of isolated sequestration ($p = 0.062$), intra- and post-operative complications ($p = 0.035$), associated neoplasm at histopathological analysis ($p = 0.014$), and sub-lobar resections ($p = 0.014$) seemed significantly related to the recurrence.

These variables were then analyzed in a univariate analysis that confirmed them as potential risk factors for symptom recurrence. The multivariate logistic regression confirmed the variables shown in Table 3 as risk factors for symptom recurrence.

The recurrence of symptoms was defined by the occurrence of productive cough, fever, hemoptysis related to pneumonia, bronchiolitis, and/or recurrent bronchitis during the follow-up period [8]. According to Calzolari et al. [10]., symptoms such asthma, recurrent wheeze, and/or respiratory distress presenting after surgery are not considered a recurrence of symptoms caused by the lesions, but symptoms related to the same congenital developmental abnormality that causes the formation of CPMs. Patients presenting with these latter symptoms were not considered affected by recurrence after treatment. In fact, lesions may not be limited to a single lung segment, but the whole respiratory structure may be affected to differing degrees, which may result in persistent respiratory symptoms after surgery that tend to regress spontaneously.

Lobectomy is more appropriate even to prevent the rare risk of malignant transformation (rhabdomyosarcoma, pulmonary blastoma), which is most frequently described in isolated or associated CCAM [21,22].

According to the literature, patients undergoing parenchyma-saving resection are likely to have early postoperative morbidities such as recurrent pulmonary infection or prolonged air leakage, and in cases of residual lesion, even malignant transformation [23]. The systematic review by Stanton et al. demonstrated a 15% rate of residual disease after segmental resection vs. 0% with lobectomy [16]. In our experience, a patient treated for CCAM by B9 segmentectomy at the age of 13 developed successive malignant transformation 14 years later (bilaterally metastatic adenocarcinoma) in the residual right lower lobe, primarily identified by respiratory symptoms occurrence (productive coughing) and radiological evidence of lung cancer abscess (Figure 3). In fact, performing subtotal lobectomy or segmentectomy or at worst, an atypical resection, would risk leaving remnants of the lesion that could later develop into lung cancer.

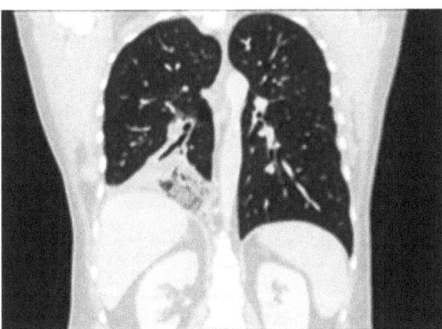

Figure 3. Lung cancer abscess in the residual right lower lobe in a patient treated with pulmonary segmentectomy for CCAM.

Our study has several limitations: data were retrospectively collected; the study population was rather small and so the power of our results is not so strong as to be conclusive; parenchyma-saving resection was performed in only selected cases (peripheral lesions, smaller than 3 cm in diameter). However, considering the rarity of the pathology, this is one of the largest studies in literature on the topic.

A prospective, randomized controlled trial would be helpful to determine if parenchyma-saving resection could be justified in patients with localized CPMs.

5. Conclusions

Surgical excision has been proven to be the treatment of choice for CPMs although a general consensus on the best type of surgery is not yet proven. To the best of our knowledge, despite the small sample size due to the rarity of the pathology described, the present multicentric study is one of the largest in literature comparing the two different surgical approaches (lobectomy vs. sub-lobar resections) for CPMs.

Despite the limits of a small sample and retrospective work, the present study aims to demonstrate the most appropriate surgical treatment for the stable remission of CPMs in both adult and paediatric patients. In conclusion, lobectomy seems to be the treatment of choice compared to sub-lobar resection, resulting in a lower or null rate of intra- and postoperative complications, a lower incidence of respiratory symptom recurrence, and preventing the rare risk of possible future malignant transformation.

Author Contributions: Conceptualization, B.T.M., C.M. and P.S.; methodology, B.T.M. and C.M.; software, S.F.; validation, E.A.R. and M.I.; formal analysis, B.T.M., C.M. and S.F.; investigation, M.T., G.N., F.M. and A.I.; resources, B.T.M. and M.T.; data curation, B.T.M., C.M. and S.F.; writing—review and editing, B.T.M. and C.M.; visualization and supervision, E.A.R., P.S. and M.I. All authors have read and agreed to the published version of the manuscript.

Funding: This research received no external funding.

Institutional Review Board Statement: The study was conducted in accordance with the Declaration of Helsinki and approved by the Institutional Review Board (or Ethics Committee) of Sant'Andrea Hospital, La Sapienza University (protocol code 188 SA/2022, 28 September 2022).

Informed Consent Statement: Informed consent was obtained from all subjects involved in the study.

Data Availability Statement: No new data were created or analyzed in this study. Data sharing is not applicable to this article.

Conflicts of Interest: The authors declare no conflict of interest.

References

1. Conran, R.M.; Stocker, J.T. Extralobar sequestration with frequently associated congenital cystic adenomatoid malformation, type 2: Report of 50 cases. *Pediatr. Dev. Pathol.* **1999**, *2*, 454–463. [CrossRef]
2. Stocker, J.T. Congenital pulmonary airway malformation: A new name and an expanded classification of congenital cystic adenomatoid malformation of the lung. *Hystopathology* **2002**, *41* (Suppl. 2), 424–431.
3. Wang, A.; D'Amico, T.; Berry, M. Surgical management of congenital pulmonary malformations after the first decade of life. *Ann. Thorac. Surg.* **2014**, *97*, 1933–1938. [CrossRef] [PubMed]
4. Sfakianaki, A.K.; Copel, J.A. Congenital cystic lesions of the lung: Congenital cystic adenomatoid malformation and bronchopulmonary sequestration. *Rev. Obstet. Gynecol.* **2012**, *5*, 85–93. [PubMed]
5. Adzick, S.; Flake, A.; Crombleholme, F. Management of congenital lung lesions. *Semin. Pediatr. Surg.* **2003**, *1*, 10–16. [CrossRef]
6. Rashmi, S.; Davenport, M. The argument for operative approach to asymptomatic lung lesions. *Semin. Pediatr. Surg.* **2015**, *24*, 187–195.
7. Kim, H.K.; Choi, Y.S. Treatment of congenital cystic adenomatoid malformations: Should lobectomy always be performed? *Ann. Thorac. Surg.* **2008**, *86*, 249–253. [CrossRef] [PubMed]
8. Trabalza Marinucci, B.; Maurizi, G.; Vanni, C.; Cardillo, G.; Poggi, C.; Pardi, V.; Inserra, A.; Rendina, E.A. Surgical treatment of pulmonary sequestration in adults and children: Long-term results. *Interact CardioVasc. Thorac. Surg.* **2020**, *31*, 71–77.
9. Lesnick, B.L.; Davis, S.D. Infant pulmonary function testing. Overview of technology and practical considerations—New current procedural terminology codes effective 2010. *Chest* **2011**, *139*, 1197–1202. [CrossRef]
10. Calzolari, F.; Braguglia, A.; Valfrè, L.; Dotta, A.; Bagolan, P.; Morini, F. Outcome of infants operated on for congenital pulmonary malformations. *Pediatr. Pulmonol.* **2016**, *51*, 1367–1372. [CrossRef]
11. Andrade, C.F.; Ferreira, H.P.C.; Fischer, G.B. Congenital lung malformations. *J. Bras Pneumol.* **2011**, *37*, 259–271. [CrossRef] [PubMed]
12. Baird, R.; Puligandla, P.; Laberge, J.M. Congenital lung malformations: Informing best practice. *Semin. Pediatr. Surg.* **2014**, *23*, 270–277. [CrossRef] [PubMed]
13. Wang, L.M.; Cao, J.L.; Hu, J. Video-assisted thoracic surgery for pulmonary sequestration: A safe alternative procedure. *J. Thorac. Dis.* **2016**, *8*, 31–36.
14. Chengwu, L.; Pu, Q.; Ma, L. Video-assisted thoracic surgery for pulmonary sequestration compared with posterolateral thoracotomy. *J. Thorac. Cardiovasc. Surg.* **2013**, *146*, 557–561.
15. Esposito, C.; Bonnard, A.; Till, H.; Leva, E.; Khen-Dunlop, N.; Zanini, A.; Montalva, L.; Sarnacki, S.; Escolino, M. Thoracoscopic Management of Pediatric Patients with Congenital Lung Malformations: Results of a European Multicenter Survey. *Laparoendosc. Adv. Surg. Tech.* **2021**, *31*, 355–362. [CrossRef]
16. Stanton, M.; Njere, I.; Ade-Ajayi, N.; Patel, S.; Davenport, M. Systematic review and meta-analysis of the postnatal management of congenital cystic lung lesions. *J. Pediatr. Surg.* **2009**, *44*, 1027–1033. [CrossRef] [PubMed]
17. Morini, F.; Zani, A.; Conforti, A.; Eaton, S.; Puri, P.; Rintala, R.; Lukač, M.; Kuebler, J.; Friedmacher, F.; Wijnen, R.; et al. Current management of congenital pulmonary airway malformations: A "European Pediatric Surgeon's Association" survey. *Eur. J. Pediatr. Surg.* **2018**, *28*, 1–5.
18. Annunziata, F.; Bush, A.; Borgia, F. Congenital lung malformations: Unresolved issues and unanswered questions. *Front. Pediatr.* **2019**, *7*, 239. [CrossRef]
19. Kyncl, M.; Koci, M.; Ptackov, A.L.; Hornofová, L.; Ondřej, F.; Šnajdauf, J.; Pychova, M. Congenital bronchopulmonary malformation: CT histopathological correlation. *Biomed. Pap. Med.* **2016**, *160*, 533–537. [CrossRef]
20. Hirose, R.; Suita, S.; Taguchi, T.; Koyanagi, T.; Nakano, H. Extralobar pulmonary sequestration mimicking cystic adenomatoid malformation in prenatal sonographic appearance and histological findings. *J. Pediatr. Surg.* **1995**, *30*, 1390–1393. [CrossRef]
21. Messinger, Y.H.; Stewart, D.R.; Priest, J.R.; Williams, G.M.; Harris, A.K.; Schultz, K.A.P.; Yang, J.; Doros, L.; Rosenberg, P.S.; Hill, D.A.; et al. Pleuropulmonary blastoma: A report on 350 central pathology-confirmed pleuropulmonary blastoma cases by the International Pleuropulomonary Blastoma Registry. *Cancer* **2015**, *121*, 276–285. [CrossRef] [PubMed]
22. Preziosi, A.; Morandi, A.; Galbiati, F.; Scanagatta, P.; Chiaravalli, S.; Fagnani, A.M.; Di Cesare, A.; Macchini, F.; Leva, E. Acute haemothorax and pleuropulmonary blastoma: Two extremely rare complications of extralobar pulmonary sequestration. *J. Pediatr. Surg.* **2022**, *80*, 102238.
23. Muller, C.; Berrebi, D.; Kheniche, A.; Bonnard, A. Is radical lobectomy required in congenital cystic adenomatoid malformation? *J. Pediatr. Surg.* **2012**, *47*, 642–664. [CrossRef] [PubMed]

Disclaimer/Publisher's Note: The statements, opinions and data contained in all publications are solely those of the individual author(s) and contributor(s) and not of MDPI and/or the editor(s). MDPI and/or the editor(s) disclaim responsibility for any injury to people or property resulting from any ideas, methods, instructions or products referred to in the content.

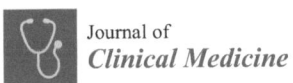

Article

Swiss Pilot Low-Dose CT Lung Cancer Screening Study: First Baseline Screening Results

Lisa Jungblut [1], Harry Etienne [2], Caroline Zellweger [1], Alessandra Matter [2], Miriam Patella [2], Thomas Frauenfelder [1] and Isabelle Opitz [2,*]

[1] Institute of Diagnostic and Interventional Radiology, University Hospital Zurich, Raemistrasse 100, CH-8091 Zurich, Switzerland
[2] Department of Thoracic Surgery, University Hospital Zurich, Raemistrasse 100, CH-8091 Zurich, Switzerland
* Correspondence: isabelle.schmitt-opitz@usz.ch; Tel.: +41-44-255-88-04

Abstract: This pilot study conducted in Switzerland aims to assess the implementation, execution, and performance of low-dose CT lung cancer screening (LDCT-LCS). With lung cancer being the leading cause of cancer-related deaths in Switzerland, the study seeks to explore the potential impact of screening on reducing mortality rates. However, initiating a lung cancer screening program poses challenges and depends on country-specific factors. This prospective study, initiated in October 2018, enrolled participants meeting the National Lung Cancer Study criteria or a lung cancer risk above 1.5% according to the PLCOm2012 lung cancer risk-model. LDCT scans were assessed using Lung-RADS. Enrollment and follow-up are ongoing. To date, we included 112 participants, with a median age of 62 years (IQR 57–67); 42% were female. The median number of packs smoked each year was 45 (IQR 38–57), and 24% had stopped smoking before enrollment. The mean PLCOm2012 was 3.7% (±2.5%). We diagnosed lung cancer in 3.6% of participants (95%, CI:1.0–12.1%), with various stages, all treated with curative intent. The recall rate for intermediate results (Lung-RADS 3,4a) was 15%. LDCT-LCS in Switzerland, using modified inclusion criteria, is feasible. Further analysis will inform the potential implementation of a comprehensive lung cancer screening program in Switzerland.

Keywords: non-small cell lung cancer (NSCLC); screening; computed tomography; diagnosis

Citation: Jungblut, L.; Etienne, H.; Zellweger, C.; Matter, A.; Patella, M.; Frauenfelder, T.; Opitz, I. Swiss Pilot Low-Dose CT Lung Cancer Screening Study: First Baseline Screening Results. *J. Clin. Med.* **2023**, *12*, 5771. https://doi.org/10.3390/jcm12185771

Academic Editor: Monica Casiraghi

Received: 4 August 2023
Revised: 29 August 2023
Accepted: 31 August 2023
Published: 5 September 2023

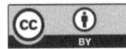

Copyright: © 2023 by the authors. Licensee MDPI, Basel, Switzerland. This article is an open access article distributed under the terms and conditions of the Creative Commons Attribution (CC BY) license (https://creativecommons.org/licenses/by/4.0/).

1. Introduction

Lung cancer is a major public health burden. In Europe, it ranks third among the most common cancers and has the highest cancer-related death rate [1]. In Switzerland, 4500 persons are diagnosed annually with lung cancer, which is the most frequent cause of cancer-related deaths with 3200 deaths [2]. A large share of this burden would be preventable through smoking cessation or early detection of suspicious lung nodules [3]. Screening for lung cancer using low-dose computed tomography (LDCT) has been proven to be effective in detecting early stage lung cancers and has been recommended by numerous professional organizations, including the National Comprehensive Cancer Network (NCCN) and the United States Preventive Services Task Force (USPSTF) [4,5]. The NELSON trial, which is the largest randomized controlled trial (RCT) on lung cancer screening in Europe, showed that lung cancer mortality can be significantly reduced over a 10-year period by using LDCT [6].

With the publication of the results of the US National Lung Screening Trial in 2011, lung cancer mortality was reduced by 20% and all-cause mortality by 6.7% (relative risk reduction) in a clearly defined high-risk cohort [7]. In absolute numbers: 13 out of 1000 screened smokers died of lung cancer in the LDCT group vs. 17 out of 1000 in the chest X-ray group. Based on these promising data, since 2015, the costs for the screening program have been reimbursed by private as well as public health insurers in America [8]. In January 2020,

Croatia became the first European country to launch a national lung cancer screening program targeting all active smokers (or those who have quit smoking in the last 15 years) between 50 and 70 years [9]. Poland has introduced a lung cancer screening program as part of its national cancer plan funded by the Ministry of Health [10,11]. The United Kingdom has also introduced regional programs; with the help of a mobile "screening truck", a very high level of adherence has been achieved, especially in remote areas [12].

According to the last published statistics from the Federal Statistic Office, 27% of the Swiss population above 15 years old are smokers, with the 6% being heavy smokers (>20 cigarettes/day) [13]. In the Zurich Canton, the prevalence of active smokers goes up to 28.2% [14]. Nevertheless, to date, there is no official screening program in Switzerland. This may be based on obstacles like lack of country-specific data or ambiguity on the cost–benefit ratio. To ensure the sustainability of a lung cancer screening program, it would be important for the screening to be covered by compulsory health insurance (KVG) in the long term. According to Art. 12d KLV (Ordinance on Health Care Services), compulsory health care insurance covers certain medical preventive measures for the early detection of diseases in certain risk groups. Each new screening measure must be assessed for its effectiveness, appropriateness, and cost-efficiency before it is covered by compulsory health insurance. However, there is rising evidence that LDCT screening is cost-effective in Switzerland [15].

The objective of this project was to assess feasibility of introducing LDCT-LCS in Switzerland and propose characteristics for its implementation.

2. Materials and Methods

2.1. Study Design

In this prospective study, starting from October 2018, asymptomatic participants aged 55–74 years with more than 30 pack years of smoking history were enrolled at a tertiary hospital in Switzerland.

2.2. Inclusion Criteria

We propose the use of the already established inclusion criteria from the national lung cancer screening study [9]:

- Age from 55 to 74 years;
- Willingness and ability to undergo LDCT;
- >30 packs years;
- Current or former smoker who quit smoking $\leq$ 15 years ago;
- No previous diagnosis of lung cancer;
- No major medical problems;
- No CT scan in the last 18 months;
- No haemoptysis or weight loss > 7 kg in the last year.

Further, individuals with a of 1.5% probability of suffering from lung cancer within the next 6 years or higher according to PLCOm2012 risk prediction model were also eligible for LDCT lung cancer screening. The PLCOm2012 risk prediction model is based on the Prostate, Lung, Colorectal, and Ovarian Cancer Screening Trial (PLCOm2012) and incorporates 15 predictors, including medical history, sociodemographic characteristics, smoking exposure, and medical history of chronic obstructive pulmonary disease (COPD) [16].

2.3. Recruitment

Participants were recruited through primary care providers (PCPs), pulmonologists, but also through newspaper articles, social media, and flyers in doctors' waiting room areas. Information about eligibility criteria as well as contact details were given. All individuals were invited for a telephone interview to check for eligibility. Further, patient information as well as smoking cessation advice and allocation to smoking cessation program were available as part of the interview. Telephone interviews were conducted by a healthcare worker (resident or medical student) employed by the radiology department.

2.4. Image Acquisition/Reporting

LDCTs were acquired using a Siemens Somatom Force, Siemens Somatom Edge Plus and a Siemens Somatom Naeotom Alpha scanner starting from October 2019 without the administration of contrast medium. For quality control, technical standards from the ESTI (European Society of Thoracic Imaging) society were obtained [12]. Each scan was read by two radiologists independently, one of whom was board certified and specialized in thoracic radiology. In all, scan nodules were automatically detected and measured by the software's built-in matching algorithm (Siemens SyngoVia MM oncology lung computer-aided detection [CAD]) and the maximum diameter was double-checked by the radiologists. Reporting was completed in a standardized way to obtain imaging parameters such as radiation dose, summary of screening findings with specific management recommendation, and additional findings. Standardized templates were used to ensure uniform reporting and guideline adherence. Nodules were classified by the Lung-RADS 1.1 reporting system [13]. Lung-RADS (Lung Imaging Reporting and Data System) is a classification for lung nodules in low-dose CT screening exams with the purpose of standardizing follow-up and management decisions. A flowchart of the screening pathway is provided in Figure 1.

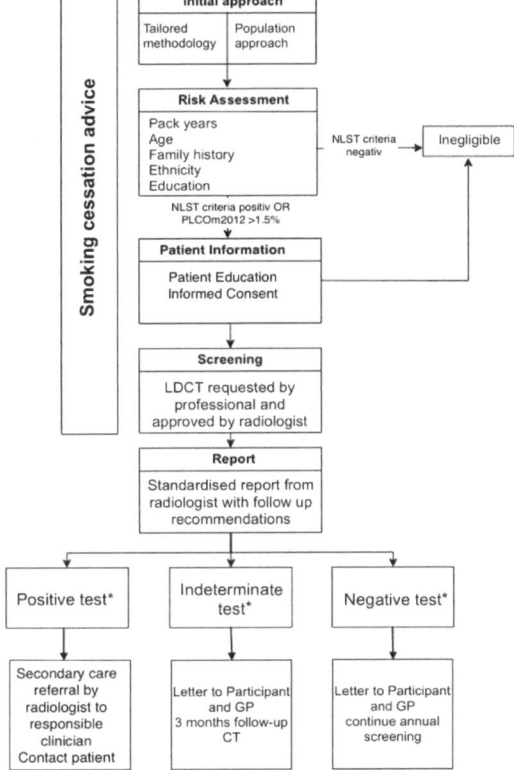

Figure 1. Screening pathway. GP, general practitioner. * positive test = lung-RADS 4, intermediate test = lung-RADS 3, negative test = lung-RADS 1 or 2.

2.5. Ethical Statement

This study respects the principles of the Declaration of Helsinki concerning human research study. This project is not subject to approval by the ethics committee of Zurich (KEK Zuständigkeitsabklärung—BASEC-Nr. Req-2017-00511).

2.6. Primary and Secondary Endpoint

The primary endpoint of this study was the incidence of lung cancer detection by screening. The second endpoint was the detection of indeterminate nodules, quantification of incidental findings, and consecutive recall rate.

2.7. Statistical Analysis

Quantitative variables were expressed as mean ± standard deviation (SD). Categorical variables were expressed as frequencies or percentages. Descriptive epidemiological summaries of data were presented with confidence intervals (CIs). For non-normally distributed continuous data, the 25th, 50th, and 75th percentiles are presented, denoting the median and interquartile range (IQR). Statistical analyses were conducted using commercially available software (IBM SPSS Statistics, release 21.0; SPSS, Chicago, IL, USA).

3. Results

3.1. Participant Cohort

A telephone interview with 150 individuals with high-risk factors was conducted. We excluded 38 participants (34 participants were not willing to sign an informed consent and 4 patients were not eligible), resulting in a final cohort of 112 participants: 65 (58%) men and 47 (42%) women. The mean age at enrollment was 62.1 (95% CI 60 to 63) years. The proportion of current smokers was 76% ($n = 85$). With regard to comorbidities, 14% ($n = 16$) of the enrolled participants had known COPD, emphysema, or bronchitis. Detailed information is shown in Table 1. Regarding the recruitment strategy, 56 (50%) of the participants became aware of the study through flyers, social media and newspapers, whereas only 28 (25%) were invited by either PCPs or other clinicians.

Table 1. Patient demographics, socioeconomic characteristics, and risk evaluation among the screened participants.

Subject Demographic/Socioeconomic Characteristic Risk Evaluation		Results
Demographics/Socioeconomics		
Gender (Number, (%))		
	Male	65 (58)
	Female	47 (42)
Age (Median, (p25–75%))		61.5 (57.0–67.0)
Ethnicity (Number, (%))		
	Black	0 (0)
	Hispanic	2 (2)
	Asian	0 (0)
	White	110 (98)
	Other (included mixed race)	0 (0)
Education Level (Number, (%))		
	Less than high-school	1 (1)
	High-school	17 (15)
	Post high-school training	35 (31)
	College degree	41 (37)
	Postgraduate/Professional	18 (16)
Risk Evaluation		
BMI (Median, (p25–75%))		25.6 (23.3–28.0)
Smoking status (Number, (%))		
	current	85 (76)
	former	27 (24)
Pack years (Median, (p25–75%))		45 (38–57)
History of COPD, Emphysema or Chron. Bronchitis (Number, (%))		16 (14)
PCLOm 2012 (Mean (SD))		3.7 (2.5)

The majority of patients (82, 73%) came from the Zurich Canton. The median distance covered to reach the University Hospital was 16.7 km (IQR: 1.3–28), and most participants (64, 57%) chose public transport. Of the participants, 92 (82%) had an educational level beyond high school graduation; 63 (56%) were currently working, and 66 (59%) had public health insurance.

3.2. Radiation Dose

The mean volume CT dose index (CTDIvol) was 0.69 ± 0.18 mGy and the dose length product (DLP) was 21.04 ± 4.36 mGy*cm.

3.3. Lung-RADS Findings

The percentage of negative tests (Lung-RADS 1 and Lung-RADS 2, respectively) was 81% ($n = 91$), whereas the prevalence of positive LDCT results (biopsy-proven carcinomas) was 3.6% ($n = 4$). Subjects with positive results were referred to thoracic surgery for immediate assessment following the baseline scan. Intermediate results (Lung-RADS 3) were found in 13% ($n = 14$) of participants. Those patients were given an outpatient appointment at the thoracic surgery consultations and were also advised for a follow-up scan considering Lung-RADS criteria [13]. Further, not all suspected lesions were biopsied or surgically extracted. Three participants were diagnosed with Lung-RADS 4a lesions (with a malignancy rate according to Lung-RADS criteria of 5–15%) and are currently under active surveillance. Taking all lesions requiring follow-up scans into account (Lung-RADS 3 and Lung-RADS 4a) resulted in a recall rate of 15%. The results are shown in Table 2.

Table 2. Screening results.

Screening Results		Results
LUNG-RADS		
0 (Number, (%))		0 (0)
1 (Number, (%))		62 (55)
2 (Number, (%))		29 (26)
3 (Number, (%))		14 (13)
4a (Number, (%))		3 (3)
4b (Number, (%))		4 (4)
Carcinomas (Number, (%))		4 (4)
	Adenocarcinoma	3 (3)
	Squamous cell carcinoma	1 (1)
Incidental Findings		
Coronary Sclerosis (Number, (%))		
	non	32 (29)
	mild	38 (34)
	moderate	32 (29)
	severe	10 (10)
Emphysema (Number, (%))		36 (32)

3.4. Detected Lung Cancer

Among the screened participants, 3.6% ($n = 4$) were diagnosed with lung cancer. Diagnosis was obtained via CT guided biopsy in all cases. One male participant (68 years-old) with a PLCOm2012 of 12.2% was diagnosed with adenocarcinoma in the left lower lobe with one metastasis in the sternal manubrium (pT3, pN0, cM1b, UICC stadium IV). The participant underwent four cycles of induction chemotherapy and radiotherapy for the osseous metastasis and subsequently underwent a video-assisted thoracoscopic lobectomy and radical mediastinal lymph node dissection. This participant is without signs of metastasis or recurrence. Another male participant (66 years-old) with a PLCOm2012 of 3.5%

was diagnosed with non-keratinizing squamous cell carcinoma in the right upper lobe and two mediastinal lymph node metastases (pT1, pN2, cM0, UICC stadium IIIA). Mediastinal lymph node metastasis (same side) was incidental and found only in histopathologic assessment post-surgery. The participant underwent robotic-assisted lobectomy and radical lymph node dissection followed by adjuvant chemotherapy with Cisplatin/Gemtacitabin. CT and PET/CT images are shown in Figure 2. After remission, the development of an osseous metastasis was found which is now under radiotherapy with a curative approach. Unfortunately, brain metastases were found at the follow-up scans and further steps are currently being discussed in multidisciplinary tumor boards. Another adenocarcinoma was found in a male patient (69 years-old) with a PLCOm2012 of 5.4%. The tumor was localized in the right upper lobe and no metastases were found (pT2a, pN0, cM0, UICC stadium IB). The participant underwent robotic-assisted lobectomy and radical lymph node dissection and is now without signs of further disease. One female participant was diagnosed with adenocarcinoma in the right lower lobe. Two lymph node metastases were found (pT3, pN2, cM0, UICC IIIA). Again, robotic-assisted lobectomy, radical lymph node dissection, as well as stereotactic radiotherapy, were performed. Positive lymph node status has not been described prior to the surgery and was confirmed via histopathological assessment. The participant is without signs of metastasis or recurrence. Further, 3% (*n* = 3) of participants are currently under active surveillance due to a highly suspicious nodule (Lung-RADS 4a).

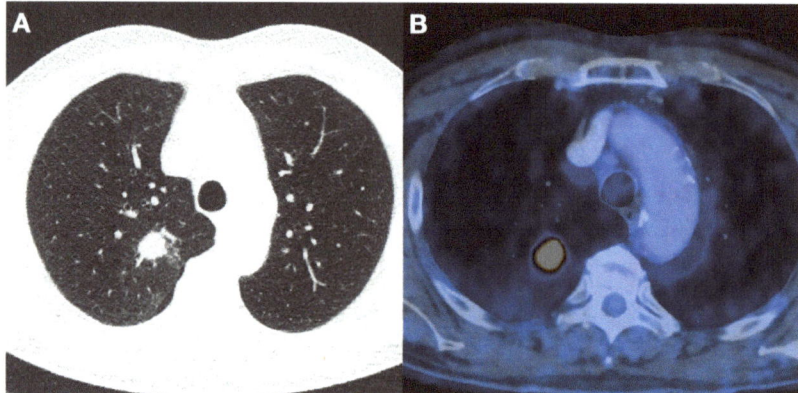

Figure 2. Low-dose CT (**A**) and FDG-PET/CT (**B**) images in axial plane of a 66-year-old male patient with stage IIIA squamous cell carcinoma in the upper right lobe. This previously asymptomatic patient underwent a lobectomy with systematic lymph node dissection and received adjuvant chemotherapy.

3.5. Incidental Findings

Incidental findings were communicated to and managed by the referring physicians. No incidental findings requiring urgent attention were found. Among the participants, 71% (*n* = 80) were diagnosed with coronary sclerosis and 32% (*n* = 36) participants were found to have emphysematous parenchymal lung changes. Further, 35% of the participants (*n* = 39) were diagnosed with bronchitis. There were also pathologies found in the partially imaged upper abdomen; none of them were in need of treatment (benign liver lesions (*n* = 14), renal cysts (*n* = 11), adrenal adenomas (*n* = 2) and cholecystolithiasis (*n* = 4)). The management of incidental findings was under the responsibility of the referring physician who received the CT report.

4. Discussion

Lung cancer is one of the leading causes of cancer-related deaths worldwide, and early detection is crucial for improving patient outcomes [6,17]. Switzerland, like many other countries, aims to implement lung cancer screening programs to ensure the detection of lung cancers in an early, curative treatable stage. To this date, we have found four curatively treated cases of lung cancer. Another three suspicious lesions are currently under active surveillance. The recall rate in our study was 15% by combining all Lung-RADS 3 and Lung-RADS 4a lesions. We found that 81% of the participants had suspected lung nodules requiring further follow-up.

Tomonaga et al. [15] have already indicated that lung screening could be cost-effective in Switzerland, a European country with a high income and a high smoking prevalence. They estimated the cost-effectiveness of LDCT screening for lung cancer to be less than EUR 50,000 per life year gained. The economic evaluation of a health care program as the lung cancer screening relies on different aspects including the life expectancy and the quality of life potentially saved. These also take into account the productivity of each individual. In our cohort, 56% of people were active workers, which means that a potential intervention would safeguard a productive subject within society.

A screening program can only be successful if it reaches as many at-risk people as possible. In our study there is an overrepresentation of high-educated participants with 92 (82%) receiving at least post-high school training. In 2017, within the portion of the Swiss population with secondary school training, 30.1% were active smokers, whereas this percentage was 23.1% within the population with a higher educational level [14]. This might mean that we are potentially missing part of the target population, and we may need to improve recruitment strategies. On the other hand, this may be attributable to the single-center design, reaching only participants in an urban area around Zurich. Within the cohort, 73% of the participants were resident in the Zurich Canton which extends for 1729 km^2, and the median distance travelled by each participant was 16.7 km, most of which was by public transport. These data are extremely important to verify the applicability of a future structured program in our country and to provide information on centralized vs. decentralized design. A more decentralized approach could lead to higher accessibility and therefore better representability of the Swiss population. Since CT density in Switzerland is estimated to be high, the degree of centralization could vary depending on the extent of pre-screening, screening, and evaluation. One possible approach is to decentralize diagnostics and organize reading and treatment centrally. A model for this would be the already mentioned "lung health checks" in Manchester, which were carried out with a mobile CT device [12].

Another aspect that must be evaluated is the enrollment strategy. In our population, half of the participants became aware of the pilot project through flyers, newspapers, or social media, and only 25% were invited by doctors. A previous study conducted in Switzerland demonstrated a better adherence to lung cancer diagnostic and treatment pathways with a more consistent involvement of primary care practitioner (PCPs) [18]. PCPs represent the frontline health care professionals with knowledge of patients' general status, behavior, and clinical history, and this relationship might be important to enhance screening adherence.

Another main issue in lung cancer screening is in defining a screening protocol associated with a low recall rate and a high detection rate. In the context of screening, the recall rate is a crucial metric that reflects the proportion of individuals who are called back for additional tests or evaluations following an initial screening, often due to the detection of suspicious findings [19]. A high recall rate can lead to increased anxiety and stress among patients who are called back for further tests. This can negatively impact their well-being and quality of life, even if they ultimately receive a negative diagnosis. Rasmussen et al. [20] evaluated the psychological impact of lung screening on patients and found that receiving a false-positive result in lung cancer screening was associated with negative short-term psychosocial consequences. The ideal recall rate can vary depending on the specific screening program, the disease being screened for, and the available resources. It is often a trade-off between achieving high sensitivity (catching more cases) and maintaining an acceptable level of specificity (avoiding unnecessary recalls). In our study we evaluated lung nodules according to Lung-RADS criteria which led to a recall rate of 15%. This value is lower compared to the NLST who used a cut off-value of 4 mm nodule size which resulted in a recall rate of 27% [7]. In breast cancer screening, the Agency for Healthcare Research and Quality has recommended a target recall rate of 10% and the American Society of Radiology (ACR) has recommended a target recall rate range of 5–12% for screening mammography [21]. To date, there are no recommended cut-off values for the recall rate in lung cancer screening. Anyhow, effort should be made towards lower recall rates which do not unnecessarily put participants under emotional stress. Currently we are evaluating the emotional stress in a prospective study (BASEC-Nr. 2022-01484).

In our pilot study, we found a cancer detection rate of 3.6% which is slightly higher than in the NELSON trial (3.2%) and higher than in the NLST (2.4%) [6,7]. This may be based on the modified inclusion criteria. In addition to the NLST criteria we also used the PLCOm2012 criteria for eligibility assessment. If patients did not have "enough" pack years or did stop smoking longer than 15 years ago we still included them if they had a PLCOm2012 higher than 1.5%. Tammemägi et al. have proven the feasibility of PLCOm2012 in a lung cancer screening setting [16]. Among others, factors like ethnicity, education, BMI, family history of cancer or COPD are taken into account in the PLCOm2012 risk evaluation.

In our study three out of four patients were diagnosed with advanced, metastatic disease. However, those patients were asymptomatic at the timepoint of screening and were treated with a curative approach.

In addition to a reduction in lung cancer-specific mortality by 20%, an all-cause mortality reduction of 6.7% could be shown in the National Lung Screening Trial [22]. The effects of smoking extend beyond cancer evolution. Smokers are also at risk of premature deaths due to chronic obstructive pulmonary disease (COPD) and coronary heart disease (CHD); both conditions can also be assessed in the context of screening [23]. For subjects in the lung cancer screening window, the relative risk of death due to ischemic heart disease is greater than three times that of a non-smoker [24]. Moreover, smoking reduces the time to development of coronary artery calcium (up to 10 years earlier for current smokers) compared with non-smokers [25]. While electrocardiogram-gated CT has been the gold standard for coronary artery quantification, there is compelling evidence that in lung cancer screening programs, a non-gated CT is a robust prognostic measure of fatal or non-fatal cardiovascular events in current and former smokers [23,26]. In our study 90% of the participants were found to have coronary artery calcification, among whom 10% were rated as severe. None of them were diagnosed with cardiovascular disease prior to participation. Further, although 14% of the participants were already diagnosed with COPD prior to our study, we found emphysematous lung changes in 32%. Those ancillary findings could contribute to risk stratification as well as health management and may lead to a reduction in mortality.

Our study has several limitations. First, the cohort is small and more participants need to be recruited for evidenced-based conclusions. There is also a lack of ethnical variety among participants (all participants were white with exception of two Hispanic participants). Anyhow, the major ethnicity in the Swiss population is white and therefore an underrepresentation of other ethnicity has to be taken into account. Given the advanced stage of three out of four detected cancers, it is important to acknowledge that this factor may have implications for the cost-effectiveness of the program. This issue warrants further attention in future projects, especially those involving a larger patient cohort. Furthermore, our pilot study is based on data from only one institution. In the future, many more sites all over Switzerland have to be included to ensure a nationwide, easily accessible screening program.

5. Conclusions

In conclusion, preliminary results from our pilot study have shown to be effective in detecting curative treatable lung cancer and improving patient outcomes. However, challenges such as limited accessibility, a lack of awareness, and the need for standardized guidelines must be addressed to ensure the program's long-term success. The continuous recruitment of participants and the involvement of further centers is necessary to guarantee easy access to screening programs and to continually evaluate the effectiveness of the screening program in Switzerland.

Author Contributions: Conceptualization, I.O. and T.F.; Methodology, A.M.; Software, A.M.; Validation, C.Z., Formal Analysis, L.J.; Investigation, L.J.; Resources, I.O.; Data Curation, A.M.; Writing—Original Draft Preparation, L.J.; Writing—Review and Editing, H.E. and M.P.; Visualization, H.E.; Supervision, M.P.; Project Administration, T.F.; Funding Acquisition, I.O. and T.F. All authors have read and agreed to the published version of the manuscript.

Funding: This research received no external funding.

Institutional Review Board Statement: This project is not subject to approval by the ethics committee of Zurich (KEK Zuständigkeitsabklärung—BASEC-Nr. Req-2017-00511).

Informed Consent Statement: Informed consent was obtained from all subjects involved in the study.

Data Availability Statement: The data presented in this study are available on request from the corresponding author. The data are not publicly available due to privacy.

Acknowledgments: Support by Innovation Grant of University Hospital Zurich and SAKF.

Conflicts of Interest: IO reports the following disclosures: Roche (Institutional Grant for Fellowship and Speakers Bureau), AstraZeneca (Advisory Board and Speakers Bureau), Medtronic (Institutional Grant), MSD, and BMS (Advisory Board), Intuitive (Proctorship). HE has no conflict of interest. TF reports the following disclosures: Bayer (Speakers Bureau), Boehringer (Speakers Bureau), and Agfa (Advisory Board). The funders had no role in the design of the study; in the collection, analyses, or interpretation of data; in the writing of the manuscript; or in the decision to publish the results.

References

1. Ferlay, J.; Colombet, M.; Soerjomataram, I.; Dyba, T.; Randi, G.; Bettio, M.; Gavin, A.; Visser, O.; Bray, F. Cancer incidence and mortality patterns in Europe: Estimates for 40 countries and 25 major cancers in 2018. *Eur. J. Cancer* **2018**, *103*, 356–387. [CrossRef] [PubMed]
2. Adamek, M.; Szablowska-Siwik, S.; Peled, N.; Rzyman, W.; Grodzki, W.; Czyzewski, D. Low-dose computed-tomography lung cancer screening: The first European recommendations from the European Society of Radiology and European Respiratory Society. *Pol. Arch. Med. Wewn.* **2015**, *125*, 607–609. [PubMed]
3. Chopra, I.; Chopra, A.; Bias, T.K. Reviewing risks and benefits of low-dose computed tomography screening for lung cancer. *Postgrad. Med.* **2016**, *128*, 254–261. [CrossRef] [PubMed]
4. Force, U.S.P.S.T. Lung cancer screening: Recommendation statement. *Ann. Intern. Med.* **2004**, *140*, 738–739. [CrossRef]
5. Jonas, D.E.; Reuland, D.S.; Reddy, S.M.; Nagle, M.; Clark, S.D.; Weber, R.P.; Enyioha, C.; Malo, T.L.; Brenner, A.T.; Armstrong, C.; et al. Screening for Lung Cancer With Low-Dose Computed Tomography: Updated Evidence Report and Systematic Review for the US Preventive Services Task Force. *JAMA* **2021**, *325*, 971–987. [CrossRef]
6. de Koning, H.J.; van der Aalst, C.M.; de Jong, P.A.; Scholten, E.T.; Nackaerts, K.; Heuvelmans, M.A.; Lammers, J.J.; Weenink, C.; Yousaf-Khan, U.; Horeweg, N.; et al. Reduced Lung-Cancer Mortality with Volume CT Screening in a Randomized Trial. *N. Engl. J. Med.* **2020**, *382*, 503–513. [CrossRef]
7. National Lung Screening Trial Research, T.; Aberle, D.R.; Adams, A.M.; Berg, C.D.; Black, W.C.; Clapp, J.D.; Fagerstrom, R.M.; Gareen, I.F.; Gatsonis, C.; Marcus, P.M.; et al. Reduced lung-cancer mortality with low-dose computed tomographic screening. *N. Engl. J. Med.* **2011**, *365*, 395–409. [CrossRef]
8. Aberle, D.R. Implementing lung cancer screening: The US experience. *Clin. Radiol.* **2017**, *72*, 401–406. [CrossRef]
9. ECHAlliance. Croatia First to Introduce Early Screening for Lung Cancer. Available online: https://echalliance.com/croatia-first-to-introduce-early-screening-for-lung-cancer/ (accessed on 20 January 2020).
10. Rzyman, W.; Didkowska, J.; Dziedzic, R.; Grodzki, T.; Orlowski, T.; Szurowska, E.; Langfort, R.; Biernat, W.; Kowalski, D.; Dyszkiewicz, W.; et al. Consensus statement on a screening programme for the detection of early lung cancer in Poland. *Adv. Respir. Med.* **2018**, *86*, 53–74. [CrossRef]
11. Nahorecki, A.; Chabowski, M.; Kuzniar, T.; Kedzierski, B.; Jazwiec, P.; Szuba, A.; Janczak, D. Low-dose computer tomography as a screening tool for lung cancer in a high risk population. *Adv. Exp. Med. Biol.* **2015**, *852*, 31–37. [CrossRef]
12. Crosbie, P.A.; Balata, H.; Evison, M.; Atack, M.; Bayliss-Brideaux, V.; Colligan, D.; Duerden, R.; Eaglesfield, J.; Edwards, T.; Elton, P.; et al. Implementing lung cancer screening: Baseline results from a community-based 'Lung Health Check' pilot in deprived areas of Manchester. *Thorax* **2019**, *74*, 405–409. [CrossRef]
13. Suisse, C. Heath-Pocket Statistics. Available online: https://www.bfs.admin.ch/bfs/en/home/statistics/health.assetdetail.2413 1868.html (accessed on 24 February 2023).

14. Observatory, S.H. Tobacco Consumption. Available online: https://ind.obsan.admin.ch/en/indicator/monam/tobacco-consumption-age-15 (accessed on 30 November 2022).
15. Tomonaga, Y.; Ten Haaf, K.; Frauenfelder, T.; Kohler, M.; Kouyos, R.D.; Shilaih, M.; Lorez, M.; de Koning, H.J.; Schwenkglenks, M.; Puhan, M.A. Cost-effectiveness of low-dose CT screening for lung cancer in a European country with high prevalence of smoking-A modelling study. *Lung Cancer* **2018**, *121*, 61–69. [CrossRef] [PubMed]
16. Tammemagi, M.C.; Ruparel, M.; Tremblay, A.; Myers, R.; Mayo, J.; Yee, J.; Atkar-Khattra, S.; Yuan, R.; Cressman, S.; English, J.; et al. USPSTF2013 versus PLCOm2012 lung cancer screening eligibility criteria (International Lung Screening Trial): Interim analysis of a prospective cohort study. *Lancet Oncol.* **2022**, *23*, 138–148. [CrossRef]
17. Field, J.K.; Duffy, S.W.; Baldwin, D.R.; Brain, K.E.; Devaraj, A.; Eisen, T.; Green, B.A.; Holemans, J.A.; Kavanagh, T.; Kerr, K.M.; et al. The UK Lung Cancer Screening Trial: A pilot randomised controlled trial of low-dose computed tomography screening for the early detection of lung cancer. *Health Technol. Assess.* **2016**, *20*, 1–146. [CrossRef] [PubMed]
18. Minerva, E.M.; Tessitore, A.; Cafarotti, S.; Patella, M. Urban-Rural Disparities in the Lung Cancer Surgical Treatment Pathway: The Paradox of a Rich, Small Region. *Front. Surg.* **2022**, *9*, 884048. [CrossRef] [PubMed]
19. Damhus, C.S.; Quentin, J.G.; Malmqvist, J.; Siersma, V.; Brodersen, J. Psychosocial consequences of a three-month follow-up after receiving an abnormal lung cancer CT-screening result: A longitudinal survey. *Lung Cancer* **2021**, *155*, 46–52. [CrossRef] [PubMed]
20. Rasmussen, J.F.; Siersma, V.; Malmqvist, J.; Brodersen, J. Psychosocial consequences of false positives in the Danish Lung Cancer CT Screening Trial: A nested matched cohort study. *BMJ Open* **2020**, *10*, e034682. [CrossRef]
21. Yankaskas, B.C.; Cleveland, R.J.; Schell, M.J.; Kozar, R. Association of recall rates with sensitivity and positive predictive values of screening mammography. *AJR Am. J. Roentgenol.* **2001**, *177*, 543–549. [CrossRef]
22. National Lung Screening Trial Research, T. Lung Cancer Incidence and Mortality with Extended Follow-up in the National Lung Screening Trial. *J. Thorac. Oncol.* **2019**, *14*, 1732–1742. [CrossRef]
23. Arcadi, T.; Maffei, E.; Sverzellati, N.; Mantini, C.; Guaricci, A.I.; Tedeschi, C.; Martini, C.; La Grutta, L.; Cademartiri, F. Coronary artery calcium score on low-dose computed tomography for lung cancer screening. *World J. Radiol.* **2014**, *6*, 381–387. [CrossRef]
24. Fan, L.; Fan, K. Lung cancer screening CT-based coronary artery calcification in predicting cardiovascular events: A systematic review and meta-analysis. *Medicine (Baltimore)* **2018**, *97*, e10461. [CrossRef] [PubMed]
25. Lu, M.T.; Onuma, O.K.; Massaro, J.M.; D'Agostino Sr, R.B.; O'Donnell, C.J.; Hoffmann, U. Lung Cancer Screening Eligibility in the Community: Cardiovascular Risk Factors, Coronary Artery Calcification, and Cardiovascular Events. *Circulation* **2016**, *134*, 897–899. [CrossRef] [PubMed]
26. Rasmussen, T.; Kober, L.; Abdulla, J.; Pedersen, J.H.; Wille, M.M.; Dirksen, A.; Kofoed, K.F. Coronary artery calcification detected in lung cancer screening predicts cardiovascular death. *Scand. Cardiovasc. J.* **2015**, *49*, 159–167. [CrossRef] [PubMed]

Disclaimer/Publisher's Note: The statements, opinions and data contained in all publications are solely those of the individual author(s) and contributor(s) and not of MDPI and/or the editor(s). MDPI and/or the editor(s) disclaim responsibility for any injury to people or property resulting from any ideas, methods, instructions or products referred to in the content.

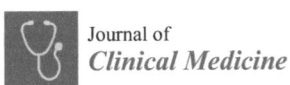

Article

Comparison of Quality of Life after Robotic, Video-Assisted, and Open Surgery for Lung Cancer

Nicole Asemota [1], Alessandro Maraschi [1], Savvas Lampridis [1], John Pilling [1], Juliet King [1], Corinne Le Reun [1] and Andrea Bille [1,2,*]

[1] Department of Thoracic Surgery, Guy's Hospital London, Great Maze Pond, London SE1 9RT, UK; corinne.lereun@yahoo.fr (C.L.R.)
[2] Division of Cancer Studies, King's College London, Guy's Hospital London, Great Maze Pond, London SE1 9RT, UK
* Correspondence: andrea.bille@gstt.nhs.uk

Abstract: Post-operative quality of life (QOL) has become crucial in choosing operative approaches in thoracic surgery. However, compared to VATS and thoracotomy, QOL results post-RATS are limited. We compared QOL before and after RATS and between RATS, VATS, and thoracotomy. We conducted a retrospective review of lung cancer surgical patients from 2015 to 2020. Patients completed validated EORTC QOL questionnaires (QLQ-C30 and QLQ-LC13). Results were analysed using the EORTC Scoring Guide, with statistical analysis. A total of 47 (94%) pre- and post-RATS questionnaires were returned. Forty-two patients underwent anatomical lung resections. In addition, 80% of patients experienced uncomplicated recovery. All global and functional QOL domains improved post-operatively, as did most symptoms (13/19). Only four symptoms worsened, including dyspnoea ($p = 0.017$), with two symptoms unchanged. Of the 148 returned questionnaires for all approaches (open-22/VATS-79/RATS-47), over 70% showed a high pre-operative performance status. Most patients underwent anatomical lung resection, with only VATS patients requiring conversion (n = 6). Complications were slightly higher in RATS, with one patient requiring re-intubation. RATS patients demonstrated the highest global and functional QOL. Physical QOL was lowest after thoracotomy ($p = 0.002$). RATS patients reported the fewest symptoms, including dyspnoea ($p = 0.046$), fatigue ($p < 0.001$), and pain ($p = 0.264$). Overall, RATS results in a significantly better post-operative QOL and should be considered the preferred surgical approach for lung cancer patients.

Keywords: quality-of-life; robotic-assisted thoracoscopic surgery (RATS); symptoms; thoracotomy; video-assisted thoracoscopic surgery (VATS)

1. Introduction

Lung cancer continues to be the most prevalent cancer globally, with surgery remaining the standard treatment for early-stage cases. Technological advancements have shifted surgical approaches from open procedures to minimally invasive surgeries, such as video-assisted thoracoscopic surgery (VATS) and robot-assisted thoracoscopic surgery (RATS) [1,2]. However, these two methods have significant differences. VATS has faced criticism for its limited manoeuvrability and reliance on a two-dimensional screen [1–4]. Consequently, RATS has gained attraction, addressing many VATS challenges by providing 360-degree articulation and a three-dimensional operating environment [1,2,5]. These advantages may offer RATS an oncological edge, facilitating improved nodal resection [1,6–8] and enabling more complex procedures, thus reducing VATS conversion rates [7,9].

The benefits of VATS compared to open surgery, including enhanced recovery and superior surgical outcomes, are well-established [1,2,6]. However, post-operative quality of life (QOL) is increasingly used to assess the true success of surgery. The VIOLET Trial [10] demonstrated that VATS led to a higher post-operative QOL and reduced adverse events

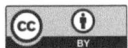

compared to open surgery without compromising oncological outcomes. QOL comparisons between VATS and open surgery are abundant, consistently favouring VATS [1,4,6,10–15]. However, QOL comparisons with RATS are not as strong currently, and tripartite comparisons of all three approaches even less so. Such comparisons are frequently limited by the lack of QOL data in RATS patients and disagreement amongst the minimal RATS QOL data available. Considering the substantial learning and financial investments required for RATS, comprehensive reviews of QOL in RATS patients are increasingly necessary.

This study will compare QOL before and after RATS and assess QOL following VATS, RATS, and open surgery in lung cancer patients after thoracic surgery.

2. Materials and Methods

We conducted a retrospective study of local patients. Patients were eligible for inclusion if they were older than 18 years, had a diagnosis of primary or secondary lung cancer, and underwent surgical resection for lung cancer at our institution between 2015 and 2020. Additional inclusion criteria were being alive without evidence of recurrence at the time of the study and not receiving adjuvant chemotherapy or radiation therapy at the time of QOL questionnaire completion. The surgical approaches included were thoracotomy (open surgery), VATS, and RATS. Acceptable types of lung resection were lobectomy, bilobectomy, segmentectomy, and wedge resection.

Patients were excluded if they died prior to study initiation, had recurrence of lung cancer, were receiving adjuvant therapy at the time of QOL assessment, underwent lung surgery for benign indications, or had surgery performed at another institution.

Eligible patients completed two QOL questionnaires designed by the European Association for Research and Treatment for Cancer (EORTC): QLQ-C30, assessing general QOL after cancer treatment, and QLQ-LC13, evaluating lung cancer-specific symptoms [16,17]. The primary endpoints of this study were changes in QOL amongst RATS patients before and after surgery, and QOL differences between RATS, VATS, and thoracotomy patients post-operatively. Secondary endpoints included differences in complication rates, ICU admission, conversion rates, and length of hospital stay.

A pictorial summary of the methods is demonstrated in Figure 1.

This study conformed to the ethical principles defined in the Declaration of Helsinki of 1964 and all subsequent revisions, and it was approved by the relevant committee of our institution as a clinical audit project (Number 7753). Written informed consent was obtained from all participants prior to inclusion.

2.1. Pre- and Post-RATS

We included only matched pre- and post-operative RATS questionnaires. The pre-operative questionnaires for RATS patients were completed in the outpatient clinic during the preadmission appointment, along with an information sheet explaining the purpose of the study. The post-operative questionnaires for all groups were administered during follow-up appointments in clinic, through postal mailings, or over the telephone by the study authors. Along with the questionnaire, patients received an information sheet describing the study and instructions for completing the survey. Completed questionnaires were returned to the study authors either in-person during a clinic visit, via post, or the answers were documented by the study authors during telephone administration. Questionnaire results were analysed according to the EORTC Scoring Guide. We categorised QLQ-C30 results into Global Health Status, Symptoms, and Functional QOL, further subdividing functional QOL into five domains: Physical, Role, Emotional, Cognitive, and Social QOL. The QLQ-LC13 questionnaire focused solely on lung symptoms.

We generated two scores for all domains: a raw score (RS), the average of scores from all contributing questions, and a final, standardised score (FS), after applying a linear transformation formula to the RS. The RS was calculated as: Raw Score = $(I1 + I2 + \ldots + In)/n$, with higher scores indicating better Global QOL and worse functional QOL/Symptoms. The FS was calculated as: Final Score = $((Rawscore - 1)/range) \times 100$

for Global Health and Symptom Scales; and Final Score = $(1 - (\text{Rawscore} - 1)/\text{range}) \times 100$ for Functional Scales. Higher Scores indicate better Global and Functional QOL and worse symptomatology. Range = Maximal–minimal possible question score. (Global Health questions = 6, All other questions = 3).

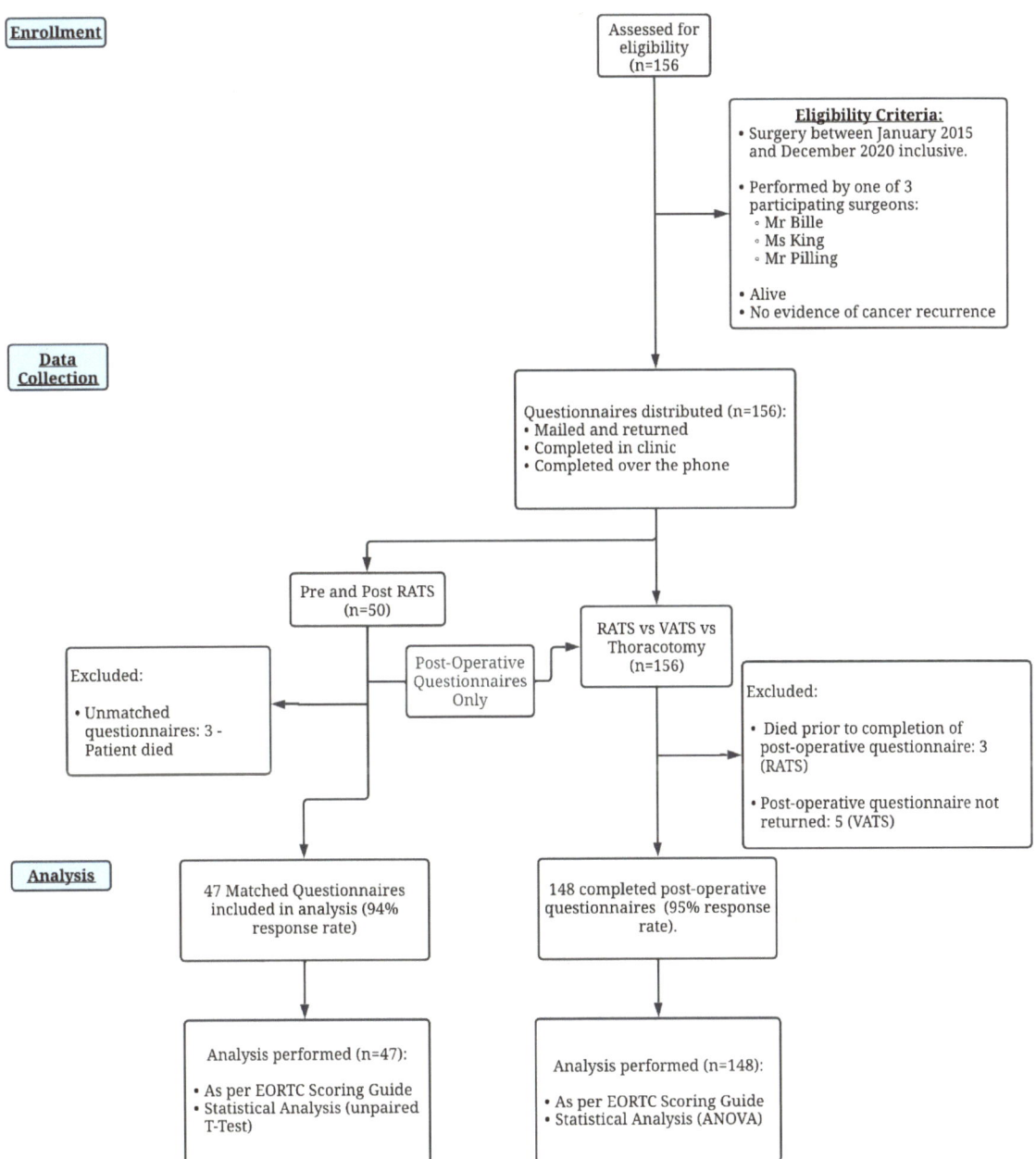

Figure 1. Overview of Methodology.

2.2. RATS, VATS, and Thoracotomy

We compared post-operative data from RATS patients against previously collected post-operative QOL data from patients who had undergone VATS and open surgery for lung cancer. We used the same questionnaires and analysis methods for all groups. Patient characteristics were described as above.

2.3. Statistical Analysis

Analysis was performed using the Stata software version 14.2 (College Station, TX, USA). Population characteristics were analysed using summary statistics (mean and standard deviation for continuous variables; frequency and percentage for categorical variables). RATS pre- and post-operative scores were compared using unpaired T tests. RS and FS between RATS, VATS, and thoracotomy were compared using one-way analysis of variance. A p-value of <0.05 was deemed to be statistically significant.

3. Results

3.1. Pre- and Post-RATS

Forty-seven patients were included in the final analysis (Figure 1). Patient characteristics are described in Table 1.

Table 1. Patient Characteristics amongst RATS patients.

		(N = 47)
Age (Median)		69.8 ± 9.1
Gender	Male	15 (34.0%)
	Female	32 (68.1%)
PS ECOG	0	12 (25.5%)
	1	23 (48.9%)
	2	12 (25.5%)
Smoking status	Non smoker	10 (25.5%)
	Ex−smoker	29 (61.7%)
	Smoker	8 (17.0%)
Comorbidities	Pulmonary	12(25.5%)
	Cardiac	26 (55.3%)
	Previous cancer	11 (23.4%)
	Of which is primary lung cancer	2 (4.3%)
	Nil	5 (10.6%)
Procedure	Lobectomy	33 (70.2%)
	Bi lobectomy	0
	Segmentectomy	10 (21.3%)
	Wedge resection	4 (8.5%)
Number of Ports	4	47 (100%)
Operating Time: Mean (±SD), mins	110.8 (±38.8)	—
Median (IQR), mins	105 (41)	—
Pre-Operative Staging	IA1	4 (8.5%)
	IA2	15 (31.9%)
	IA3	12 (25.5%)
	IB	1 (2.1%)
	IIA	2 (4.3%)
	IIB	2 (4.3%)
	IIIA	2 (4.3%)
	IVB [1]	1 (2.1%)
	Secondary Lung Metastases	7 (14.9%)
	No Pre-op Staging	1 (2.1%)

Table 1. Cont.

		(N = 47)
Post-Operative Staging	IA1	2 (4.3%)
	IA2	13 (27.7%)
	IA3	10 (21.3%)
	IB	6 (12.8%)
	IIA	1 (2.1%)
	IIB	5 (10.6%)
	IIIA	2 (4.3%)
	IIIB	1 (2.1%)
	No Staging (Secondary Metastasis)	7 (14.9%)
Post-Operative Histology	Adenocarcinoma	33 (70.2%)
	Squamous Cell Carcinoma	3 (6.4%)
	Metastasis	7 (14.9%)
	Carcinoid	4 (8.5%)
Complications	Inpatient complications	17 (36.2%)
	Of which:	
	COVID	2 (4.3%)
	Prolonged AL (>7 days)	5 (10.6%)
	AF	3 (6.4%)
	Atelectasis/sputum plug/bronchoscopy	3 (6.4%)
	Hospital Acquired Pneumonia (HAP)	4 (8.5%)
	Pleural effusion/empyema	2 (4.3%)
	Pneumothorax—new drain insertion	1 (2.1%)
Clavien–Dindo	0	30 (63.8%)
	1	9 (19.2%)
	2	5 (10.6%)
	3	0
	3a	2 (4.3%)
	4a	1 (2.1%)

[1] Patient who was originally staged as M1C and restaged after chemotherapy and immunotherapy with residual disease in the lung and no evidence of metastatic disease.

Most patients were female (68%), with an average age of 69 years. Most patients had a performance status (PS) of 0 or 1. Twenty-nine (61.7%) were ex-smokers, with a median of 21 pack years. Almost all patients had co-morbidities, particularly cardiac (n = 26; 55%) and lung (n = 12; 25.5%) diseases. A total of 43 patients (91%) underwent anatomical lung resections, most commonly lobectomy (70.2%, n = 33). All RATS procedures were performed by a single surgeon (AB). All four non-anatomical wedge resections performed were for lung metastases.

In total, 82.9% of patients had an uncomplicated recovery [Clavien–Dindo = 0 (n = 30) or 1 (n = 9)]. The most common complication was prolonged air leak (>7 days) and pneumonia, occurring in five patients (10.6%) and four patients (8.5%), retrospectively. Two patients (4.3%) developed COVID-19. One patient (2.1%) had a Clavien–Dindo score of 4, experiencing pneumonia and respiratory failure that required admission to critical care and re-intubation. Post-operative questionnaires were completed with an average interval period of 7 months (range, 5–9). Notably, 83.3% of patients returned to baseline health within 2 to 3 months.

Quality of Life Results

The complete QOL results are displayed in Figures 2 and 3 and Supplemental Table S1. Global QOL (Figure 2A) appears to have improved post-RATS ($p = 0.113$). There was an improvement in functional QOL in all five domains post-RATS, with a statistically significant improvement in emotional functioning (FS: increase of (+) 9, $p < 0.001$) (Figure 2B). Importantly, patients demonstrated a mild improvement in physical health post-RATS (FS: +1.42).

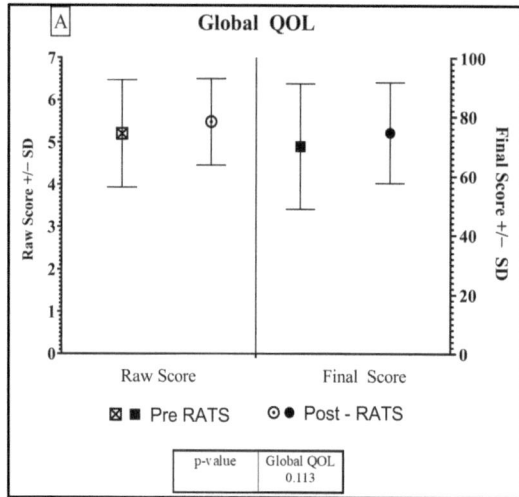
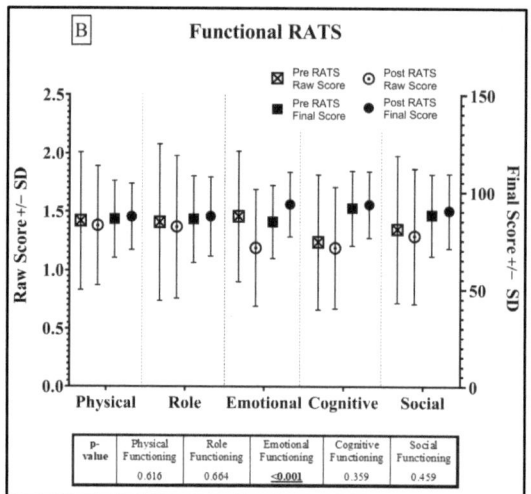

Figure 2. Global (**A**) and Function (**B**) QOL Results—Pre- and Post-RATS. Standard deviation shown in bars.

Symptoms assessed in the QLQ-C30 questionnaire (Figure 3A,B) showed an improvement in six out of nine symptoms, although these were not statistically significant. Nausea/vomiting and diarrhoea appeared to worsen post-RATS (FS: +1.42 and +0.71, respectively). Results from QLQ-LC13 (Figure 3C,D) were similar, with an improvement in most symptoms, but statistically significant only in alopecia (FS decrease of (−) 2.84, $p = 0.044$).

Dyspnoea and pain were the only QOL measures that appeared in both questionnaires. In both questionnaires, dyspnoea appeared to worsen post-RATS. However, this was only statistically significant in QLQ-C30 (FS: +11.34, $p = 0.017$), with a much smaller FS increase of 1.19 in QLQ-LC13. In both questionnaires, pain was overall lower post-RATS, although not statistically significant.

3.2. RATS vs. VATS vs. Thoracotomy

We included 148 patients in the analysis: VATS, n = 79; RATS, n = 47; and open surgery, n = 22. Patient characteristics are described in Table 2.

VATS patients were, on average, 5.8 years older (75.6 years) than thoracotomy (68.2 years) and RATS (69.8 years) patients ($p < 0.001$). Sex was more evenly split in VATS (58.2% female) and thoracotomy patients (50% each) than in RATS patients (68.1% female). A PS of 0 or 1 was reported in over 70% of all groups. Most patients were ex-smokers (median of 21 pack years).

Table 2. Patient Characteristics amongst thoracotomy, VATS, and RATS patients.

		Thoracotomy (N = 22)	VATS (N = 79)	RATS (N = 47)	*p*-Value
Age		68.2 ± 8.8	75.6 ± 9.6	69.8 ± 9.1	<0.001
Gender	Male	11 (50.0%)	33 (41.8%)	15 (31.9%)	0.32
	Female	11 (50.0%)	46 (58.2%)	32 (68.1%)	
PS ECOG	0	6 (27.3%)	15 (19.0%)	12 (25.5%)	0.86
	1	11 (50.0%)	45 (57.0%)	23 (48.9%)	
	2	5 (22.7%)	19 (24.0%)	12 (25.5%)	
Smoking Status	Non-Smoker	2 (9.1%)	9 (11.4%)	12 (25.5%)	0.24
	Ex-smoker	16 (72.7%)	58 (73.4%)	27 (57.5%)	
	Smoker	4 (18.2%)	12 (15.2%)	8 (17.0%)	

Table 2. Cont.

		Thoracotomy (N = 22)	VATS (N = 79)	RATS (N = 47)	p-Value
Co-morbidities	Pulmonary	7 (31.8%)	28 (35.4%)	12 (25.5%)	0.51
	Cardiac	11 (50.0%)	54 (68.4%)	26 (55.3%)	0.17
	Renal	—	4 (5.1%)	1 (2.1%)	0.57
	Previous cancer	6 (27.3%)	25 (31.6%)	11 (23.4%)	0.61
	Previous primary lung cancer	2 (9.1%)	2 (2.5%)	2 (4.3%)	0.29
Pre-Operative Staging	IA1	0 (0%)	12 (15.2%)	4 (8.5%)	
	IA2	2 (9.1%)	27 (34.2%)	15 (31.9%)	
	IA3	1 (4.5%)	8 (10.1%)	12 (25.5%)	
	IB	2 (9.1%)	14 (17.7%)	1 (2.1%)	
	IIA	1 (4.5%)	4 (5.1%)	2 (4.3%)	
	IIB	6 (27.3%)	8 (10.1%)	2 (4.3%)	
	IIIA	4 (18.2%)	0	2 (4.3%)	
	IIIB	2 (9.1%)	1 (1.3%)	0	
	IIIC	1 (4.5%)	0	0	
	IV	3 (13.6%)	0	1 (2.1%)	
	Secondary Metastasis		3 (3.8%)	7 (14.9%)	
	No Staging (No Pre-op Staging)		2 (2.5%)	1 (2.1%)	
Procedure	Lobectomy	15 (68.2%)	50 (63.3%)	33 (70.2%)	
	Pneumonectomy	2 (9.1%)	0	0	
	Segmentectomy	2 (9.1%)	17 (21.5%)	10 (21.3%)	
	Wedge resection	3 (13.6%)	12 (15.2%)	4 (8.5%)	
Number of Ports	3	—	79 (100%)	0	
	4	—	0	47 (100%)	
Operating Time: Mean (+/−SD), mins Median (IQR), mins		143.2 (±38.4) 142 (60)	116.1 (±32.2) 120 (51.25)	110.8 (±38.8) 105 (41)	
Conversion	Yes	N/A	6 (7.6%)	0	
	No	N/A	73 (92.4%)	47 (100%)	
Final Staging	IA1	0	4 (5.1%)	2 (4.3%)	
	IA2	0	18 (22.8%)	13 (27.7%)	
	IA3	0	9 (11.4%)	10 (21.3%)	
	IB	3 (13.6%)	17 (21.5%)	6 (12.8%)	
	IIA	2 (9.1%)	5 (6.3%)	1 (2.1%)	
	IIB	5 (22.7%)	11 (13.9%)	5 (10.6%)	
	IIIA	5 (22.7%)	6 (7.6%)	2 (4.3%)	
	IIIB	2 (9.1%)	1 (1.3%)	1 (2.1%)	
	0 (no staging)	1 (4.5)	0	0	
	Secondary Metastasis	4 (18.2%)	5 (6.3%)	7 (14.9%)	
	Benign Disease	0	1 (1.3%)	0	
	Carcinoid	0	1 (1.3%)	0	
	TNM Staging Not Applicable [1]	0	1 (1.3%)	0	
Complications	In-hospital complications	6 (27.3%)	21 (26.6%)	17 (36.2%)	0.50
	COVID	0	0	2 (4.3%)	0.22
	Prolonged air leak (>7 days)	2 (9.1%)	3 (3.8%)	5 (10.6%)	0.23
	AF	0	9 (11.4%)	3 (6.4%)	0.24
	Airway complications	1 (4.5%)	4 (5.1%)	3 (6.4%)	>0.99
	HAP	4 (18.2%)	12 (15.2%)	4 (8.5%)	0.48
	Pleural effusion/empyema	0	1 (1.3%)	2 (4.3%)	0.73
	Surgical emphysema	0	2 (2.5%)	0	0.66
	Pneumothorax—new drain insertion	0	1 (1.3%)	1 (2.1%)	>0.99
Clavien–Dindo	0	16 (72.7%)	58 (73.4%)	30 (63.8%)	
	1	2 (9.1%)	3 (3.8%)	9 (19.1%)	
	2	3 (13.6%)	15 (19%)	5 (10.6%)	0.083
	3	1 (4.5%)	2 (2.5%)	0	
	3a	0	1 (1.3%)	2 (4.3%)	
	4a	0	0	1 (2.1%)	

[1]—Final Histology: Angiosarcoma; therefore, Lung TNM staging not applicable.

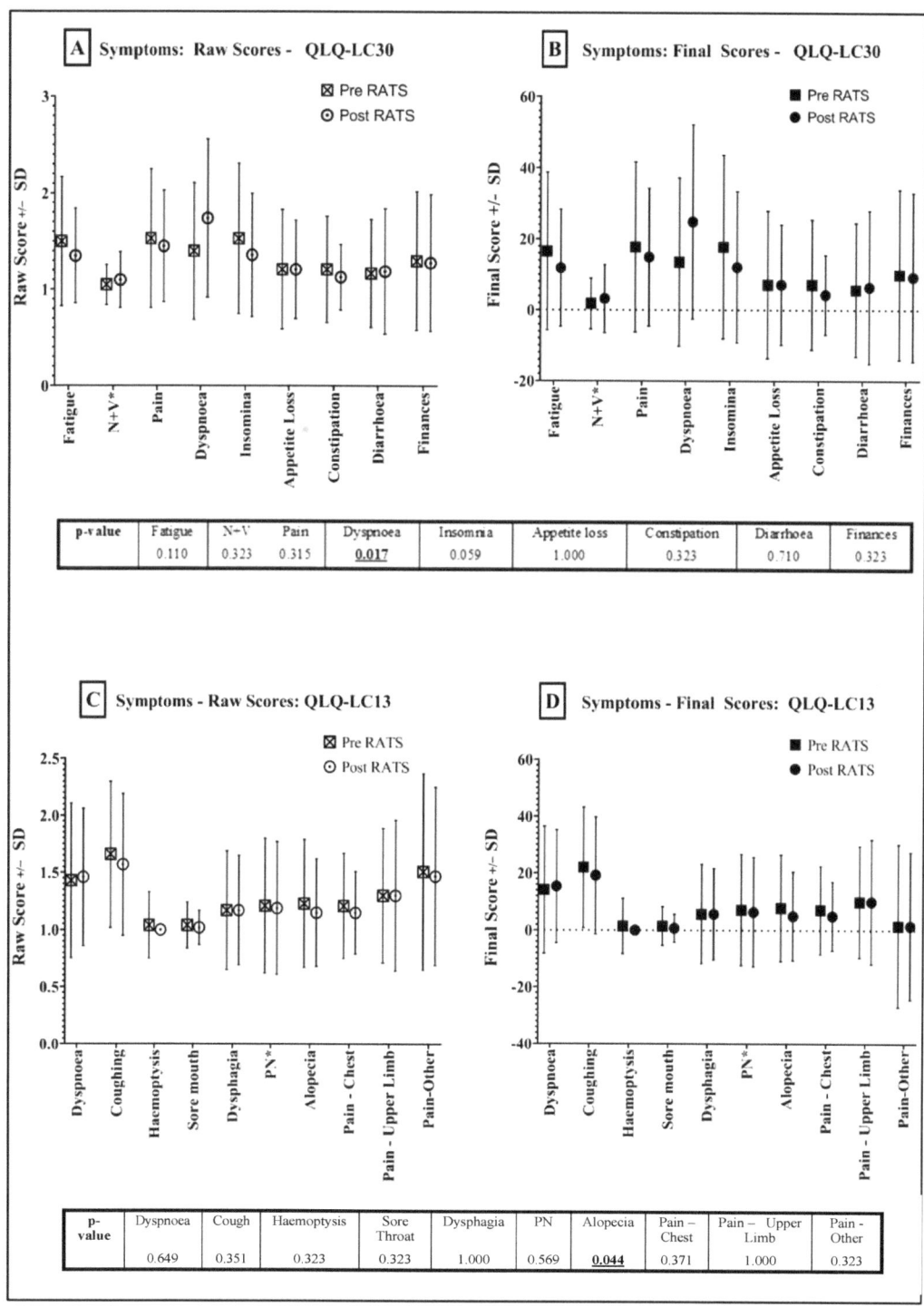

Figure 3. Symptom Scores—Pre- and Post-RATS. QLQ-C30 Results = (**A**) (RS) and (**B**) (FS). LC13 Results = (**C**) (RS) and (**D**) (FS). Standard deviation shown in bars.

Only 8% of all patients had no additional co-morbidities (VATS, n = 9; thoracotomy, n = 3). The most common co-morbidities in all groups were pulmonary (thoracotomy, 31.8%; VATS, 35.4%; RATS, 25.5%) and cardiac (thoracotomy, 50%; VATS, 68.4%; RATS, 55.3%) diseases. Previous lung cancer was most common in the VATS group (31.6%). The average pre-operative staging was higher in the thoracotomy group (Stage II and III at 32% each) compared to the VATS and RATS group (Stage I—77% (VATS) and 68% (RATS)).

Most patients underwent anatomical lung resection (>80% for all groups, $p = 0.251$). AB, JK, and JP all contributed to VATS and thoracotomy procedures. Segmentectomies were at least five times more common in VATS and RATS patients compared to thoracotomy. Conversion to thoracotomy occurred only in VATS patients (n = 6, 7.9%). Inpatient complications occurred at a higher proportion after RATS (36.2% vs. 26.6%—VATS vs. 27.3%—thoracotomy, $p = 0.504$). Hospital-Acquired Pneumonia (HAP) was the most common complication in all groups. Although more VATS patients developed HAP (n = 12), this was proportionally smaller compared to thoracotomy (15.2% vs. 18.2%), but almost double compared to RATS (15.2% vs. 8.5%) patients. Most patients had Clavien–Dindo scores of 0 or 1. Only 1 RATS patient had a score of 4 (described above).

Quality of Life Results

All QOL results are shown in Figures 4–6 and Supplement Table S2. Questionnaires were completed with an average interval period of 7 months amongst RATS patients and 10 months amongst VATS and open patients. Global QOL (Figure 4) was equal between thoracotomy and VATS patients (FS: 66.67 and 66.24), but higher amongst RATS patients (FS: 73.76, $p = 0.176$).

Functional QOL (Figure 5) was highest amongst RATS patients in all subdomains. FS was similar between open and VATS patients in all subdomains. VATS patients had the lowest scores in all sub-domains, except physical functioning where thoracotomy patients were lowest (FS:73.94—open vs. 79.95—VATS and 86.1—RATS, $p = 0.02$). Differences in all sub-domains, except role functioning, were statistically significant.

RATS patients were least symptomatic in almost all QLQ-C30 domains (Figure 6A,B), with statistically significant results in fatigue ($p < 0.001$) and dyspnoea ($p = 0.046$). VATS patients reported the least diarrhoea and least financial difficulties ($p = 0.863$) after surgery.

QLQ-LC13 lung-specific symptoms were low, with an average RS of <2 in all patients (Figure 6C,D). RATS patients were less symptomatic in all domains except alopecia (VATS patients with lowest FS: 3.56 vs. 7.94—thoracotomy, 6.38—RATS) and dysphagia (thoracotomy patients with lowest FS—3.17 vs. 6.22—VATS and 6.38—RATS). Coughing and sore throat were the only statistically significant scores ($p = 0.036$ and $p = 0.047$, respectively), with RATS patients the least symptomatic.

Dyspnoea scores appeared to differ between questionnaires. RATS patients reported the lowest dyspnoea across both questionnaires, but with a larger and more statistically significant difference in QLQ-C30 (Figure 6A,B) compared to non-RATS patients than in the QLQ-LC13 (Figure 6C,D). RATS patients reported the least overall pain in both questionnaires. VATS patients reported the highest overall QLQ-C30 pain score ($p = 0.264$) (Figure 6A,B). Area-specific pain, in QLQ-LC13 (Figure 6C,D), was worst amongst thoracotomy patients in the arm/shoulder ($p = 0.837$) and chest (0.073), with only pain elsewhere appearing worse amongst VATS patients ($p = 0.233$).

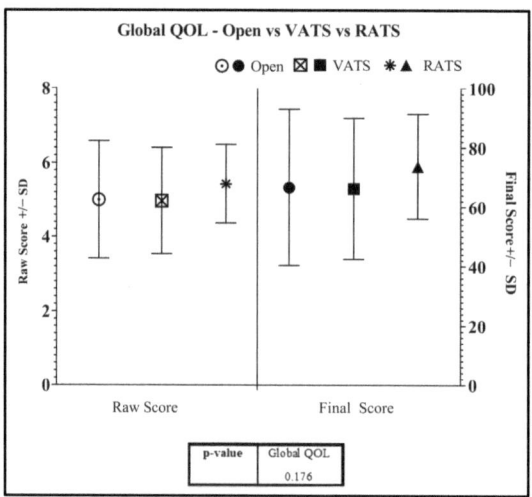

Figure 4. Global QOL Scores—RATS vs. VATS vs. Open. Standard deviation shown in bars.

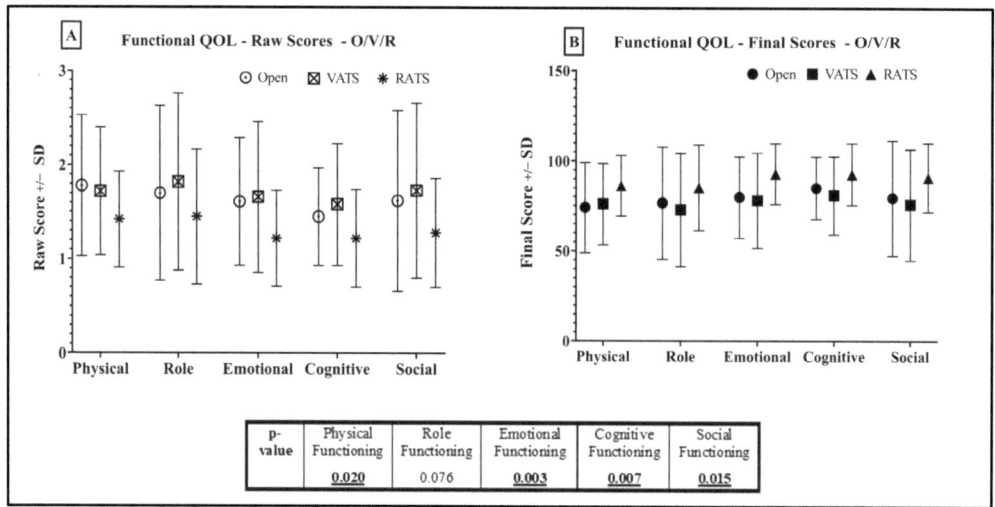

Figure 5. Functional QOL—RATS (R) vs. VATS (V) vs. Open (O). Raw Scores (RS) = (**A**), Final Scores (FS) = (**B**). Standard deviation shown in bars.

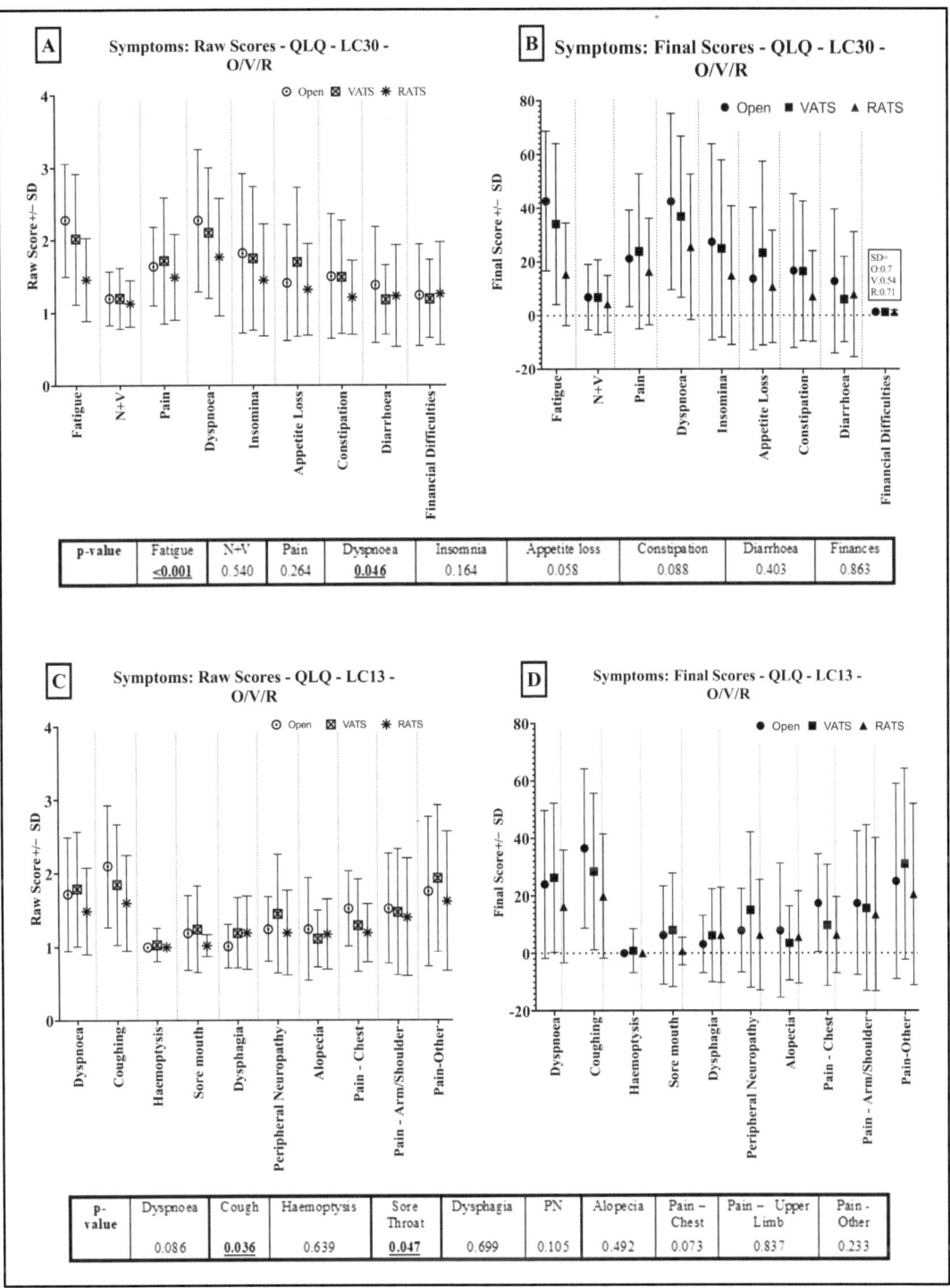

Figure 6. Symptom Scores—RATS (R) vs. VATS (V) vs. Open (O). QLQ-C30 Results = (**A**) (RS) and (**B**) (FS). LC13 Results = (**C**) (RS) and (**D**) (FS). Standard deviation shown in bars.

4. Discussion

The present study provides robust evidence that QOL is higher amongst RATS patients, both in direct comparison before and after surgery, and when compared with VATS and open surgery. This finding corroborates the existing literature that demonstrates improved QOL among RATS patients [7,14,18,19].

However, notable discrepancies exist in the assessment of QOL in RATS patients within the literature [2,8,20]. These inconsistencies arise primarily from variations in study protocols, such as the surgical approaches compared (RATS only [2,19] vs. VATS [5,8,10,20] or vs. thoracotomy [7,19]) and the substantial differences in patient numbers. The present study addresses these limitations by utilising a single cohort to examine temporal changes in QOL in RATS patients while comparing them to VATS and thoracotomy patients. Moreover, the study benefits from being conducted at a single institution with a single surgeon (AB) performing all RATS operations, thereby mitigating the influence of the surgical learning curve for robotic surgery [7] and variable post-operative protocols, such as pain control. Consequently, our results suggest that the observed improvements in QOL are more likely attributable to RATS rather than alternative factors.

To the best of our knowledge, this study is the only clinical investigation that examines QOL in VATS, RATS, and thoracotomy patients simultaneously. Although recent meta-analyses and systematic reviews have attempted similar three-way comparisons, they have been hindered by the scarcity of the RATS QOL literature [6]. As a result, many studies group RATS and VATS into a 'minimally invasive' category, comparing them against thoracotomy [1,18]. This approach fails to demonstrate the specific superiority of RATS, including over VATS. Therefore, the present study is essential in illustrating the QOL differences between all three approaches independently.

Existing evidence suggests that the QOL benefits of RATS decrease over time, with a return to baseline after four months [18,21]. However, our study found that RATS patients maintained their higher QOL scores after seven months, indicating that these benefits may persist for a longer duration [18].

Prior studies have suggested that patients with a higher pre-operative PS are less symptomatic pre-operatively and thus exhibit higher overall QOL scores [14]. In our cohort, significant differences in QOL were observed across all three approaches despite over 75% of all patients having high PS scores (0 or 1). Therefore, as QOL results were different despite a largely similar PS amongst all patients, a pre-operative PS is unlikely to have had a significant impact in our results. However, further studies directly assessing PS on QOL are required.

When compared to pre-operative assessments and non-RATS patients post-operatively, post-operative functional QOL was highest among RATS patients. Multiple studies have emphasised the advantages of minimally invasive surgery on physical functioning [13,14,20]. In our study, we observed no change in physical functioning before and after RATS surgery. This may be attributed to patient selection, as most RATS patients had a high PS and minimal symptoms pre-operatively, which may have rendered them less likely to notice significant changes post-operatively. However, RATS patients demonstrated a significantly higher physical QOL compared to VATS and thoracotomy patients. Thoracotomy patients, likely due to the larger incision, exhibited the lowest physical functioning QOL, which is consistent with the existing literature [13,14,20]. Emotional functioning was found to be significantly lower after RATS in both parts of the study. This supports current evidence and may be attributed to the smaller scar, reduced hospital stay, and enhanced post-operative recovery associated with RATS, leading to improved mental health.

Overall, symptoms were fewer among patients who underwent RATS. Pain was significantly lower in RATS patients compared to VATS and thoracotomy patients, both in our study group and within the current literature [6,13,18,20,21]. Nausea, vomiting, and constipation were also lowest in RATS patients. These findings may be partly attributed to side effects from post-operative pain medications, especially nausea and constipation from opioid use [6,13,18,20,21]. As such, it is plausible that the reduced pain experienced by RATS patients led to lower opioid use, and subsequently fewer drug-related side effects [7,22]. Interestingly, VATS patients reported more pain than thoracotomy patients, despite having a smaller incision. This might be due to the increased pressure from leverage exerted on the rib and intercostal bundle, [7] a phenomenon less noted in RATS (due to superior articulation) and open surgery.

Dyspnoea is an important symptom amongst lung cancer patients. Overall, post-operative dyspnoea scores were worse in RATS patients compared to the baseline, but still lower when compared to non-RATS patients. The current literature suggests that patients with a higher pre-operative PS may report worse shortness of breath (SOB) symptoms post-operatively [14] as these patients will have had minimal pre-operative dyspnoea, will be less tolerant of small SOB changes, and may over-estimate the extent of change when asked. This may explain the worsening SOB post-RATS compared to the baseline in our cohort, in whom the pre-operative PS was high for the majority of RATS patients. However, this does not account for the clear dyspnoea difference noted amongst VATS, RATS, and thoracotomy patients despite a relatively equal pre-operative PS. Ultimately, further studies utilising a single dyspnea evaluation are needed to obtain a definitive answer [18,20].

A challenge in comparing the QOL literature lies in the numerous assessment methods available [4,7,23]. In this study, we used the highly validated EORTC questionnaires for the assessment of QOL [21,24] and, specifically, the QLQ-LC13, which is tailored to lung cancer patients. Additional questionnaires used in the literature include the 12-item Short Form Survey (SF12) [22], 36-item Short Form Survey (SF36) [12], and VAS pain score [4]. However, to our knowledge, the EORTC questionnaires are the most commonly used and validated QOL questionnaires [11,13,14,18,20,25]. Despite their widespread use, these questionnaires are not exempt from error, as demonstrated by the significant disparity when comparing dyspnea scores, the only identical symptom present on both questionnaires. Similar studies on QOL have also shown conflicting results within the same population group [20]. This underlines the subjective nature of questionnaires and the need for increased QOL data to validate results.

This study has some limitations. First, the QLQ-LC13 questionnaire has been recently updated to include questions specifically related to QOL after lung cancer surgery [26]. However, we used the older version of the QLQ-LC13 to facilitate the comparison of RATS results with pre-collected VATS and thoracotomy data that utilised the original LC13 questionnaire. Future QOL studies could consider using the updated questionnaire [6,27]. Second, the number of patients per group was unequal, with the number of thoracotomy patients (n = 22) being less than a third of those in the VATS group (n = 79). This was unavoidable as VATS is the predominant approach in most institutions. In future studies, equal, propensity-matched groups would allow for a more accurate comparison of QOL.

A key limitation of this study was the lack of pre-operative QOL data for the VATS and thoracotomy groups. Without this baseline data, we could not definitively determine if the surgical approaches had equivalent impacts on QOL compared to each patient's pre-operative status. While we prospectively obtained matched pre- and post-operative QOL assessments for RATS patients, the retrospective nature of the VATS and thoracotomy data precluded gathering pre-operative QOL information. The lack of baseline QOL data for all groups is a limitation, as we cannot exclude the possibility that pre-operative QOL variability influenced the differences seen post-operatively. Future prospective studies should incorporate pre-operative QOL assessments for all surgical groups to better evaluate the impact of each approach compared to the baseline.

Another recognised limitation in this study is the different timeframes for post-operative assessment between groups, with RATS post-op questionnaires completed at 7 months, and the VATS and thoracotomy patients completed at 10 months. It is possible that the QOL for RATS patients may have continued to improve further in the 3-month difference. Standardised timeframes would have strengthened our results, likely further highlighting the higher QOL for RATS compared to VATS and thoracotomy. Lastly, the QOL questionnaires are inherently subjective and specific to the patient cohort, making it challenging to generalise these results to the broader population. Further studies on QOL are needed for a more accurate assessment of post-operative QOL.

5. Conclusions

In conclusion, RATS appears to result in a minimal impact on quality of life when compared to pre-operative QOL and significantly improved QOL post-operatively when compared directly to VATS and open surgery in many categories, particularly in functional QOL. RATS demonstrated improved dyspnoea and reduced post-operative pain compared to VATS and thoracotomy. Therefore, RATS is likely to become the preferred operative approach, especially if QOL, length of stay (LOS), and operative outcomes can be balanced against its cost.

The findings of this study contribute to the growing body of evidence supporting the use of RATS in surgical practice, while highlighting the need for further research to validate and expand upon these results. By carefully considering the limitations and challenges associated with QOL assessments and addressing them in future studies, researchers can continue to advance our understanding of the impact of different surgical approaches on patient outcomes. Ultimately, these insights will help guide clinical decision making and ensure that patients receive the most effective and appropriate care for their individual needs.

Supplementary Materials: The following supporting information can be downloaded at: https://www.mdpi.com/article/10.3390/jcm12196230/s1, Table S1: Full QOL Results (Pre and Post RATS), Table S2: Full QOL Results (RATS vs. VATS vs. Thoracotomy).

Author Contributions: Conceptualisation, N.A., A.M., S.L., J.P., J.K., C.L.R. and A.B. Methodology: N.A., A.M., S.L., J.P., J.K., C.L.R. and A.B. Software: N/A Validation: N.A., A.M., S.L., J.P., J.K., C.L.R. and A.B. Formal Analysis: N.A., J.P., J.K., C.L.R. and A.B. Investigation: N.A., A.M., S.L., J.P., J.K., C.L.R. and A.B. Resources: N.A., C.L.R. and A.B. Data Curation: N.A., A.M., S.L., J.P., J.K., C.L.R. and A.B. Writing—Original Draft Preparation: N.A., C.L.R. and A.B. Writing—Review and Editing: N.A., A.M., S.L., J.P., J.K., C.L.R. and A.B. Visualisation: N.A., A.M., S.L., J.P., J.K., C.L.R. and A.B. Supervision: J.P., J.K. and A.B. Project Administration: N.A., S.L. and A.B. All authors have read and agreed to the published version of the manuscript.

Funding: This research received no external funding.

Institutional Review Board Statement: The study was conducted according to the guidelines of the Declaration of Helsinki and approved by the Institutional Clinical Audit Team of Guys and St Thomas' NHS Foundation Trust as a clinical audit project (Number 7753).

Informed Consent Statement: Informed consent was obtained from all subjects involved in the study.

Data Availability Statement: The data presented in this study are available on request from the corresponding author. The data are not publicly available due to privacy concerns.

Conflicts of Interest: Andrea Bille is a Proctor for Intuitive Surgical.

References

1. Young, A.; Gallesio, J.M.A.; Sewell, D.B.; Carr, R.; Molena, D. Outcomes of robotic esophagectomy. *J. Thorac. Dis.* **2021**, *13*, 6163–6168. [CrossRef] [PubMed]
2. Lazzaro, R.S.; Patton, B.D.; Wasserman, G.A.; Karp, J.; Cohen, S.; Inra, M.L.; Scheinerman, S.J. Robotic-assisted tracheobronchoplasty: Quality of life and pulmonary function assessment on intermediate follow-up. *J. Thorac. Cardiovasc. Surg.* **2021**, *164*, 278–286. [CrossRef] [PubMed]
3. Suda, T. Transition from video-assisted thoracic surgery to robotic pulmonary surgery. *J. Vis. Surg.* **2017**, *3*, 55. [CrossRef] [PubMed]
4. Veronesi, G.; Galetta, D.; Maisonneuve, P.; Melfi, F.; Schmid, R.A.; Borri, A.; Vannucci, F.; Spaggiari, L. Four-arm robotic lobectomy for the treatment of early-stage lung cancer. *J. Thorac. Cardiovasc. Surg.* **2010**, *140*, 19–25. [CrossRef]
5. Flores, R.M.; Alam, N. Video-Assisted Thoracic Surgery Lobectomy (VATS), Open Thoracotomy, and the Robot for Lung Cancer. *Ann. Thorac. Surg.* **2008**, *85*, S710–S715. [CrossRef]

6. Ng, C.S.H.; MacDonald, J.K.; Gilbert, S.; Khan, A.Z.; Kim, Y.T.; Louie, B.E.; Marshall, M.B.; Santos, R.S.; Scarci, M.; Shargal, Y.; et al. Optimal Approach to Lobectomy for Non-Small Cell Lung Cancer: Systemic Review and Meta-Analysis. *Innov. Technol. Tech. Cardiothorac. Vasc. Surg.* **2019**, *14*, 90–116. [CrossRef]
7. Louie, B.E.; Farivar, A.S.; Aye, R.W.; Vallières, E. Early Experience with Robotic Lung Resection Results in Similar Operative Outcomes and Morbidity when Compared with Matched Video-Assisted Thoracoscopic Surgery Cases. *Ann. Thorac. Surg.* **2012**, *93*, 1598–1605. [CrossRef]
8. Yang, H.X.; Woo, K.M.; Sima, C.S.; Bains, M.S.; Adusumilli, P.S.; Huang, J.; Finley, D.J.; Rizk, N.P.; Rusch, V.W.; Jones, D.R.; et al. Long-Term Survival Based on the Surgical Approach to Lobectomy for Clinical Stage I Non-Small Cell Lung Cancer: Comparison of Robotic, Video Assisted Thoracic Surgery, and Thoracotomy Lobectomy. *Ann Surg.* **2017**, *265*, 431. [CrossRef]
9. Cerfolio, R.J.; Bryant, A.S.; Skylizard, L.; Minnich, D.J. Initial consecutive experience of completely portal robotic pulmonary resection with 4 arms. *J. Thorac. Cardiovasc. Surg.* **2011**, *142*, 740–746. [CrossRef]
10. Veronesi, G.; Abbas, A.E.-S.; Muriana, P.; Lembo, R.; Bottoni, E.; Perroni, G.; Testori, A.; Dieci, E.; Bakhos, C.T.; Car, S.; et al. Perioperative Outcome of Robotic Approach Versus Manual Videothoracoscopic Major Resection in Patients Affected by Early Lung Cancer: Results of a Randomized Multicentric Study (ROMAN Study). *Front. Oncol.* **2021**, *11*, 726408. [CrossRef]
11. Fang, W.T.; Chen, T.B.; Luo, J.Z.; Ji, C.Y.; Yao, F. Minimally invasive surgery for centrally located lung cancers. *Zhonghua Wai Ke Za Zhi* **2020**, *58*, 57–60. [PubMed]
12. Lim, E.; Batchelor, T.J.; Dunning, J.; Shackcloth, M.; Anikin, V.; Naidu, B.; Belcher, E.; Loubani, M.; Zamvar, V.; Harris, R.A.; et al. Video-Assisted Thoracoscopic or Open Lobectomy in Early-Stage Lung Cancer. *NEJM Evid.* **2022**, *1*. [CrossRef]
13. Balduyck, B.; Hendriks, J.; Lauwers, P.; Van Schil, P. Quality of life evolution after lung cancer surgery: A prospective study in 100 patients. *Lung Cancer* **2007**, *56*, 423–431. [CrossRef] [PubMed]
14. Handy, J.R., Jr.; Asaph, J.W.; Douville, E.C.; Ott, G.Y.; Grunkemeier, G.L.; Wu, Y. Does video-assisted thoracoscopic lobectomy for lung cancer provide improved functional outcomes compared with open lobectomy? *Eur. J. Cardiothorac. Surg.* **2010**, *37*, 451–455. [CrossRef]
15. Bendixen, M.; Jørgensen, O.D.; Kronborg, C.; Andersen, C.; Licht, P.B. Postoperative pain and quality of life after lobectomy via video-assisted thoracoscopic surgery or anterolateral thoracotomy for early stage lung cancer: A randomised controlled trial. *Lancet Oncol.* **2016**, *17*, 836–844. [CrossRef]
16. Aaronson, N.K.; Ahmedzai, S.; Bergman, B.; Bullinger, M.; Cull, A.; Duez, N.J.; Filiberti, A.; Flechtner, H.; Fleishman, S.B.; De Haes, J.C.J.M.; et al. The European Organization for Research and Treatment of Cancer QLQ-C30: A Quality-of-Life Instrument for Use in International Clinical Trials in Oncology. *J. Natl. Cancer Inst.* **1993**, *85*, 365–376. [CrossRef]
17. Bergman, B.; Aaronson, N.; Ahmedzai, S.; Kaasa, S.; Sullivan, M.; EORTC Study Group on Quality of Life. The EORTC QLQ-LC13: A modular supplement to the EORTC core quality of life questionnaire (QLQ-C30) for use in lung cancer clinical trials. *Eur. J. Cancer* **1994**, *30*, 635–642. [CrossRef]
18. Marzorati, C.; Mazzocco, K.; Monzani, D.; Pavan, F.; Casiraghi, M.; Spaggiari, L.; Monturano, M.; Pravettoni, G. One-Year Quality of Life Trends in Early-Stage Lung Cancer Patients After Lobectomy. *Front. Psychol.* **2020**, *11*, 534428. [CrossRef]
19. Pompili, C. Quality of life after lung resection for lung cancer. *J. Thorac. Dis.* **2015**, *7* (Suppl. S2), S138–S144. [CrossRef]
20. Singer, E.S.; Kneuertz, P.J.; Nishimura, J.; D'souza, D.M.; Diefenderfer, E.; Moffatt-Bruce, S.D.; Merritt, R.E. Effect of operative approach on quality of life following anatomic lung cancer resection. *J. Thorac. Dis.* **2020**, *12*, 6913–6919. [CrossRef]
21. Cao, C.; Manganas, C.; Ang, S.C.; Yan, T.D. A systematic review and meta-analysis on pulmonary resections by robotic video-assisted thoracic surgery. *Ann. Cardiothorac. Surg.* **2012**, *1*, 3. [CrossRef] [PubMed]
22. Lacroix, V.; Kahn, D.; Matte, P.; Pieters, T.; Noirhomme, P.; Poncelet, A.; Steyaert, A. Robotic-Assisted Lobectomy Favors Early Lung Recovery versus Limited Thoracotomy. *Thorac. Cardiovasc. Surg.* **2021**, *69*, 557–563. [CrossRef] [PubMed]
23. Lacroix, V.; Nezhad, Z.M.; Kahn, D.; Steyaert, A.; Poncelet, A.; Pieters, T.; Noirhomme, P. Pain, Quality of Life, and Clinical Outcomes after Robotic Lobectomy. *Thorac. Cardiovasc. Surg.* **2016**, *65*, 344–350. [CrossRef] [PubMed]
24. Williams, A.M.; Zhao, L.; Grenda, T.R.; Kathawate, R.G.; Biesterveld, B.E.; Bhatti, U.F.; Carrott, P.W.; Lagisetty, K.H.; Chang, A.C.; Lynch, W.; et al. Higher Long-term Quality of Life Metrics After Video-Assisted Thoracoscopic Surgery Lobectomy Com-pared With Robotic-Assisted Lobectomy. *Ann. Thorac. Surg.* **2020**, *113*, 1591–1597. [CrossRef]
25. Worrell, S.G.; Dedhia, P.; Gilbert, C.; James, C.; Chang, A.C.; Lin, J.; Reddy, R.M. The cost and quality of life outcomes in developing a robotic lobectomy program. *J. Robot. Surg.* **2019**, *13*, 239–243. [CrossRef]
26. Koller, M.; Hjermstad, M.; Tomaszewski, K.; Tomaszewska, I.; Hornslien, K.; Harle, A.; Arraras, J.; Morag, O.; Pompili, C.; Ioannidis, G.; et al. An international study to revise the EORTC questionnaire for assessing quality of life in lung cancer patients. *Ann. Oncol.* **2017**, *28*, 2874–2881. [CrossRef]
27. Pompili, C.; Koller, M.; Velikova, G. Choosing the right survey: The lung cancer surgery. *J. Thorac. Dis.* **2020**, *12*, 6892–6901. [CrossRef]

Disclaimer/Publisher's Note: The statements, opinions and data contained in all publications are solely those of the individual author(s) and contributor(s) and not of MDPI and/or the editor(s). MDPI and/or the editor(s) disclaim responsibility for any injury to people or property resulting from any ideas, methods, instructions or products referred to in the content.

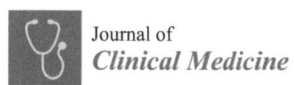

Article

Long-Term Oncologic Outcomes in Robot-Assisted and Video-Assisted Lobectomies for Non-Small Cell Lung Cancer

Giulia Fabbri [1,2,*], Federico Femia [1,2], Savvas Lampridis [1], Eleonora Farinelli [1,3], Alessandro Maraschi [1], Tom Routledge [1] and Andrea Bille [1]

[1] Department of Thoracic Surgery, Guy's and St. Thomas' NHS Trust Foundation, London SE1 9RT, UK; federico.femia@nhs.net (F.F.); savvas.lampridis@nhs.net (S.L.); eleonora.farinelli@studio.unibo.it (E.F.); alessandro.maraschi1@nhs.net (A.M.); tom.routledge@nhs.net (T.R.); andrea.bille@gstt.nhs.uk (A.B.)
[2] AOU Città della Salute e della Scienza di Torino, University of Turin, 10124 Turin, Italy
[3] St. Orsola-Malpighi University Hospital, University of Bologna, 40126 Bologna, Italy
* Correspondence: giulia.fabbri@edu.unito.it

Abstract: This study compares long-term outcomes in patients undergoing video-assisted thoracic surgery (VATS) and robotic-assisted thoracic surgery (RATS) lobectomy for non-small cell lung cancer (NSCLC); all consecutive patients who underwent RATS or VATS lobectomy for NSCLC between July 2015 and December 2021 in our center were enrolled in a single-center prospective study. The primary outcomes were overall survival (OS), disease-free survival (DFS), and recurrence rate. The secondary outcomes were complication rate, length of hospitalization (LOS), duration of chest tubes (LOD), and number of lymph node stations harvested. A total of 619 patients treated with RATS (n = 403) or VATS (n = 216) were included in the study. There was no significant difference in OS between the RATS and VATS groups (3-year OS: 75.9% vs. 82.3%; 5-year OS: 70.5% vs. 68.5%; p = 0.637). There was a statistically significant difference in DFS between the RATS and VATS groups (3-year DFS: 92.4% vs. 81.2%; 5-year DFS: 90.3% vs. 77.6%; p < 0.001). Subgroup analysis according to the pathological stage also demonstrated a significant difference between RATS and VATS groups in DFS in stage I (3-year DFS: 94.4% vs. 88.9%; 5-year DFS: 91.8% vs. 85.2%; p = 0.037) and stage III disease (3-year DFS: 82.4% vs. 51.1%; 5-year DFS: 82.4% vs. 37.7%; p = 0.024). Moreover, in multivariable Cox regression analysis, the surgical approach was significantly associated with DFS, with an HR of 0.46 (95% CI 0.27–0.78, p = 0.004) for RATS compared to VATS. VATS lobectomy was associated with a significantly higher recurrence rate compared to RATS (21.8% vs. 6.2%; p < 0.001). LOS and LOD, as well as complication rate and in-hospital and 30-day mortality, were similar among the groups. RATS lobectomy was associated with a higher number of lymph node stations harvested compared to VATS (7 [IQR:2] vs. 5 [IQR:2]; p < 0.001). In conclusion, in our series, RATS lobectomy for lung cancer led to a significantly higher DFS and significantly lower recurrence rate compared to the VATS approach. RATS may allow more extensive nodal dissection, and this could translate into reduced recurrence.

Keywords: non-small cell lung cancer (NSCLC); minimally invasive surgery; robotic surgery; long-term survival

1. Introduction

Lung cancer is the leading cause of cancer death worldwide [1]. For early-stage disease, surgical resection is currently considered the gold standard treatment. Recently, the VIOLET trial proved that the thoracoscopic minimally invasive approach is a feasible and effective approach for the surgical treatment of early-stage cancer since it is associated with improved postoperative short-term outcomes, namely less postoperative pain, fewer complications, and shorter length of hospitalization, without affecting the long-term oncological outcomes when compared to the open approach [2].

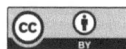

In recent years, the robotic approach has been increasingly used for lung resection surgery because of its advantageous technical features, such as a three-dimensional visualization and multi-wristed instruments that allow a more precise and efficient dissection. Numerous studies have suggested that robotic surgery might be associated with similar or even better perioperative outcomes [3–7] compared to the thoracoscopic approach, and a higher mean number of lymph node stations harvested [4,8,9]. However, there is a lack of robust long-term oncological data for the robotic approach, and hence it is still a matter of debate whether or not robotic surgery gives any advantage in patients' survival [9–11].

Therefore, the aim of our study is to compare long-term outcomes, namely overall survival (OS) and disease-free survival (DFS), and perioperative outcomes in patients who underwent video-assisted thoracic surgery (VATS) and robotic-assisted thoracic surgery (RATS) lobectomy for primary lung cancer.

2. Materials and Methods

2.1. Patient Selection

All consecutive patients from a prospective database who underwent minimally invasive lobectomy for non-small cell lung cancer (NSCLC) performed by two board-certified surgeons at Guy's Hospital (Guy's and St. Thomas' NHS Foundation Trust, London, UK) between July 2015 and December 2021 were included in this study. Patients with other concurrent or previous primary cancers, patients with Small-Cell Lung Cancer (SCLC) or with pathological stage IV metastatic disease (according to the 8th edition of the TNM classification of malignant tumors) [12], patients without complete pathological resection, and patients who underwent a procedure other than lobectomy, namely segmentectomy, wedge resection, pneumonectomy, and chest wall resection, were excluded from the study (Figure 1).

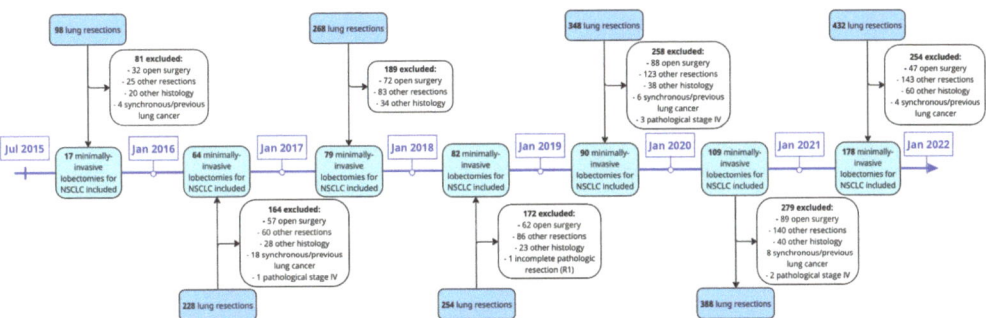

Figure 1. Flowchart of our lung resections' surgical series collected between 2015 and 2021 answering to inclusion and exclusion criteria.

Patients operated on before the adoption of the 8th edition of the TNM classification of malignant tumors were restaged according to the 8th edition [12].

Patients were characterized according to demographic variables, including age, sex, smoking history (never, former, and current smokers), clinical variables, namely performance status (<2 or ≥2), comorbidities, previous neoadjuvant therapy, forced expiratory volume in 1 s (FEV1), diffusing capacity of the lungs for carbon monoxide (DLCO), and clinical and pathological stage (I, II, III).

Patients were divided into two groups according to surgical approach: the RATS group and the VATS group.

2.2. Outcomes

The primary outcomes of this study were overall survival (OS), recurrence rate, and disease-free survival (DFS) 3 and 5 years after the surgery. A subgroup analysis comparing OS and DFS in RATS and VATS lobectomies according to the pathological stage of disease was performed. Secondary outcomes of this study were complication rate, length of hospitalization (LOS), duration of chest tubes (LOD), and number of lymph node stations harvested.

2.3. Follow-Up

Patients were followed up after surgery according to institutional guidelines. Follow-up visits were scheduled every 6 months for the first 2 years after surgery, then annually thereafter. At each follow-up visit, patients underwent a physical examination and thoracic computed tomography. Positron emission tomography integrated with computed tomography was performed if recurrence was suspected based on symptoms or other imaging findings. Patients were defined as lost to follow-up when they did not return for at least two consecutive follow-ups and the study team was unable to reach them.

Recurrence was defined as the presence of new lesions on imaging consistent with metastatic disease along with a biopsy confirmation if possible. Sites and dates of the first recurrence were recorded. OS was determined as the time from surgery until death from any cause or loss to follow-up. Patients who did not die during the observation period were censored at the date of the last available follow-up. DFS was defined as the time from surgery until recurrence or death from any cause.

2.4. Surgical Technique

All the surgical procedures were performed by two board-certified surgeons in our center. RATS lobectomies were performed using a Da Vinci Xi Surgical Robot (Intuitive Surgical, Inc., Santa Clara, CA, USA) via 4 robotic ports (two 8 mm ports and two 12 mm ports) plus an additional port for bedside assistance and specimen retrieval. CO_2 at a pressure of 6–8 cm H_2O was used to perform the robotic procedure. Regarding VATS lobectomies, we used a 3-ports anterior approach according to the Copenhagen technique, as reported by Henrik J. Hansen and René H. Petersen [13].

Lymph node dissection was performed in accordance with the NCCN guidelines for NSCLC [14].

The perioperative management was similar for all the patients. We used one single postoperative drain measuring either 24 or 28 Fr. Locoregional analgesia was administered via intercostal or paravertebral blocks.

2.5. Statistical Analysis

The characteristics of this study's population are reported using numbers and percentages or median and interquartile range (IQR). Between-group differences were evaluated using the Chi-square test for categorical variables and the Wilcoxon–Mann–Whitney test for continuous variables.

OS and DFS were estimated using the Kaplan–Meier method, with differences among groups assessed with a log-rank test and compared across groups using multivariate Cox proportional hazard models in the full cohort.

All statistical tests were two-tailed, and p values < 0.05 were considered statistically significant. All analyses were carried out using GraphPad Prism version 9.5.1 (528).

3. Results

3.1. Patients' Characteristics

A total of 619 patients were included in the study: 403 were treated with RATS lobectomy, and 216 with VATS lobectomy. The mean age of the entire population was 70 years (± 10 years), and 62.2% ($n = 385$) of the patients were women. Patient demographics, comorbidities, and tumor characteristics are listed in Table 1. The majority of patients were pathological stage I, and the predominant histologic type was adenocarcinoma in both groups. Within the RATS group, 1.5% ($n = 6$) of patients received neoadjuvant therapy, while in the

VATS group, 1.9% (n = 4) received neoadjuvant therapy. Chemotherapy was the primary neoadjuvant treatment given, followed by combined or sequential chemo-radiotherapy.

Table 1. Patient characteristics.

Patient Characteristics	Total	VATS	RATS	p
Age (±SD [1])	70 ± 10	69 ± 10	70 ± 10	0.059
Women	62.2% (n = 385)	64.4% (n = 139)	61% (n = 246)	0.435
Smoking habits				
Never	14.4% (n = 89)	11.6% (n = 25)	15.9% (n = 64)	0.152
Former	68.8% (n = 426)	69.9% (n = 151)	68.2% (n = 275)	0.716
Current	16.2% (n = 100)	18.5% (n = 40)	14.9% (n = 60)	0.253
unknown	0.6% (n = 4)	0.0% (n = 0)	1.0% (n = 4)	0.304
Performance status				0.591
<2	81.1% (n = 502)	82.4% (n = 178)	80.4% (n = 324)	
≥2	18.9% (n = 117)	17.6% (n = 38)	19.6% (n = 79)	
Comorbidities				
COPD [2]	20.7% (n = 128)	25.0% (n = 54)	18.4% (n = 74)	0.061
AF [3]	6.0% (n = 37)	5.6% (n = 12)	6.2% (n = 25)	0.860
CAD/IHD [4]	13.4% (n = 83)	14.4% (n = 31)	12.9% (n = 52)	0.622
CKD [5]	4.2% (n = 26)	3.7% (n = 8)	4.5% (n = 18)	0.834
DM [6]	11.8% (n = 73)	14.4% (n = 31)	10.4% (n = 42)	0.153
TIA/CVA [7]	2.7% (n = 17)	1.9% (n = 4)	3.2% (n = 13)	0.441
Respiratory function				
FEV1 [8] (median; IQR [9])	91% (IQR [9]: 30)	92% (IQR [9]: 30)	90% (IQR [9]: 30)	0.195
DLCO [10] (median; IQR [9])	73% (IQR [9]: 26)	71% (IQR [9]: 25)	76% (IQR [9]: 26)	0.001
Tumor location				
Right				
Upper	33.6% (n = 208)	35.2% (n = 76)	32.8% (n = 132)	0.592
Middle	11.3% (n = 70)	12.1% (n = 26)	10.9% (n = 44)	0.691
Lower	21.0% (n = 130)	19.4% (n = 42)	21.8% (n = 88)	0.535
Left				
Upper	18.3% (n = 113)	17.1% (n = 37)	18.9% (n = 76)	0.663
Lower	15.8% (n = 98)	16.2% (n = 35)	15.6% (n = 63)	0.908
Tumor size (mean; ±SD [1])	28 ± 18 mm	28 ± 16 mm	29 ± 19 mm	0.979
Tumor histology				
Adenocarcinoma	76.4% (n = 473)	74.1% (n = 160)	77.7% (n = 313)	0.322
Squamous cell carcinoma	20.0% (n = 124)	21.7% (n = 47)	19.1% (n = 77)	0.461
Large cell carcinoma	3.6% (n = 22)	4.2% (n = 9)	3.2% (n = 13)	0.649
Clinical stage				
I	78.8% (n = 488)	83.8% (n = 181)	76.2% (n = 307)	0.03
II	14.6% (n = 90)	13.0% (n = 28)	15.4% (n = 62)	0.473
III	5.8% (n = 36)	3.2% (n = 7)	7.2% (n = 29)	0.048
Unknown	0.8% (n = 5)	0.0% (n = 0)	1.2% (n = 5)	0.169
Pathological stage				
I	65.6% (n = 406)	63.9% (n = 138)	66.5% (n = 268)	0.535
II	20.5% (n = 127)	22.2% (n = 48)	19.6% (n = 79)	0.466
III	13.9% (n = 86)	13.9% (n = 30)	13.9% (n = 56)	>0.999
Final nodal status				
N1	9.5% (n = 59)	8.3% (n = 18)	10.2% (n = 41)	0.556
N2	9.4% (n = 58)	10.6% (n = 23)	8.7% (n = 35)	0.470
Neoadjuvant therapy	1.6% (n = 10)	1.9% (n = 4)	1.5% (n = 6)	0.746
Chemotherapy	1.5% (n = 9)	1.4% (n = 3)	1.5% (n = 6)	>0.999
Chemo-radiotherapy	0.2% (n = 1)	0.5% (n = 1)	0.0% (n = 0)	0.349

[1] Standard deviation; [2] chronic obstructive pulmonary disease; [3] atrial fibrillation; [4] coronary artery disease/ischemic heart disease; [5] chronic kidney disease; [6] diabetes mellitus; [7] transient ischemic attack/cerebral vascular accident; [8] forced expiratory volume in the 1st second; [9] interquartile range; [10] diffusing capacity of the lungs for carbon monoxide.

The average preoperative pulmonary function (DLCO percentage) was better in the RATS group than in the VATS group (76.2% vs. 71%; $p = 0.001$). For 70 patients in the RATS cohort, the respiratory function was not retrievable.

Excluding the aforementioned differences, patients' characteristics were similar in terms of comorbidities, respiratory function, tumor location, tumor size, histologic characteristics, pathological stage, and neoadjuvant therapy.

3.2. Overall Survival

The mean follow-up period was 37 months in the whole series (29 months and 52 months for the RATS group and VATS group, respectively). Complete follow-up was achieved for all patients in the cohort, with no patients lost to follow-up. At the end of the follow-up, 481 (77.7%) patients were still alive. Out of the 138 deaths, 67 in the VATS cohort and 71 in the RATS cohort, 30 deaths were lung cancer related (14 in the RATS group and 16 in the VATS group), 11 were related to another type of cancer (6 in the RATS group and 5 in the VATS group), 81 were non-cancer related (41 in the RATS group and 40 in the VATS group), while for a total of 16 patients, the cause of death was non-retrievable (10 in the RATS group and 6 in the VATS group).

There was no statistically significant difference between RATS and VATS groups in overall survival (3-year OS: 75.9% vs. 82.3%; 5-year OS: 70.5% vs. 68.5%, respectively; $p = 0.637$). Subgroup analysis according to the pathological stage also did not show significant differences in OS between the RATS and VATS approaches (Table 2, Figure 2). These results were confirmed by the multivariate analysis, in which the surgical approach (RATS vs. VATS) was not independently associated with OS, with a hazard ratio of 1.23 (95% CI: 0.83–1.81; $p = 0.293$) for RATS compared to VATS, suggesting no significant difference in OS between RATS and VATS after adjusting for confounders. Higher pathological stage (stage II and III), as well as worse pulmonary function (DLCO), older age, and male sex, were strong predictors of worse OS, as shown in Table 3A.

Table 2. Long-term survivals at 3 and 5 years following VATS and RATS lobectomy for NSCLC.

Survival	VATS	RATS	p
Overall Survival			0.637
3 years	82.3%	75.9%	
5 years	68.5%	70.5%	
OS [1] stage I			0.436
3 years	86.8%	86.3%	
5 years	75.7%	83.4%	
OS [1] stage II			0.070
3 years	77.0%	58.2%	
5 years	68.7%	51.7%	
OS [1] stage III			0.412
3 years	70.0%	48.5%	
5 years	33.7%	24.3%	
Disease-free Survival			<0.001
3 years	81.2%	92.4%	
5 years	77.6%	90.3%	
DFS [2] stage I			0.037
3 years	88.9%	94.4%	
5 years	85.2%	91.8%	
DFS [2] stage II			0.105
3 years	77.7%	92.6%	
5 years	73.4%	92.6%	

Table 2. Cont.

Survival	VATS	RATS	p
DFS [2] stage III			0.024
3 years	51.1%	82.4%	
5 years	37.7%	82.4%	

[1] Overall survival; [2] disease-free survival.

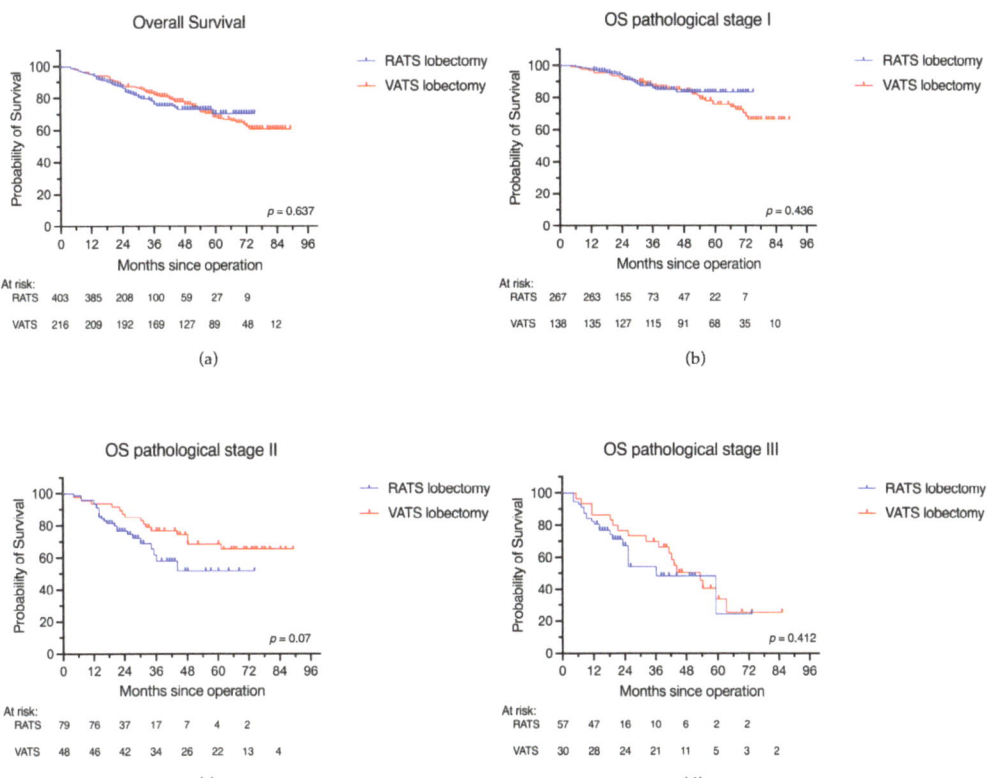

Figure 2. Overall survival after robotic and videothoracoscopic lobectomy for NSCLC. (a) Overall survival in the complete cohort; (b) overall survival for stage I disease after RATS and VATS lobectomy; (c) overall survival for stage II disease after RATS and VATS lobectomy; (d) overall survival for stage III disease after RATS and VATS lobectomy.

Table 3. (A). Multivariate analysis of prognostic factors for death. (B). Multivariate analysis of prognostic factors for recurrence or death.

(A)				
	Variable	HR [1]	95% CI [2]	p
Approach				
	VATS	Reference	-	-
	RATS	1.23	0.83–1.81	0.293
Sex				
	Female	Reference	-	-
	Male	1.62	1.09–2.37	0.015
	Age (continuous)	1.05	1.03–1.08	<0.001

Table 3. *Cont.*

(A)			
Variable	**HR** [1]	**95% CI** [2]	***p***
Pathology			
Adenocarcinoma	Reference	-	-
Squamous cell carcinoma	1.01	0.64–1.55	0.963
Large cell carcinoma	1.26	0.52–2.57	0.570
Pathological stage			
I	Reference	-	-
II	1.8	1.13–2.82	0.011
III	4.54	2.93–6.97	<0.001
Induction therapy			
no	Reference	-	-
yes	2.29	0.56–6.21	0.165
Comorbidities			
Pulmonary [3]	0.99	0.64–1.50	0.960
Cardiovascular [4]	1.12	0.76–1.66	0.572
Diabetes	1.11	0.69–1.72	0.663
Renal failure	0.36	0.11–0.89	0.051
Respiratory function			
FEV1 [5] (continuous)	0.99	0.99–1.00	0.168
DLCO [6] (continuous)	0.98	0.97–0.99	0.015
(B)			
Variable	**HR** [1]	**95% CI** [2]	***p***
Approach			
VATS	Reference	-	-
RATS	0.46	0.27–0.78	0.004
Sex			
Female	Reference	-	-
Male	2.02	1.20–3.37	0.008
Age (continuous)	0.99	0.96–1.01	0.205
Pathology			
Adenocarcinoma	Reference	-	-
Squamous cell carcinoma	0.48	0.22–0.96	0.052
Large cell carcinoma	0.99	0.24–2.72	0.989
Pathological stage			
I	Reference	-	-
II	2.27	1.12–4.45	0.02
III	6.44	2.82–14.12	<0.001
Induction therapy			
no	Reference	-	-
yes	1.44	0.23–4.92	0.625
Nodal upstaging			
no	Reference	-	-
yes	1.23	0.60–2.56	0.582

[1] Hazard ratio; [2] 95% confidence interval; [3] pulmonary complications: chronic obstructive pulmonary disease, asthma, interstitial lung disease, pulmonary embolism, obstructive sleep apnea syndrome, pulmonary hypertension; [4] cardiovascular complications: hypertension, ischemic heart disease, atrial fibrillation, previous cardiac surgery; peripheral vascular disease; deep venous thrombosis; cerebral vascular disease; [5] forced expiratory volume in the 1st second; [6] diffusing capacity of the lungs for carbon monoxide.

3.3. Disease-Free Survival

There was a statistically significant difference in DFS between RATS and VATS groups, favoring the robotic patients (3-year DFS: 92.4% vs. 81.2%; 5-year DFS: 90.3% vs. 77.6%, respectively; $p < 0.001$). The subgroup analysis according to the pathological stage also demonstrated a significant difference between RATS and VATS in DFS in stage I (3-year DFS: 94.4% vs. 88.9%; 5-year DFS: 91.8% vs. 85.2%, respectively; $p = 0.037$) and stage III disease (3-year DFS: 82.4% vs. 51.1%; 5-year DFS: 82.4% vs. 37.7%, respectively; $p = 0.024$). Patients in the RATS group with pathological stage II disease showed a trend of better DFS compared to those in the VATS group, but the difference was not statistically significant (3-year DFS: 92.6% vs. 77.7%; 5-year DFS: 92.6% vs. 73.4%, $p = 0.105$) (Table 2, Figure 3). In multivariable Cox regression analysis, the surgical approach (RATS vs. VATS) was significantly associated with disease-free survival, with a hazard ratio of 0.46 (95% CI 0.27–0.78; $p = 0.004$) for RATS compared to VATS. This indicates that RATS was associated with significantly better DFS compared to VATS after adjusting for other factors. Higher pathological stage (stage II and III) and male sex were significantly associated with worse DFS, as illustrated in Table 3B.

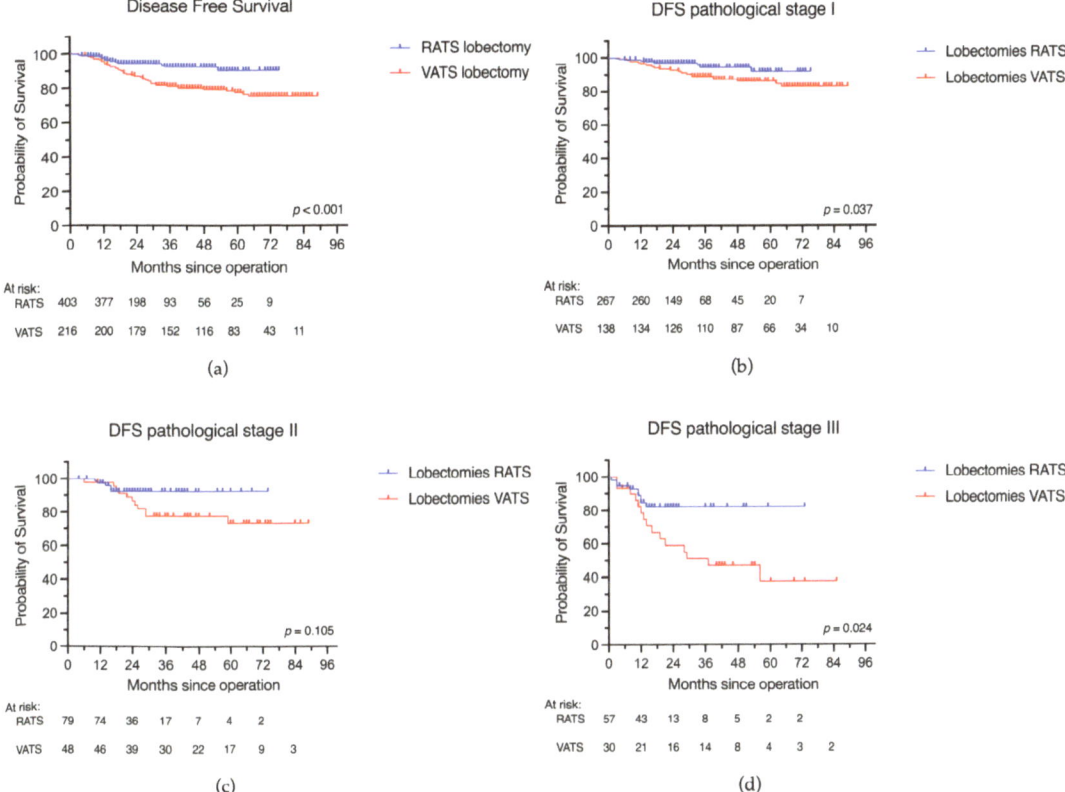

Figure 3. Disease-free survival after robotic and videothoracoscopic lobectomy for NSCLC. (**a**) Disease-free survival in the complete cohort; (**b**) disease-free survival for stage I disease after RATS and VATS lobectomy; (**c**) disease-free survival for stage II disease after RATS and VATS lobectomy; (**d**) disease-free survival for stage III disease after RATS and VATS lobectomy.

3.4. Recurrence Rate

A total of 72 patients (11.6%) had a recurrence, 25 (6.2%) in the RATS group and 47 (21.8%) in the VATS group, with a statistically significant difference between the groups ($p < 0.001$) (Table 4). Moreover, subgroup analysis according to pathological stage showed that patients who underwent a VATS lobectomy had a significantly higher recurrence rate in each staging group compared to RATS, as illustrated in Table 4. VATS was also associated with a significantly higher number of both local (7.4% vs. 1.2%; $p < 0.001$) and distant recurrences (11.6% vs. 4.5%; $p = 0.001$) compared to RATS.

Table 4. Recurrence rate following VATS and RATS lobectomy.

	VATS	RATS	p
Recurrence rate			
Overall	21.8% ($n = 47$)	6.2% ($n = 25$)	<0.001
Stage I	12.3% ($n = 17$)	4.1% ($n = 11$)	<0.001
Stage II	27.1% ($n = 13$)	6.3% ($n = 5$)	<0.001
Stage III	56.7% ($n = 17$)	15.8% ($n = 9$)	<0.001
Recurrence site			
local	7.4% ($n = 16$)	1.2% ($n = 5$)	<0.001
distant	11.6% ($n = 25$)	4.5% ($n = 18$)	0.001
both	2.8% ($n = 6$)	0.5% ($n = 2$)	0.024
Stage I			
local	3.6% ($n = 5$)	0.7% ($n = 2$)	0.048
distant	6.5% ($n = 9$)	3.0% ($n = 8$)	0.117
both	2.2% ($n = 3$)	0.4% ($n = 1$)	0.117
Stage II			
local	6.3% ($n = 3$)	0.0% ($n = 0$)	0.052
distant	16.7% ($n = 8$)	6.3% ($n = 5$)	0.075
both	4.2% ($n = 2$)	0.0% ($n = 0$)	0.141
Stage III			
local	26.7% ($n = 8$)	5.3% ($n = 3$)	0.007
distant	26.7% ($n = 8$)	8.8% ($n = 5$)	0.054
both	3.3% ($n = 1$)	1.8% ($n = 1$)	>0.999

The distant recurrences in the RATS and VATS groups occurred mainly in the brain ($n = 17$), bones ($n = 16$), contralateral lung ($n = 8$), liver ($n = 1$), adrenal gland ($n = 2$), and in the skin ($n = 1$).

3.5. Surgery-Related Outcomes

Postoperative length of stay (LOS) and length of chest drain (LOD), as well as complication rate and in-hospital, 30-day, and 90-day mortality, were similar among the RATS and VATS groups (Table 5). There were no intraoperative deaths. In the RATS cohort, one patient died in hospital (0.25%) of acute respiratory distress syndrome (ARDS).

Table 5. Surgery-related outcomes.

	VATS	RATS	p
LOS [1] (median; IQR [3])	5 days (IQR [3]: 5)	5 days (IQR [3]: 5)	0.453
LOD [2] (median; IQR [3])	2 days (IQR [3]: 3)	2 days (IQR [3]: 3)	0.818
Complication rate	38.4% ($n = 83$)	34.0% ($n = 137$)	0.291
In-hospital mortality	0.0% ($n = 0$)	0.25% ($n = 1$) *	>0.999
30-day mortality	0.0% ($n = 0$)	0.25% ($n = 1$) *	>0.999
90-day mortality	0.0% ($n = 0$)	0.25% ($n = 1$) *	>0.999
Nodal stations harvested (median; IQR)			
Overall	5 (IQR [3]: 2)	7 (IQR [3]: 2)	<0.001
Mediastinal (N2)	3 (IQR [3]: 1)	4 (IQR [3]: 1)	<0.001
Hilar or intrapulmonary (N1)	2 (IQR [3]: 1)	3 (IQR [3]: 1)	<0.001
Upstaging rate	27.8% ($n = 60$)	18.6% ($n = 75$)	0.001
Nodal upstaging	16.7% ($n = 36$)	13.2% ($n = 53$)	0.233
T–upstaging	26.4% ($n = 57$)	22.6% ($n = 91$)	0.322

[1] Length of hospital stay; [2] length of chest drain; [3] interquartile range. * Patient died of hospital-acquired pneumonia and ARDS.

Compared to the thoracoscopic approach, the robotic approach was associated with a higher median number of lymph node stations harvested overall (5 [IQR:2] vs. 7 [IQR:2], respectively; $p < 0.001$), mediastinal (3 [IQR:1] vs. 4 [IQR:1]; $p < 0.001$) and hilar (2 [IQR:1] vs. 3 [IQR:1]; $p < 0.001$) (Table 5, Figure 4). However, the nodal upstaging rate did not differ between the RATS and VATS groups (13.2% vs. 16.7%; $p < 0.233$). There was a statistically significant difference in the upstaging rate between the RATS and VATS groups (18.6% vs. 27.8%; $p = 0.001$).

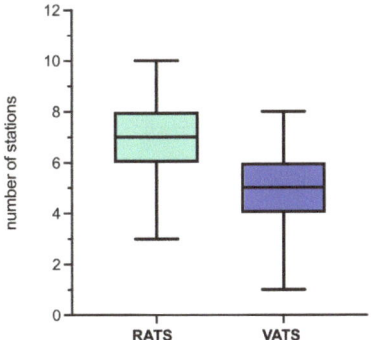

Figure 4. Difference in the median number of nodal stations harvested with the two approaches.

4. Discussion

In recent years, robotic lobectomy has been proven to be a feasible minimally invasive approach, with similar or, in some reports, even improved perioperative outcomes compared to VATS and the traditional open approach [3–7]. However, whether there is any difference in long-term outcomes between the robotic and thoracoscopic minimally invasive approaches is still a subject of debate.

In the current literature, there is a lack of robust data about survival comparison between robotic and VATS lobectomy in patients with NSCLC. A large propensity score study made by Kneuertz et al. [10] reported a similar locoregional and distant recurrence rate among VATS, RATS, and open lobectomy ($p = 0.9$), as well as equivalent 5-year overall survival among the groups (55%, 63%, and 65%, respectively; $p = 0.56$). A previous study made by Yang et al. [9] compared RATS, VATS, and open lobectomy with similar 5-year OS (77.6%, 73.5%, and 77.9%, respectively) and DFS (72.7%, 69%, and 65.5%, respectively), and no association was found between surgical approach and long-term survival in multivariate analysis. Our results partially support these findings, since we did not find any significant differences in OS between RATS and VATS lobectomy. However, in our series, RATS lobectomy was associated both with a significantly improved DFS and with a lower recurrence rate compared to VATS (6.2% vs. 21.8%, $p < 0.001$). In particular, the VATS approach was associated with a higher number of local recurrences compared to RATS (16 vs. 5; $p < 0.001$). Moreover, in the multivariate analysis, the RATS surgical approach was associated with significantly better DFS compared to VATS, after adjusting for other factors (HR: 0.46; 95% CI 0.27–0.78; $p = 0.004$), suggesting that there might be specific factors related to the RATS surgical approach that might confer an advantage in patients' survival.

In several studies, the robotic approach was associated with a higher lymph node yield compared to VATS [4,8,9]. Nelson et al. [4] have reported a significantly higher mean of N2 and N1 lymph node stations collected with RATS (3.1 ± 1 and 2.5 ± 0.9, respectively) compared with both open (2.7 ± 0.9 and 1.8 ± 0.7, respectively) and VATS (2.4 ± 0.9 and 1.8 ± 0.6, respectively) ($p < 0.001$). Our findings are in line with the aforementioned results, with a median number of mediastinal and hilar lymph node stations harvested with the robotic approach of 4 [IQR:1] and 3 [IQR:1], respectively, compared with a median N2 and N1 stations collected with VATS of 3 [IQR:1] and 2 [IQR:1], respectively ($p < 0.001$). The hypothesis behind these results is that the robotic approach, due to its advantageous features, such as 3D vision, stable camera platform, and improved instrument articulation, could allow a more thorough and meticulous lymphadenectomy. The European Association of Thoracic Surgeons (ESTS) guidelines recommend a systematic nodal dissection in all cases in order to ensure a complete resection and a correct postoperative staging of the disease [15]. The International Association for the Study of Lung Cancer (IASLC)'s definition of systematic nodal dissection is the excision of ≥ 6 lymph nodes and ≥ 3 nodal stations, including the subcarinal station [16]. In several studies, a higher lymph node yield was associated with better long-term survival [17,18]; Wu et al. [19] conducted a randomized trial to investigate whether systematic nodal dissection was superior to mediastinal lymph nodal sampling in the treatment of NSCLC. They found that systematic lymphadenectomy was associated with a significantly improved 5-year survival. An adequate lymphadenectomy is essential in lung cancer surgery to obtain an accurate staging so as to identify patients who need adjuvant therapies [20]. However, in our series, the difference in the extensiveness of the robotic nodal dissection did not translate into a difference between the two approaches in nodal upstaging. The lack of difference in nodal upstaging between our series' cohorts raises questions about whether the more extensive RATS lymphadenectomy fully explains the DFS results we obtained. One of the potential reasons for which the higher lymph node yield with RATS may contribute to better DFS, even without differences in nodal upstaging, is that the technical aspects of robotic surgery could allow for more meticulous dissection, with the removal of additional nodes not as easily reachable by VATS. This may potentially lead to the removal of micrometastatic disease, not necessarily detected in standard pathology, that could later progress to recurrence if not resected. Numerous studies have demonstrated the association between the presence of these lymph node micrometastases, detected by ancillary histopathological and molecular techniques, and a poorer OS and DFS compared to patients without nodal micrometastases, as evidenced in a systematic review and meta-analysis by Hüyük, M et al. [21]. Another meta-analysis showed that nodal micrometastases were detected in 25.3% of 2026 NSCLC cases without nodal disease in histologic examination, and that the presence of nodal micrometastases was significantly correlated with a higher recurrence rate and worse survival [22]. Considering the aforementioned evidence, the association we found in our study between RATS and both a longer DFS and a lower recurrence rate, especially of local recurrences, might be explained by a more thorough lymphadenectomy. It must be said that, in our series, there may have been underlying group differences or selection biases that favored the RATS group independently from the nodal dissection extent.

Some studies have shown that RATS is associated with less morbidity and mortality than VATS [6,7], whereas others have shown similar results among the two approaches [3–5]. In our series, we observed that VATS and RATS approaches were comparable in terms of LOS, LOD, complication rate, as well as in-hospital, 30-day, and 90-day mortality. These results might show that RATS is at least as feasible and safe as the video-assisted approach to perform a lobectomy.

Strengths and Limitations of the Study

One of the main strengths of this study is the large cohort of 619 patients who underwent minimally invasive lung cancer surgery. The median follow-up time was 37 months, allowing for a robust assessment of long-term oncological outcomes, including overall survival and disease-free survival. Importantly, complete follow-up was achieved for all patients in the cohort, with no patients lost to follow-up. These complete follow-up data enhance the reliability and validity of the survival and recurrence results observed in our study sample.

The limitations of this study must also be considered. First, there might be a selection bias among the groups due to the retrospective assignment of the patients to surgical arms, and due to its single-center nature. Secondly, the lack of randomization in this study means that the two groups could differ both on measured and unmeasured factors. Finally, the length of surveillance may not be consistent among the groups. In fact, the median follow-up overall was 37 months, but the median follow-up of the patients who underwent a VATS lobectomy was almost twice as long as the one for those who had undergone a RATS lobectomy (52 months vs. 29 months, respectively). This is due to the fact that in our center, the robotic approach has been adopted since 2017, while the videothoracoscopic approach has been used since long before that. For this reason, we believe that a longer follow-up period is necessary to update the survival results in the future. Moreover, since the robotic approach was more recently adopted in our center, the RATS cohort encompasses the surgeons' learning curve experience, whereas the VATS cohort does not, given the surgeons' substantial prior experience of over 5 years with VATS at the study's inception.

Despite the fact that our results are in line with similar studies published in scientific literature, large multicentric and possibly randomized trials are warranted to consolidate this evidence.

5. Conclusions

In our study, robotic lobectomy for NSCLC was associated with significantly improved disease-free survival and lower recurrence rate compared to VATS, while there was no significant difference in OS between surgical approaches. RATS was associated with a higher lymph node yield compared to VATS, but there was no difference among the approaches in nodal upstaging; hence, the robotic approach may allow more extensive nodal dissection, and this could translate into a reduced recurrence rate.

RATS and VATS showed comparable postoperative complications, hospital stay, and duration of chest drain. Our results support the continued adoption of the robotic techniques, but further studies are warranted to confirm these results and if RATS provides a durable DFS benefit over RATS.

Author Contributions: Conceptualization, A.B., F.F. and G.F.; methodology, G.F.; software, G.F.; validation, A.B., F.F. and S.L.; formal analysis, G.F.; investigation, A.M., G.F. and E.F.; resources, A.B. and T.R.; data curation, A.M. and G.F.; writing—original draft preparation, G.F.; writing—review and editing, F.F. and S.L.; visualization, G.F., F.F. and S.L.; supervision, A.B.; project administration, A.B. All authors have read and agreed to the published version of the manuscript.

Funding: This research received no external funding.

Institutional Review Board Statement: The study conformed to the ethical principles defined in the Declaration of Helsinki of 1964 and all subsequent revisions, and it was approved by the relevant committee of our institution (Guy's and St. Thomas NHS Foundation Trust) as a service evaluation project.

Informed Consent Statement: Informed consent was obtained from all subjects involved in the study.

Data Availability Statement: The data presented in this study are available on request from the corresponding author. The data are not publicly available.

Conflicts of Interest: The authors declare no conflict of interest.

References

1. Siegel, R.L.; Miller, K.D.; Fuchs, H.E.; Jemal, A. Cancer statistics, 2022. *CA Cancer J. Clin.* **2022**, *72*, 7–33. [CrossRef]
2. Lim, E.; Batchelor, T.J.P.; Dunning, J.; Shackcloth, M.; Anikin, V.; Naidu, B.; Belcher, E.; Loubani, M.; Zamvar, V.; Harris, R.A.; et al. Video-Assisted Thoracoscopic or Open Lobectomy in Early-Stage Lung Cancer. *NEJM Evid.* **2022**, *1*. [CrossRef]
3. Louie, B.E.; Wilson, J.L.; Kim, S.; Cerfolio, R.J.; Park, B.J.; Farivar, A.S.; Vallières, E.; Aye, R.W.; Burfeind, W.R., Jr.; Block, M.I. Comparison of Video-Assisted Thoracoscopic Surgery and Robotic Approaches for Clinical Stage I and Stage II Non-Small Cell Lung Cancer Using The Society of Thoracic Surgeons Database. *Ann. Thorac. Surg.* **2016**, *102*, 917–924. [CrossRef]
4. Nelson, D.B.; Mehran, R.J.; Mitchell, K.G.; Rajaram, R.; Correa, A.M.; Bassett, R.L., Jr.; Antonoff, M.B.; Hofstetter, W.L.; Roth, J.A.; Sepesi, B.; et al. Robotic-Assisted Lobectomy for Non-Small Cell Lung Cancer: A Comprehensive Institutional Experience. *Ann. Thorac. Surg.* **2019**, *108*, 370–376. [CrossRef]
5. Lee, B.E.; Korst, R.J.; Kletsman, E.; Rutledge, J.R. Transitioning from video-assisted thoracic surgical lobectomy to robotics for lung cancer: Are there outcomes advantages? *J. Thorac. Cardiovasc. Surg.* **2014**, *147*, 724–729. [CrossRef]

6. Adams, R.D.; Bolton, W.D.; Stephenson, J.E.; Henry, G.; Robbins, E.T.; Sommers, E. Initial multicenter community robotic lobectomy experience: Comparisons to a national database. *Ann. Thorac. Surg.* **2014**, *97*, 1893–1898; discussion 1899–1900. [CrossRef]
7. Kent, M.; Wang, T.; Whyte, R.; Curran, T.; Flores, R.; Gangadharan, S. Open, video-assisted thoracic surgery, and robotic lobectomy: Review of a national database. *Ann. Thorac. Surg.* **2014**, *97*, 236–242; discussion 242–244. [CrossRef]
8. Novellis, P.; Maisonneuve, P.; Dieci, E.; Voulaz, E.; Bottoni, E.; Di Stefano, S.; Solinas, M.; Testori, A.; Cariboni, U.; Alloisio, M.; et al. Quality of Life, Postoperative Pain, and Lymph Node Dissection in a Robotic Approach Compared to VATS and OPEN for Early Stage Lung Cancer. *J. Clin. Med.* **2021**, *10*, 1687. [CrossRef]
9. Yang, H.X.; Woo, K.M.; Sima, C.S.; Bains, M.S.; Adusumilli, P.S.; Huang, J.; Finley, D.J.; Rizk, N.P.; Rusch, V.W.; Jones, D.R.; et al. Long-term Survival Based on the Surgical Approach to Lobectomy for Clinical Stage I Nonsmall Cell Lung Cancer: Comparison of Robotic, Video-assisted Thoracic Surgery, and Thoracotomy Lobectomy. *Ann. Surg.* **2017**, *265*, 431–437. [CrossRef]
10. Kneuertz, P.J.; D'Souza, D.M.; Richardson, M.; Abdel-Rasoul, M.; Moffatt-Bruce, S.D.; Merritt, R.E. Long-Term Oncologic Outcomes After Robotic Lobectomy for Early-stage Non-Small-cell Lung Cancer Versus Video-assisted Thoracoscopic and Open Thoracotomy Approach. *Clin. Lung Cancer* **2020**, *21*, 214–224.e2. [CrossRef]
11. Sesti, J.; Langan, R.C.; Bell, J.; Nguyen, A.; Turner, A.L.; Hilden, P.; Leshchuk, K.; Dabrowski, M.; Paul, S. A Comparative Analysis of Long-Term Survival of Robotic Versus Thoracoscopic Lobectomy. *Ann. Thorac. Surg.* **2020**, *110*, 1139–1146. [CrossRef]
12. Nicholson, A.G.; Chansky, K.; Crowley, J.; Beyruti, R.; Kubota, K.; Turrisi, A.; Eberhardt, W.E.; van Meerbeeck, J.; Rami-Porta, R.; Staging and Prognostic Factors Committee, Advisory Boards, and Participating Institutions. The International Association for the Study of Lung Cancer Lung Cancer Staging Project: Proposals for the Revision of the Clinical and Pathologic Staging of Small Cell Lung Cancer in the Forthcoming Eighth Edition of the TNM Classification for Lung Cancer. *J. Thorac. Oncol.* **2016**, *11*, 300–311. [CrossRef] [PubMed]
13. Hansen, H.J.; Petersen, R.H. Video-assisted thoracoscopic lobectomy using a standardized three-port anterior approach—The Copenhagen experience. *Ann. Cardiothorac. Surg.* **2012**, *1*, 70–76. [CrossRef] [PubMed]
14. Ettinger, D.S.; Wood, D.E.; Aisner, D.L.; Akerley, W.; Bauman, J.; Chirieac, L.R.; D'Amico, T.A.; DeCamp, M.M.; Dilling, T.J.; Dobelbower, M.; et al. Non-Small Cell Lung Cancer, Version 5.2017, NCCN Clinical Practice Guidelines in Oncology. *J. Natl. Compr. Canc. Netw.* **2017**, *15*, 504–535. [CrossRef] [PubMed]
15. Lardinois, D.; De Leyn, P.; Van Schil, P.; Porta, R.R.; Waller, D.; Passlick, B.; Zielinski, M.; Lerut, T.; Weder, W. ESTS guidelines for intraoperative lymph node staging in non-small cell lung cancer. *Eur. J. Cardiothorac. Surg.* **2006**, *30*, 787–792. [CrossRef]
16. Asamura, H.; Chansky, K.; Crowley, J.; Goldstraw, P.; Rusch, V.W.; Vansteenkiste, J.F.; Watanabe, H.; Wu, Y.L.; Zielinski, M.; Ball, D.; et al. The International Association for the Study of Lung Cancer Lung Cancer Staging Project: Proposals for the Revision of the N Descriptors in the Forthcoming 8th Edition of the TNM Classification for Lung Cancer. *J. Thorac. Oncol.* **2015**, *10*, 1675–1684. [CrossRef]
17. Dong, S.; Du, J.; Li, W.; Zhang, S.; Zhong, X.; Zhang, L. Systematic mediastinal lymphadenectomy or mediastinal lymph node sampling in patients with pathological stage I NSCLC: A meta-analysis. *World J. Surg.* **2015**, *39*, 410–416. [CrossRef]
18. Wu, Y.C.; Lin, C.F.; Hsu, W.H.; Huang, B.S.; Huang, M.H.; Wang, L.S. Long-term results of pathological stage I non-small cell lung cancer: Validation of using the number of totally removed lymph nodes as a staging control. *Eur. J. Cardiothorac. Surg.* **2003**, *24*, 994–1001. [CrossRef]
19. Wu, Y.L.; Huang, Z.F.; Wang, S.Y.; Yang, X.N.; Ou, W. A randomized trial of systematic nodal dissection in resectable non-small cell lung cancer. *Lung Cancer* **2002**, *36*, 1–6. [CrossRef]
20. D'Andrilli, A.; Venuta, F.; Rendina, E.A. The role of lymphadenectomy in lung cancer surgery. *Thorac. Surg. Clin.* **2012**, *22*, 227–237. [CrossRef]
21. Hüyük, M.; Fiocco, M.; Postmus, P.E.; Cohen, D.; von der Thüsen, J.H. Systematic review and meta-analysis of the prognostic impact of lymph node micrometastasis and isolated tumour cells in patients with stage I–IIIA non-small cell lung cancer. *Histopathology* **2023**, *82*, 650–663. [CrossRef] [PubMed]
22. Jeong, J.H.; Kim, N.Y.; Pyo, J.S. Prognostic roles of lymph node micrometastasis in non-small cell lung cancer. *Pathol. Res. Pract.* **2018**, *214*, 240–244. [CrossRef] [PubMed]

Disclaimer/Publisher's Note: The statements, opinions and data contained in all publications are solely those of the individual author(s) and contributor(s) and not of MDPI and/or the editor(s). MDPI and/or the editor(s) disclaim responsibility for any injury to people or property resulting from any ideas, methods, instructions or products referred to in the content.

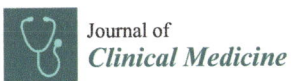

Article

Enhancing Immune Response in Non-Small-Cell Lung Cancer Patients: Impact of the 13-Valent Pneumococcal Conjugate Vaccine

Jolanta Smok-Kalwat [1], Paulina Mertowska [2,*], Izabela Korona-Głowniak [3], Sebastian Mertowski [2], Paulina Niedźwiedzka-Rystwej [4], Dominika Bębnowska [4], Krzysztof Gosik [2], Andrzej Stepulak [5], Stanisław Góźdź [1,6], Jacek Roliński [7], Zofia Górecka [8], Jan Siwiec [9] and Ewelina Grywalska [2]

1. Department of Clinical Oncology, Holy Cross Cancer Centre, 3 Artwinskiego Street, 25-734 Kielce, Poland; jolantasm@onkol.kielce.pl (J.S.-K.); stanislawgo@onkol.kielce.pl (S.G.)
2. Department of Experimental Immunology, Medical University of Lublin, 4a Chodzki Street, 20-093 Lublin, Poland; sebastian.mertowski@umlub.pl (S.M.); krzysztof.gosik@umlub.pl (K.G.); ewelina.grywalska@umlub.pl (E.G.)
3. Department of Pharmaceutical Microbiology, Medical University of Lublin, 1 Chodzki Street, 20-093 Lublin, Poland; iza.glowniak@umlub.pl
4. Institute of Biology, University of Szczecin, Felczaka 3c, 71-412 Szczecin, Poland; paulina.niedzwiedzka-rystwej@usz.edu.pl (P.N.-R.); dominika.bebnowska@usz.edu.pl (D.B.)
5. Department of Biochemistry and Molecular Biology, Medical University of Lublin, 1 Chodzki Street, 20-093 Lublin, Poland; andrzej.stepulak@umlub.pl
6. Institute of Medical Science, Collegium Medicum, Jan Kochanowski University of Kielce, IX Wieków Kielc 19A, 25-317 Kielce, Poland
7. Department of Clinical Immunology, Medical University of Lublin, 4a Chodzki Street, 20-093 Lublin, Poland; jacek.rolinski@umlub.pl
8. Department of Plastic and Reconstructive Surgery and Microsurgery, Medical University of Lublin, 8 Jaczewskiego Street, 20-090 Lublin, Poland; zfgrecka@gmail.com
9. Department of Pneumonology, Oncology and Allergology, Medical University of Lublin, 8 Jaczewskiego Street, 20-090 Lublin, Poland; jan.siwiec@umlub.pl
* Correspondence: paulina.mertowska@umlub.pl

Abstract: Background: Non-small-cell lung cancer (NSCLC) is one of the most frequently diagnosed diseases among all types of lung cancer. Infectious diseases contribute to morbidity and mortality by delaying appropriate anti-cancer therapy in patients with NSCLC. **Methods:** The study aimed to evaluate the effectiveness of vaccination with the 13-valent pneumococcal conjugate vaccine (PCV13) in 288 newly diagnosed NSCLC patients. The analysis of the post-vaccination response was performed after vaccination by assessing the frequency of plasmablasts via flow cytometry and by assessing the concentration of specific anti-pneumococcal antibodies using enzyme-linked immunosorbent assays. **Results:** The results of the study showed that NSCLC patients responded to the vaccine with an increase in the frequencies of plasmablasts and antibodies but to a lesser extent than healthy controls. The immune system response to PCV13 vaccination was better in patients with lower-stage NSCLC. We found higher antibody levels after vaccination in NSCLC patients who survived 5 years of follow-up. **Conclusions:** We hope that our research will contribute to increasing patients' and physicians' awareness of the importance of including PCV13 vaccinations in the standard of oncological care, which will extend the survival time of patients and improve their quality of life.

Keywords: non-small-cell lung cancer; immune system; 13-valent pneumococcal conjugate vaccine; *Streptococcus pneumoniae*; vaccination

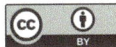

1. Introduction

Non-small-cell lung cancer (NSCLC) is one of the most commonly diagnosed entities of lung cancer [1,2]. Numerous interdisciplinary studies are currently investigating factors contributing to the development and progression of this particular form of cancer, including the influence of environmental factors, genetics, and, significantly, the immune system's involvement in its pathogenesis [3–5]. The involvement of microorganisms in pathogenesis, particularly changes in the lung microbiome, and the development of infections were widely reported [6–11]. Infections may be one of the most common causes of lung cancer progression, associated with decreased patient response to treatment, poorer prognosis, and increased mortality [10,11]. One of the newer research areas observed in recent years is the discussion of the role and involvement of *Streptococcus pneumoniae* (not only in the progression of lung cancer but also in its participation in the process of carcinogenesis itself) [12–15]. This is related to the increased susceptibility to infections caused by these Gram-positive bacteria, which can cause invasive and non-invasive pneumococcal disease, observed among cancer patients. Infection caused by *S. pneumoniae* may promote the pathomechanism of the carcinogenesis process by increasing the proliferation and migration of neoplastic cells in the course of NSCLC, and their increased number observed in studies correlates with the development of cancer [12–14]. The increased incidence of pneumococcal infections among NSCLC patients is an extremely difficult therapeutic challenge and significantly affects the survival rates of cancer patients [16–18]. Database analysis showed that out of 105,060 articles on NSCLC, only 691 deal with the occurrence of pneumonia, and only 3 highlight the importance of vaccination. To protect oncology patients, especially those with NSCLC, from the harmful effects of *S. pneumoniae* infections, it is essential to use preventive vaccinations. Previous studies performed with the 23-valent pneumococcal polysaccharide vaccine (PPSV23) demonstrated that the immunogenicity of pneumococcal vaccines in cancer patients could induce adequate immune responses in patients undergoing chemotherapy [19,20]. Moreover, a recent study reported that the 13-valent pneumococcal conjugate vaccine (PCV13) is safe and immunogenic in children who completed cancer treatment [21]. However, data on PCV13 use in adult cancer patients are still scarce.

This study aimed to assess the post-vaccination response of patients diagnosed with NSCLC after administration of the PCV13 vaccine concerning their survival rate and cancer stage. Our understanding of vaccine response will be crucial in introducing a successful, customized approach to infection prevention, referring to leading complications in these patients and potentially decreasing associated morbidity and mortality.

2. Materials and Methods

2.1. Characteristics of the Patients with NSCLC Included in the Study and the Control Group

The study included 288 patients from the Świętokrzyskie province (Poland) diagnosed with NSCLC at various stages of cancer (Figure 1). Patients were admitted for treatment to the Holycross Cancer Center in Kielce (Poland) in the years 2014–2015. The mean age of the patients in the study group was 52.36 ± 9.12 (Table 1). This study focused on patients diagnosed with NSCLC who had not previously received any treatment for the disease, including chemotherapy and immunotherapy. Blood samples were taken from these patients to analyze NSCLC grade and stage. Certain exclusion criteria were established to ensure accurate results, including prior vaccination against *S. pneumoniae*, medication affecting the immune system, recent infection, blood transfusion history, autoimmune disease, cancer, allergies, and pregnancy or lactation within the past year. The patients had not been diagnosed with other diseases or were taking any medications that could affect the results of the study before and 30 days after vaccination. Anti-cancer treatment was initiated in all patients 30 days after the vaccination, just after the blood was collected for the tests that are the subject of this study. The implemented treatment depended on the cancer stage and included standard methods: surgery, radiotherapy, chemotherapy, molecularly targeted drugs, immunotherapy, and combined methods. There were no differences in post-vaccination response or infection rates depending on the applied anti-cancer therapy. All study participants and a control group of healthy individuals matched in age. None of the study participants had COVID-19 or received any preventive vaccinations other than PCV13 during follow-up. After giving consent, 52.43% of patients were vaccinated against pneumococci. The control group consisted of 69 people, age-matched to the study group (53.47 ± 10.14), who voluntarily underwent pneumococcal vaccination. The control group's health was verified through regular diagnostic evaluations conducted during visits to a general practitioner. Among the control group, 49.27% of the patients recruited for the study received a protective vaccine against pneumococcus.

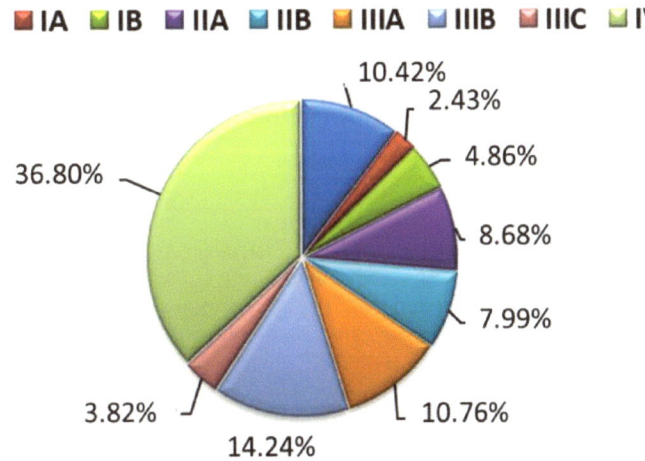

Figure 1. Tumor staging of NSCLC patients at admission based on the TNM scale.

Table 1. Characteristics of patients from the control and study groups.

	Research Group (*n* = 288)	**Control Group (*n* = 69)**
Age	Mean ± SD 52.36 ± 9.12 Median (Range) 54.24 (45.00–84.00)	Mean ± SD 53.47 ± 10.14 Median (Range) 55.12 (43.00–79.00)
Sex	156 (54.16%) men 132 (45.8%) women	36 (52.17%) men 33 (47.8%) women
Other vaccinations	18.99% of people were vaccinated against influenza (53 people)	20% of patients were additionally vaccinated against influenza
Smoking	7.88% of patients were non-smokers 92.11% of patients smoked cigarettes	9% of patients were non-smokers 91% of patients smoked cigarettes
Surgical procedure	12.19% of patients underwent surgery 87.81% of patients did not undergo surgery	100% of patients did not undergo surgery

2.2. Research Material

For each patient in the control and study groups, we collected peripheral blood (PB) from the basilic vein at three different times: before vaccination, 7 days after vaccination, and 30 days after. The collected blood was used to perform the following tests: (1) measure the level of specific anti-pneumococcal antibodies in the serum before and 30 days after vaccination (3 mL of PB was collected into coagulation factor tubes); (2) determine the percentage of plasmablasts, identified as CD19+/IgD2/CD27++, at three specific time intervals (5 mL of PB collected in tubes with EDTA anticoagulant); and (3) concentration of IgG in serum and IgG1, IgG2, IgG3, and IgG4 at three time points (5 mL of PB collected in tubes with coagulation activator). In addition, a blood count was performed each time with an additional biochemical determination of C-reactive protein (CRP). Samples of serum were kept at −80 °C until analysis of the level of specific anti-pneumococcal antibodies. We assessed the percentage of plasmablasts in fresh PB samples from both NSCLC patients and healthy volunteers. Additionally, the level of IgG and its subclasses was measured in fresh serum samples. We conducted further examinations of patients in the study group at 1, 2, 3, 4, and 5 years after vaccination or diagnosis of NSCLC to monitor changes in post-vaccination response over time.

2.3. Vaccine

Patients diagnosed with NSCLC and a control group received a 13-valent subunit conjugate vaccine (PCV13) called Prevenar13, made by Pfizer. The vaccine contains polysaccharide antigens from various pneumococcal serotypes, including 1, 3, 4, 5, 6A, 6B, 7F, 9V, 14, 18C, 19A, 19F, and 23F. The vaccine was given to all patients once through an intramuscular injection according to the manufacturer's instructions. None of the patients in either group had received a pneumococcal vaccine before.

2.4. Plasmablasts Evaluation

To prepare for testing, the blood samples were mixed with a solution of phosphate-buffered saline that contained no calcium or magnesium. This mixture was then layered onto a substance called Gradisol L (Aqua Medica, Poznań, Poland) and spun in a centrifuge for 20 min. The resulting cells (PBMC) were collected and washed twice with the same calcium and magnesium-free solution. After that, the cells were counted, and their vitality was checked using trypan blue (0.4% Trypan Blue Solution, Sigma Aldrich, Darmstadt, Germany). To test the response to the 13-valent pneumococcal conjugate vaccine in patients, PBMCs were separated using density gradient centrifugation and labeled with monoclonal antibodies according to the manufacturer's instructions. Each sample was incubated with 20 μL of antibodies at room temperature for 20 min before being washed twice with PBS and analyzed using the FACSCalibur flow cytometer. We used the FACS Diva Software 6.1.3 system in the data acquisition process and the CellQuest Pro software for data analysis, both from Becton Dickinson. To exclude erythrocytes, platelets, dead cells, and cell fragments from analysis, 30,000 events were collected in the lymphocyte gate in a forward-scatter (FSC)/side-scatter (SSC) dot plot for each sample. Labeled cells were recorded based on the created lymphocyte gate, and the results were presented as a percentage of CD45+ cells stained with the antibody. To conduct our study, we utilized a variety of monoclonal antibodies that were conjugated with appropriate fluorochromes. These included FITC-mouse anti-human IgM, FITC-mouse anti-human IgD, PE-mouse anti-human CD19, PE-mouse anti-human CD38, PE-Cy5-mouse anti-human CD19, and APC-mouse anti-human CD27 (all from Becton Dickinson, Holdrege, NE, USA). To ensure accuracy, we also utilized mouse isotype controls, including FITC Mouse IgG1k, Isotype Control, Clone MOPC-21, FITC Mouse IgG2a k, Isotype Control, Clone G155-178, PE Mouse IgG1 k, Isotype Control, Clone MOPC-21, and APC Mouse IgG1k, Isotype Control, respectively. We evaluated the proportion of plasmablasts in the peripheral blood on the day of vaccination and 7 and 30 days following vaccination.

2.5. Serum Pneumococcal Antibody Assessment

Before and after vaccination, all subjects underwent a serum pneumococcal antibody assessment. This involved measuring the amount of anti-capsular-polysaccharides antibody specific for 23 different pneumococcal serotypes (1, 2, 3, 4, 5, 6B, 7F, 8, 9N, 9V, 10A, 11A, 12F, 14, 15B, 17F, 18C, 19A, 19F, 20, 22F, 23F, and 33F) using a commercial ELISA test (ELIZEN Pneumococcus IgG Assay, Zentech, Liège, Belgium). To increase the test's specificity, each serum sample was pre-adsorbed with 10 mg/mL polysaccharide C (C-PS, Statens Serum Institute, København, Denmark) for 1 h at 37 °C. The manufacturer's instructions were followed during the evaluation process, and a VICTOR3 reader (Perkin Elmer, Waltham, MA, USA) was used for result interpretation.

2.6. Assessment of IgG Subclasses

The IgG subclasses (IgG1, IgG2, IgG3, and IgG4) were evaluated using a nephelometer BN2 (Dade Behring, Marburg, Germany) through nephelometric techniques. The process was carried out following the instructions provided by the manufacturer.

2.7. Statistical Analysis

Statistical information about continuous variables was presented, including the median, minimum, and maximum values, arithmetic means, and standard deviations (SD). We used methods such as the Mann–Whitney U test and Spearman rank order correlations to compare between groups. Logistic regression models were fitted to identify factors associated with NSCLC patient's survival. Separate multivariate models were constructed for three periods of time (before vaccination, 7 days, and 30 days after vaccination). The variance inflation factor (VIF) was calculated to estimate a multicollinearity of each predictor with all the other predictors. A backward elimination model including blood parameters examined in respective time periods was built, and nonsignificant variables were removed sequentially until only those significant at $p < 0.1$ remained. From these models, adjusted odds ratios (OR) and 95% confidence intervals were derived; corresponding p- values were from Wald's test. The goodness-of-fit was checked using Hosmer and Lemeshow's test. We performed all calculations using Statistica 13 (StatSoft, Tulsa, OK, USA) and considered a significance level of $p < 0.05$.

3. Results

3.1. Evaluation of Post-Vaccination Response to PCV13 in NSCLC Patients and Controls

When patients were recruited for the NSCLC and the control groups, an analysis of selected parameters of PB counts and the level of the C-reactive protein (CRP) was performed. The obtained test results are presented in Table 2. Patients from the study group had higher levels of WBC (1.58 times), MON (1.65 times), NEU (2.04 times), and PLT (1.24 times) than the patients in the control group. Additionally, patients with NSCLC had CRP values more than 12 times higher than those of healthy volunteers. Moreover, these patients also had reduced levels of RBC, hemoglobin, and hematocrit. Considering the heterogeneity of the NSCLC group, the differences in blood parameters among patients in the early stages of the disease—0 to II stage—and patients in late stages—III and IV—were established (Table 2). The tested blood parameters showed no significant differences among patients in these groups, but the WBC and neutrophil accounts were significantly higher in patients with advanced NSCLC ($p = 0.002$ and $p = 0.012$, respectively).

Table 2. Analysis of selected parameters of peripheral blood count and CRP protein level in NSCLC patients and healthy volunteers before.

Parameters	NSCLC Group (n = 288)		Control Group (n = 69)		p-Value	NSCLC Group (0–II Stages) (n = 103)		NSCLC Group (III–IV Stages) (n = 182)		p-Value
	Mean ± SD	Median (Range)	Mean ± SD	Median (Range)		Mean ± SD	Median (Range)	Mean ± SD	Median (Range)	
WBC [10^3/mm^3]	10.10 ± 3.47	9.57 (3.96–30.3)	6.40 ± 1.62	5.95 (3.99–12.63)	<0.0001	9.23 ± 2.5	9.2 (8.7–5.2)	10.63 ± 3.8	9.98 (4.0–30.3)	0.002
LYM [10^3/mm^3]	1.86 ± 0.77	1.70 (0.44–4.91)	2.06 ± 0.63	1.94 (0.97–3.76)	0.0055	1.92 ± 0.8	1.68 (0.7–4.9)	1.84 ± 0.7	1.7 (0.4–4.8)	0.71
MON [10^3/mm^3]	0.84 ± 0.34	0.76 (0.34–2.5)	0.51 ± 0.15	0.51 (0.24–1.08)	<0.0001	0.81 ± 0.3	0.73 (0.3–2.5)	0.85 ± 0.3	0.8 (0.4–2.0)	0.15
NEU [10^3/mm^3]	7.19 ± 3.24	6.57 (1.8–24.94)	3.53 ± 1.21	3.3 (1.63–8.48)	<0.0001	6.53 ± 2.5	6.2 (2.9–15.2)	7.60 ± 3.6	6.9 (1.8–24.9)	0.012
EOS [10^3/mm^3]	0.20 ± 0.19	0.15 (0.0–1.5)	0.20 ± 0.15	0.15 (0.0–0.79)	0.99	0.20 ± 0.2	0.15 (0.0–1.1)	0.2 ± 0.19	0.15 (0.0–1.5)	0.99
BAS [10^3/mm^3]	0.04 ± 0.03	0.04 (0.0–0.15)	0.04 ± 0.02	0.04 (0.0–0.11)	0.46	0.04 ± 0.03	0.03 (0.01–0.1)	0.04 ± 0.03	0.04 (0.0–0.2)	0.71
RBC [10^6/mm^3]	4.55 ± 0.50	4.58 (3.27–6.02)	4.79 ± 0.41	4.83 (3.36–5.5)	<0.0001	4.60 ± 0.5	4.63 (3.3–5.7)	4.52 ± 0.5	4.5 (3.3–6.0)	0.21
HGB [g/dL]	13.26 ± 1.64	13.4 (8.5–17.5)	14.52 ± 1.26	14.6 (11.2–16.8)	<0.0001	13.48 ± 1.5	13.4 (9.3–16.8)	13.12 ± 1.7	13.3 (8.5–17.5)	0.11
HCT [%]	40.30 ± 4.63	40.8 (22.8–56.6)	42.97 ± 3.45	43.3 (31.7–49.9)	<0.0001	40.68 ± 4.8	41.2 (22.8–56.6)	40.04 ± 4.5	40.7 (27.9–56.5)	0.23
PLT [10^3/mm^3]	304.72 ± 83.95	307.5 (47.0–529.0)	244.96 ± 58.29	248.0 (117.0–370.0)	<0.0001	300.33 ± 80.2	290.0 (124.0–496.0)	307.68 ± 86.0	312.5 (47.0–529.0)	0.28
CRP [mg/L]	26.77 ± 17.47	23.84 (0.4–89.7)	2.09 ± 2.25	1.26 (0.23–14.4)	<0.0001	25.35 ± 14.8	23.7 (0.9–79.3)	27.75 ± 18.8	24.5 (0.4–89.7)	0.60

Abbreviations: WBC—white blood cells; LYM—lymphocytes; MON—monocytes; NEU—neutrophils; EOS—eosinophils; BAS—basophils; RBC—red blood cells; HGB—hemoglobin; HCT—hematocrit; PLT—pellets; CRP—C-reactive protein.

Of the 288 patients diagnosed with NSCLC, 151 patients were voluntarily vaccinated with PCV13 (52.43%), and 34 (49.27%) were in the control group. To evaluate the response to the vaccine, we analyzed the levels of anti-pneumococcal IgG antibodies and subclasses of IgG antibodies, as well as the percentage of plasmablasts (IgD-CD19+CD27+++) before vaccination, 7 days after vaccination, and 30 days after vaccination. The test results are chronologically presented in Table 3, Figures 2 and 3.

NSCLC patients already had significantly lower levels of anti-pneumococcal antibodies at the time of recruitment compared to healthy volunteers (Figure 2). In addition, we observed that patients from the NSCLC group were also characterized by lower levels of IgG1, IgG2, and IgG3 subclasses, selective deficiency associated with susceptibility to viral and bacterial infections, and especially capsulated bacteria, which include *S. pneumoniae*. According to the data reported in the other studies, a decrease in the value of IgG2 and IgG3 is observed in patients with recurrent infections of the upper and lower respiratory tract [22,23] (Table 3). Changes in the level of anti-pneumococcal antibodies and the level of individual IgG subclasses were checked after 7 and 30 days from the moment of vaccination (Table 3). At the first time point, the antibody level increased by 25.04% for vaccinated NSCLC patients and was 18.02% higher than in the case of unvaccinated patients, for whom there was a slight fluctuation in antibody values. Despite the increase in the level of anti-pneumococcal antibodies in NSCLC patients, the recorded values were significantly lower than the post-vaccination response of healthy volunteers. There was a more than 2-fold increase in antibody levels, which was 4.71-fold higher than in vaccinated lung cancer patients (Figure 2). All observed differences between individual groups of patients were statistically significant.

At the second time point, i.e., 30 days after vaccination, the level of anti-pneumococcal antibodies in vaccinated patients from the NSCLC group was, on average, 4.92 times higher than before vaccination and 3.17 times higher than after 7 days. The observed values were more than 4-fold higher than in unvaccinated lung cancer patients (Figure 2). In the case of patients in the control group, the mean anti-pneumococcal antibody level 30 days after vaccination increased by nearly 8-fold compared to the values recorded before vaccination and 3.69-fold compared to the values after 7 days (Figure 2).

In addition, the level of individual IgG subclasses, which protect the body against bacterial infections, was also analyzed. For both groups of patients who received the vaccination, IgG2 and IgG3 values increased both on the 7th and 30th days after vaccination. In the case of NSCLC patients, the increase in mean IgG2 and IgG3 levels 30 days after vaccination was 1.59-fold and 1.65-fold, respectively. Despite the increase in their levels, the observed values were more than 1.5 times (for IgG2) and 2 times (for IgG3) lower than in the case of healthy subjects (Table 3).

The observed trends of changes in the level of antibodies in individual groups of patients were also reflected in the percentage of peripheral blood plasmablasts. The increase in CD19+ and IgD-CD19+CD27+++ plasmablasts (both CD19+ and total) was significantly higher in vaccinated patients in comparison to the non-vaccinated in both groups tested (Figure 3). Moreover, the rise in plasmablasts was higher in all analyzed cases of healthy patients than in patients diagnosed with NSCLC, which may indicate defects in the functioning of the immune system and show plasmablasts impact on the formation of a normal post-vaccination response (Figure 3). For a broader perspective, Table S1 presents the changes in selected parameters of peripheral blood and CRP levels in NSCLC patients and healthy volunteers in the process of time after vaccination.

Moreover, the point was to estimate if there was a difference in immunological response between patients with early stages of NSCLC and advanced NSCLC (III-IV stages). It turned out that patients from the first group had significantly higher levels of anti-pneumococcal IgG 7 and 30 days after vaccination (Table 4), as well as that the tested plasmablasts revealed significantly higher frequency in cases of patients in early NSCLC at least 30 days after vaccination. Additionally, Table S2 presents the changes in selected parameters of peripheral blood and CRP levels in NSCLC patients divided into two stages of disease groups after vaccination.

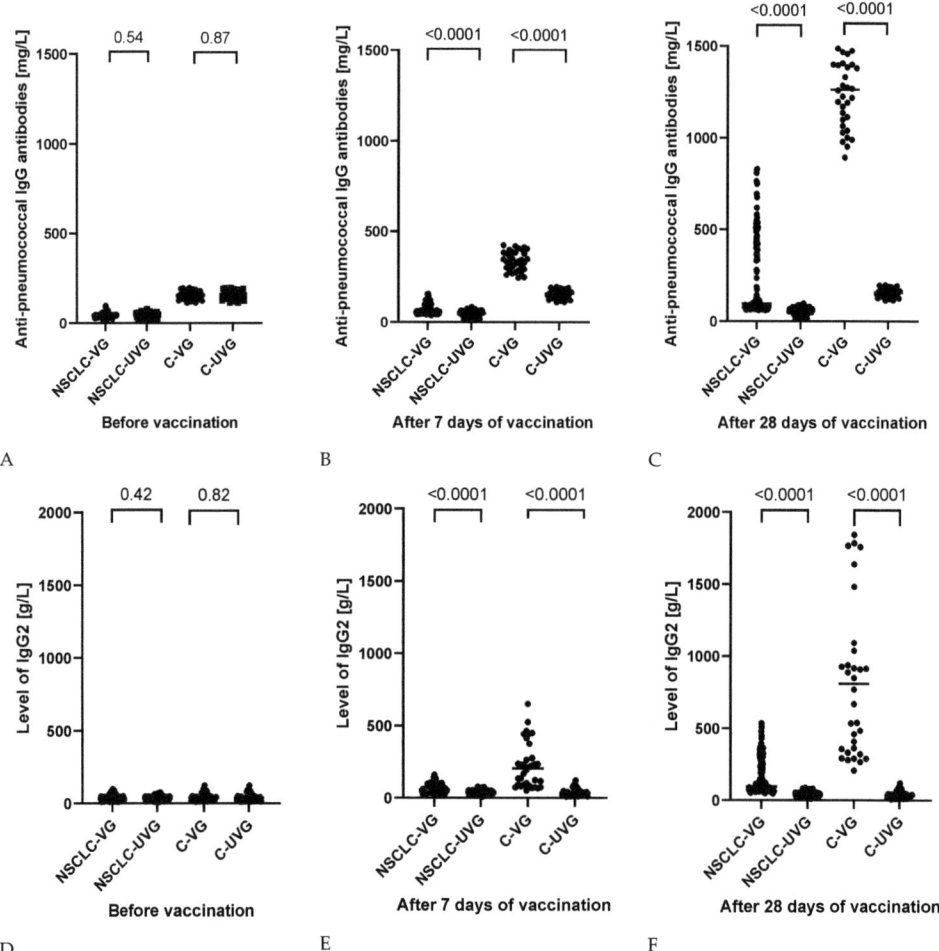

Figure 2. Changes in the level of anti-pneumococcal IgG antibodies (**A**–**C**) and the level of individual IgG2 subclass (**D**–**F**) before and after 7 and 30-day periods from the moment of vaccination (NSCLC-VG—NSCLC vaccinated group, NSCLC-UVG—NSCLC unvaccinated group, C-VG—control vaccinated group, and C-UVG—control unvaccinated group).

Table 3. Evaluation of anti-pneumococcal IgG antibodies and IgG subclasses in NSCLC patients and controls after PCV13 vaccination at three time points (before vaccination and at the 7th and 30th days after vaccination).

		NSCLC Group (n = 288)			Control Group (n = 69)		p-Value		
		Vaccinated (Group 1) (n = 151)	Unvaccinated (Group 2) (n = 137)	Vaccinated (Group 3) (n = 34)	Unvaccinated (Group 4) (n = 35)	1 vs. 2	3 vs. 4	1 vs. 3
Level of IgG1 [g/L]	Before vaccination	Mean ± SD Median (Range)	5.04 ± 1.03 4.89 (2.69–8.06)	5.21 ± 1.26 4.97 (3.02–7.12)	6.23 ± 2.06 6.22 (3.29–9.14)	6.19 ± 1.95 6.15 (3.32–8.84)	0.069	0.79	0.041
	After 7 days	Mean ± SD Median (Range)	5.16 ± 1.47 4.92 (2.79–7.99)	5.29 ± 1.55 4.83 (2.94–6.83)	7.33 ± 2.15 7.26 (5.13–10.84)	6.22 ± 1.73 6.11 (3.12–7.53)	0.071	0.032	0.0001
	After 30 days	Mean ± SD Median (Range)	5.31 ± 1.33 5.02 (3.07–7.57)	5.37 ± 1.47 4.79 (2.73–6.37)	7.68 ± 2.34 7.58 (5.73–10.9)	6.15 ± 1.68 6.21 (3.56–7.62)	0.97	0.027	0.0001
Level of IgG2 [g/L]	Before vaccination	Mean ± SD Median (Range)	1.69 ± 0.63 1.63 (0.88–2.65)	1.66 ± 0.48 1.62 (0.99–2.34)	2.04 ± 0.68 2.04 (1.08–3.01)	2.03 ± 0.64 2.02 (1.09–2.92)	0.84	0.96	0.032
	After 7 days	Mean ± SD Median (Range)	1.78 ± 0.71 1.86 (0.92–2.73)	1.62 ± 0.51 1.63 (0.83–2.06)	3.63 ± 0.56 3.59 (2.17–4.93)	2.08 ± 0.69 2.05 (1.16–2.84)	0.041	0.0001	0.0001
	After 30 days	Mean ± SD Median (Range)	2.68 ± 0.62 2.53 (1.31–4.27)	1.67 ± 0.49 1.65 (0.73–1.85)	4.27 ± 0.43 4.37 (2.84–5.64)	2.18 ± 0.54 2.10 (1.34–2.62)	0.0001	0.0001	0.0001
Level of IgG3 [g/L]	Before vaccination	Mean ± SD Median (Range)	0.21 ± 0.23 0.293 (0.121–0.464)	0.23 ± 0.11 0.29 (0.11–0.41)	0.741 ± 0.250 0.74 (0.39–1.10)	0.73 ± 0.23 0.74 (0.4–1.06)	0.81	0.83	0.0001
	After 7 days	Mean ± SD Median (Range)	0.297 ± 0.183 0.305 (0.136–0.513)	0.23 ± 0.12 0.26 (0.10–0.39)	0.78 ± 0.30 0.78 (0.41–1.16)	0.73 ± 0.22 0.73 (0.40–0.99)	0.037	0.044	0.00001
	After 30 days	Mean ± SD Median (Range)	0.35 ± 0.13 0.35 (0.263–0.615)	0.23 ± 0.16 0.23 (0.13–0.40)	0.80 ± 0.14 0.79 (0.44–1.53)	0.73 ± 0.19 0.73 (0.31–0.84)	0.01	0.037	0.0001
Level of IgG4 [g/L]	Before vaccination	Mean ± SD Median (Range)	0.337 ± 0.215 0.29 (0.21–0.53)	0.34 ± 0.2 0.27 (0.21–0.56)	0.38 ± 0.19 0.27 (0.25–0.69)	0.36 ± 0.29 0.27 (0.15–0.4)	0.77	0.36	0.087
	After 7 days	Mean ± SD Median (Range)	0.35 ± 0.2 0.28 (0.23–0.52)	0.35 ± 0.17 0.28 (0.21–0.54)	0.37 ± 0.14 0.27 (0.24–0.67)	0.36 ± 0.22 0.27 (0.15–0.41)	0.52	0.44	0.19
	After 30 days	Mean ± SD Median (Range)	0.34 ± 0.17 0.29 (0.19–0.48)	0.34 ± 0.16 0.28 (0.17–0.46)	0.37 ± 0.19 0.28 (0.20–0.49)	0.37 ± 0.18 0.27 (0.16–0.43)	0.54	0.37	0.82

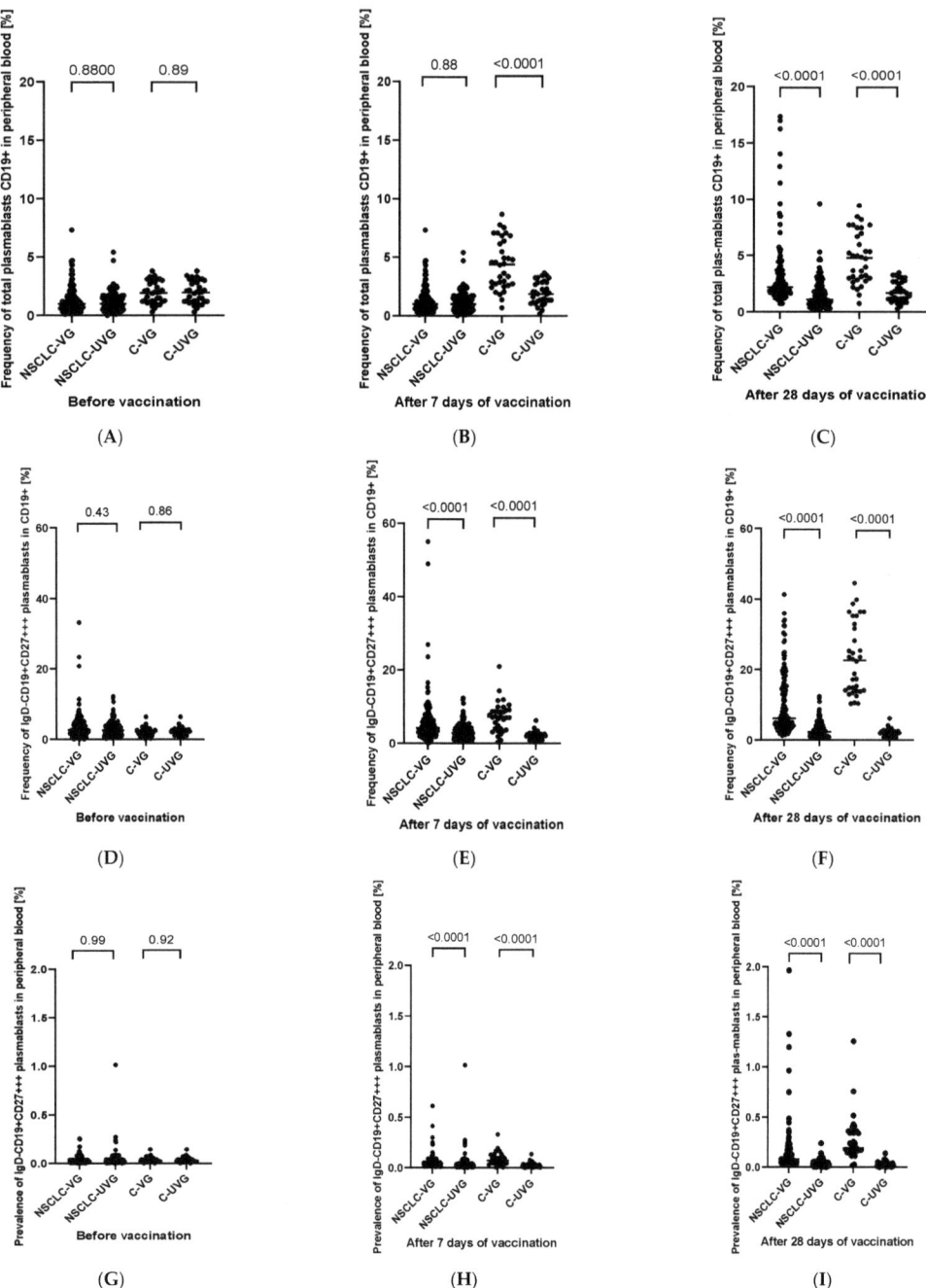

Figure 3. Frequency of total plasmablasts CD19+ in peripheral blood (**A–C**); frequency of IgD-CD19+CD27+++ plasmablasts in CD19+ (**D–F**) and prevalence of IgD-CD19+CD27+++ plasmablasts in peripheral blood (**G–I**) in vaccinated versus non-vaccinated patients in both groups tested before and after 7 and 30-days periods from the moment of vaccination. (NSCLC-VG—NSCLC vaccinated group, NSCLC-UVG—NSCLC unvaccinated group, C-VG—control vaccinated group, and C-UVG—control unvaccinated group).

Table 4. Evaluation of anti-pneumococcal response in vaccinated NSCLC patients divided regarding the stage of the disease tested before and after 7 and 30 days from the moment of vaccination.

Parameters		NSCLC Group (0–II Stages) (n = 103)		NSCLC Group (III–IV Stages) (n = 182)		p-Value				
		Vaccinated (Group 1) (n = 67)	Unvaccinated (Group 2) (n = 36)	Vaccinated (Group 3) (n = 83)	Unvaccinated (Group 4) (n = 99)	1 vs. 2	3 vs. 4	1 vs. 3	2 vs. 4	
Level of IgG [g/L]	Before vaccination	Mean ± SD	44.71 ± 11.3	46.07 ± 9.51	47.44 ± 11.8	43.25 ± 13.8	0.4	0.18	0.46	0.21
		Median (Range)	44.6 (16.7–70.0)	47.7 (28.5–59.3)	44.4 (38.1–98.6)	43.8 (12.5–79.7)				
	After 7 days	Mean ± SD	91.38 ± 31.6	51.7 ± 9.6	56.3 ± 13.1	46.7 ± 14.1	<0.0001	<0.0001	<0.0001	0.045
		Median (Range)	92.8 (37.2–156.0)	51.7 (32.4–66.6)	54.6 (42.2–110.9)	47.3 (15.0–83.8)				
	After 30 days	Mean ± SD	407.9 ± 213.6	69.44 ± 15.6	83.4 ± 16.1	51.8 ± 17.8	<0.0001	<0.0001	<0.0001	<0.0001
		Median (Range)	421.5 (60.8–829.6)	72.8 (33.1–90.7)	78.1 (61.0–142.2)	51.1 (15.3–96.0)				
Frequency of total plasmablasts CD19+ in peripheral blood	Before vaccination	Mean ± SD	1.40 ± 1.3	1.06 ± 0.6	1.21 ± 0.93	1.2 ± 0.9	0.55	0.88	0.72	0.56
		Median (Range)	1.0 (0.2–7.3)	0.95 (0.3–2.3)	1.0 (0.1–4.7)	1.0 (0.0–5.4)				
	After 7 days	Mean ± SD	3.13 ± 3.13	1.3 ± 0.74	1.80 ± 0.96	1.32 ± 1.0	<0.0001	0.0001	0.027	0.68
		Median (Range)	2.12 (0.5–17.2)	1.11 (0.4–3.1)	1.5 (0.6–5.4)	1.03 (0.0–5.6)				
	After 30 days	Mean ± SD	4.81 ± 4.9	1.77 ± 1.32	2.23 ± 0.9	1.42 ± 1.3	<0.0001	<0.0001	0.0004	0.17
		Median (Range)	2.9 (0.7–26.9)	1.15 (0.3–4.7)	1.96 (1.1–5.7)	1.10 (0.2–9.6)				
Frequency of IgD-CD19+CD27+++ plasmablasts in CD19+	Before vaccination	Mean ± SD	4.16 ± 5.4	2.9 ± 1.65	3.09 ± 1.88	3.06 ± 2.3	0.67	0.56	0.87	0.81
		Median (Range)	2.76 (0.1–33.1)	2.6 (0.4–7.0)	2.69 (0.1–8.3)	2.59 (0.3–12.1)				
	After 7 days	Mean ± SD	9.02 ± 12.6	3.24 ± 1.8	4.01 ± 1.9	3.31 ± 2.3	<0.0001	0.0034	0.0005	0.68
		Median (Range)	6.04 (0.2–78.0)	2.8 (0.5–7.4)	3.6 (0.8–9.6)	2.8 (0.5–12.4)				
	After 30 days	Mean ± SD	17.38 ± 9.1	1.80 ± 1.5	4.46 ± 1.9	3.12 ± 2.3	<0.0001	<0.0001	<0.0001	0.0002
		Median (Range)	15.5 (1.7–41.3)	1.6 (0.4–7.2)	4.07 (1.2–10.0)	2.59 (0.44–12.3)				
Prevalence of IgD-CD19+CD27+++ plasmablasts in peripheral blood	Before vaccination	Mean ± SD	0.07 ± 0.3	0.02 ± 0.02	0.04 ± 0.04	0.05 ± 0.1	0.96	0.80	0.33	0.38
		Median (Range)	0.02 (0.01–2.4)	0.03 (0.05–0.06)	0.03 (0.01–0.3)	0.03 (0.002–1.0)				
	After 7 days	Mean ± SD	0.16 ± 0.7	0.03 ± 0.02	0.05 ± 0.04	0.05 ± 0.1	<0.0001	0.0008	0.20	0.45
		Median (Range)	0.05 (0.01–5.7)	0.03 (0.01–0.07)	0.04 (0.01–0.25)	0.03 (0.02–1.0)				
	After 30 days	Mean ± SD	0.48 ± 2.2	0.03 ± 0.02	0.06 ± 0.06	0.04 ± 0.04	<0.0001	<0.0001	<0.0001	0.28
		Median (Range)	0.12 (0.03–18.2)	0.03 (0.01–0.07)	0.05 (0.01–0.26)	0.03 (0.0–0.3)				

3.2. Monitoring the Number of Respiratory Infections and Survival Stage of NSCLC Patients after Receiving PCV13 Vaccine

Due to the commencement of treatment at the Holycross Cancer Center, patients diagnosed with NSCLC included in this study were monitored for the number of upper and lower respiratory tract infections caused by *S. pneumoniae* during 5 consecutive years. Unfortunately, over time, 65.62% of patients recruited for the study did not survive the assumed 5-year period. Figure 4 shows the change in the number of patients analyzed each year. All recorded deaths concerned patients whose cancer was in stage III or IV at the time of recruitment for the study. Irrespective of the adoption of the protective anti-pneumococcal vaccination and the applied treatment, these patients could not be saved.

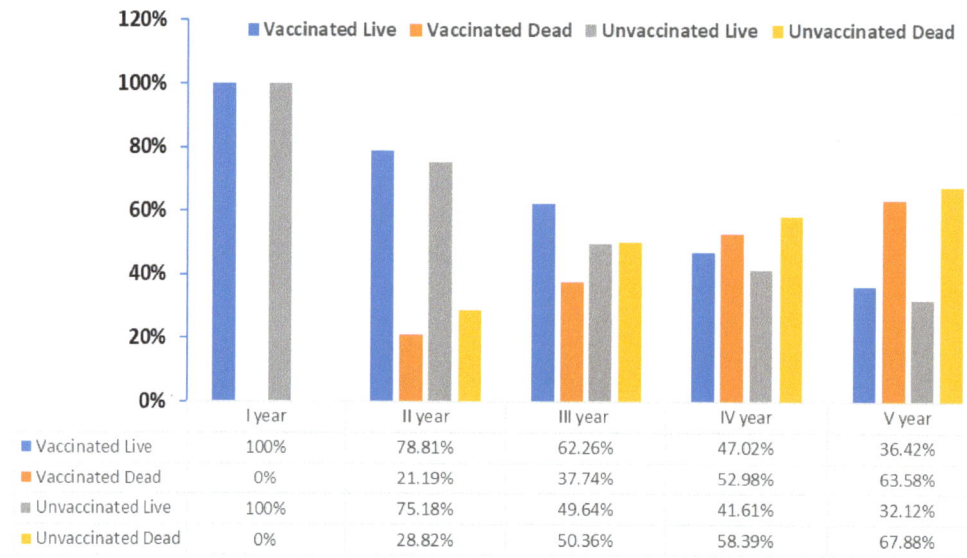

Figure 4. Changes in the number of patients diagnosed with NSCLC over the 5-year study period.

When analyzing the count of upper and lower respiratory tract infections caused by various infectious agents in patients who were vaccinated and unvaccinated with the PCV13 vaccine, we observed that among vaccinated patients with NSCLC, the number of infections per year did not exceed two throughout the study period, while in the case of unvaccinated patients, the number of infections ranged between three and six per year. Detailed analysis showed that among unvaccinated NSCLC patients, the rate of upper and lower respiratory tract infections increased over time elapsed since NSCLC diagnosis, being 23.18% after the first year, 30.85% in the second year, 45.07% in the third year, and reaching 58.18% in the fifth year.

An additional aspect of our research was to follow up on the post-vaccination response of NSCLC patients every year for 5 years. The results obtained are presented in Table 5. The breakdown of patients with NSCLC, both PCV13-vaccinated and unvaccinated, was received, together with the survival status of the patients. Live vaccinated patients had a significantly higher post-vaccination response than the vaccinated patients who did not survive, who preceded non-vaccinated patients. In the process of time, both the level of anti-pneumococcal antibodies and the percentage of peripheral blood plasmablasts gradually decreased in all groups of analyzed patients. The differences in the potency of response were observed in the level of anti-pneumococcal IgG antibodies, frequency of total plasmablasts CD19+ in peripheral blood, and the frequency of IgD-CD19+CD27+++ plasmablasts in CD19+ after 7 and 30 days after vaccination yet (Figure 5). This observation would be important as a survival prediction factor.

Table 5. Evaluation of the post-vaccination response of NSCLC patients after receiving PCV13 and unvaccinated patients by their survival during the 5 years of follow-up.

		Dead NSCLC Patients		Alive NSCLC Patients		*p*-Value					
Parameters		Vaccinated (Group 1)	Unvaccinated (Group 2)	Vaccinated (Group 3)	Unvaccinated (Group 4)	1 vs. 2	3 vs. 4	1 vs. 3	2 vs. 4
Anti-pneumococcal IgG antibodies [mg/L]									
Before vaccination	Mean ± SD	46.89 ± 11.18	43.48 ± 13.87	44.96 ± 12.43	45.12 ± 10.20	0.44	0.94	0.75	0.46
	Median (Range)	44.39 (38.05–98.55)	44.12 (12.54–79.71)	44.56 (16.69–69.97)	44.34 (26.00–64.44)				
After 1 year	Mean ± SD	81.51 ± 15.13	47.15 ± 14.29	478.16 ± 151.10	75.80 ± 10.16	<0.0001	<0.0001	<0.0001	<0.0001
	Median (Range)	76.72 (59.32–147.22)	48.29 (15.27–85.51)	453.04 (170.09–812.62)	74.38 (54.78–93.21)				
After 2 years	Mean ± SD	79.47 ± 12.63	45.12 ± 14.25	466.05 ± 147.30	71.15 ± 9.64	<0.0001	<0.0001	<0.0001	<0.0001
	Median (Range)	74.81 (56.88–143.95)	47.25 (14.29–79.69)	449.50 (161.22–794.33)	73.44 (52.49–90.09)				
After 3 years	Mean ± SD	73.82 ± 5.13	42.36 ± 11.82	415.93 ± 85.21	69.43 ± 9.27	<0.0001	<0.0001	<0.0001	0.047
	Median (Range)	70.19 (55.14–98.24)	43.29 (11.29–75.16)	420.71 (151.36–698.34)	68.89 (50.94–86.37)				
After 4 years	Mean ± SD	67.80 ± 8.59	42.87 ± 10.55	403.28 ± 71.23	68.37 ± 8.74	<0.0001	<0.0001	<0.0001	0.039
	Median (Range)	62.04 (48.96–81.45)	41.28 (12.36–69.38)	397.69 (136.98–654.71)	67.22 (51.29–85.48)				
After 5 years	Mean ± SD	54.29 ± 7.13	42.36 ± 9.77	396.58 ± 56.33	66.29 ± 7.26	0.039	<0.0001	<0.0001	0.042
	Median (Range)	52.44 (44.69–75.63)	41.79 (13.26–64.78)	387.15 (132.44–597.36)	66.47 (48.33–77.12)				
Frequency of total plasmablasts CD19+ in peripheral blood [%]									
Before vaccination	Mean ± SD	1.20 ± 0.88	1.20 ± 0.89	1.47 ± 1.42	1.11 ± 0.67	0.95	0.74	0.83	0.74
	Median (Range)	1.00 (0.10–4.70)	1.00 (0.05–5.40)	1.00 (0.020–7.30)	1.04 (0.28–2.40)				
After 1 year	Mean ± SD	2.21 ± 0.9	1.33 ± 1.28	5.42 ± 5.24	1.88 ± 1.20	<0.0001	<0.0001	<0.0001	0.036
	Median (Range)	1.95 (1.10–5.74)	0.90 (0.20–9.60)	3.69 (0.74–26.94)	1.70 (0.20–4.60)				
After 2 years	Mean ± SD	2.03 ± 0.99	1.24 ± 0.91	5.28 ± 5.11	1.75 ± 0.63	<0.0001	0.001	0.001	0.001
	Median (Range)	1.91 (1.45–3.68)	1.30 (0.39–2.20)	5.09 (1.83–9.00)	1.81 (1.29–2.22)				
After 3 years	Mean ± SD	1.89 ± 0.40	1.17 ± 0.76	4.71 ± 2.95	1.71 ± 0.61	<0.0001	<0.0001	<0.0001	0.047
	Median (Range)	1.79 (1.41–2.51)	1.19 (0.31–2.07)	4.77 (1.71–7.91)	1.69 (1.25–2.12)				
After 4 years	Mean ± SD	1.73 ± 0.68	1.18 ± 0.67	4.57 ± 2.47	1.68 ± 0.57	<0.0001	<0.0001	<0.0001	0.037
	Median (Range)	1.58 (1.25–2.08)	1.14 (0.34–1.91)	4.51 (1.55–7.42)	1.65 (1.26–2.10)				
After 5 years	Mean ± SD	1.39 ± 0.56	1.17 ± 0.63	4.49 ± 1.95	1.63 ± 0.48	<0.0001	<0.0001	<0.0001	0.034
	Median (Range)	1.34 (1.14–1.93)	1.15 (0.36–1.79)	4.39 (1.50–6.77)	1.63 (1.19–1.89)				

Table 5. *Cont.*

Parameters		Dead NSCLC Patients		Alive NSCLC Patients		*p*-Value				
		Vaccinated (Group 1)	Unvaccinated (Group 2)	Vaccinated (Group 3)	Unvaccinated (Group 4)	1 vs. 2	3 vs. 4	1 vs. 3	2 vs. 4
Frequency of IgD-CD19+CD27+++ plasmablasts in CD19+ [%]	Before vaccination	Mean ± SD	3.56 ± 3.85	3.01 ± 2.14	2.19 ± 1.24	2.25 ± 1.15	0.43	0.85	0.021	0.072
		Median (Range)	2.69 (0.10–33.07)	2.59 (0.26–12.13)	2.20 (0.11–6.39)	2.23 (0.57–6.39)				
	After 1 year	Mean ± SD	10.37 ± 7.12	3.26 ± 1.93	24.15 ± 9.19	3.77 ± 1.07	0.0001	0.0001	0.0001	0.16
		Median (Range)	7.83 (0.32–26.33)	3.34 (1.06–5.92)	24.26 (1.21–45.46)	3.71 (2.73–4.65)				
	After 2 years	Mean ± SD	6.19 ± 5.21	3.12 ± 2.20	22.70 ± 14.69	3.56 ± 1.09	0.0001	0.0001	0.0001	0.059
		Median (Range)	5.82 (4.50–11.18)	3.27 (0.98–5.52)	21.89 (7.85–37.81)	3.66 (2.61–4.49)				
	After 3 years	Mean ± SD	5.60 ± 1.63	2.93 ± 1.82	20.26 ± 8.50	3.46 ± 1.04	0.0001	0.0001	0.0001	0.073
		Median (Range)	5.33 (4.18–7.46)	2.99 (0.78–5.21)	20.49 (7.37–34.02)	3.43 (2.43–4.31)				
	After 4 years	Mean ± SD	5.14 ± 1.95	2.57 ± 1.27	19.64 ± 7.10	3.26 ± 0.98	0.0001	0.0001	0.0001	0.031
		Median (Range)	4.71 (2.72–5.18)	2.45 (0.86–4.80)	19.37 (6.67–31.89)	3.21 (2.44–4.26)				
	After 5 years	Mean ± SD	4.12 ± 2.45	2.33 ± 0.51	19.32 ± 5.62	3.30 ± 0.82	0.0001	0.0001	0.0001	0.059
		Median (Range)	3.98 (3.39–5.74)	2.27 (0.91–4.48)	18.86 (6.45–29.09)	3.31 (2.41–3.84)				

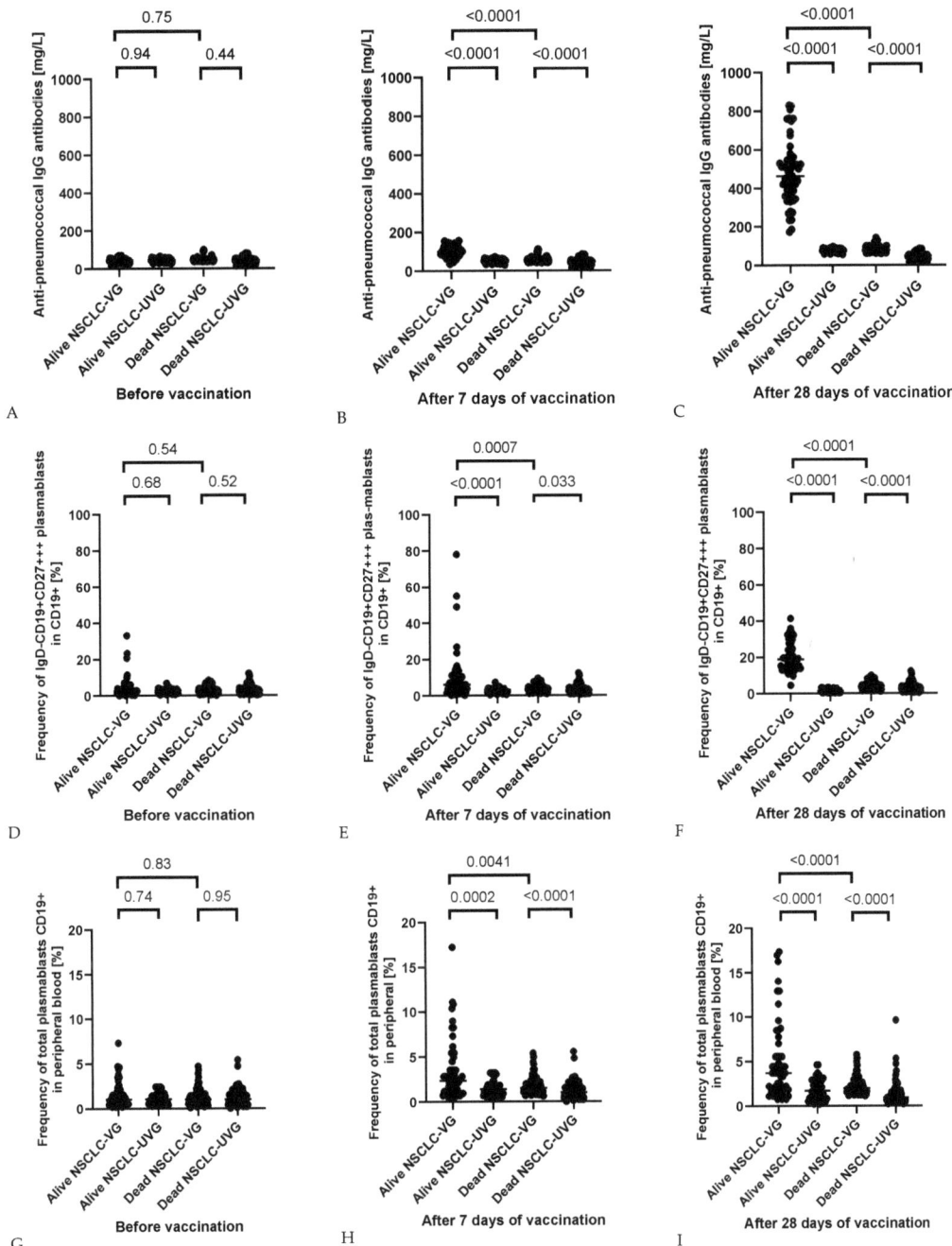

Figure 5. Evaluation of the post-vaccination response of NSCLC patients after receiving PCV13 and unvaccinated NSCLC patients by their survival before vaccination and at the 7th and 30th days after vaccination. Level of anti-pneumococcal IgG antibodies (**A–C**); frequency of IgD-CD19+CD27+++ plasmablasts in CD19+ (**D–F**) and frequency of total plasmablasts CD19+ in peripheral blood (**G–I**). (NSCLC-VG—NSCLC vaccinated group and NSCLC-UVG—NSCLC unvaccinated group).

The vast majority of patients who survived the follow-up period were vaccinated and diagnosed at stage 0 or IIA or IIB (RR 1.7, 95%CI 1.3–2.2, $p < 0.0001$), while the patients who died were predominately grade IV (both vaccinated and non-vaccinated, RR 1.1, 95%CI 0.5–2.5, $p = 0.82$). Moreover, multivariate analyses of the association between various clinical characteristics and overall survival were carried out in three periods of time, namely before and at the 7th and 30th days after vaccination. It showed that in the model built for parameters examined 7 days after vaccination, other than an improvement of selected parameters of peripheral blood in time after vaccination, lower NSCLC staging was a statistically significant factor associated with patients' survival (Table 6). In the multivariate analysis at 30 days after the vaccination period, we observed that patients with lower monocyte and lymphocyte levels but higher hemoglobin, platelet, and leukocyte levels and higher anti-pneumococcal IgG antibody levels had better survival rates.

Table 6. Multivariate analyses of the association between various clinical characteristics and overall survival stage before vaccination and at the 7th and 30th days after vaccination.

Period	Parameters	Wald Stat.	Odds Ratio (95%CI)	p-Value
Before vaccination	Intercept	6.42	19.99 (1.96–204.29)	0.012
	Lymphocyte	4.38	1.45 (1.03–2.03)	0.031
	NSCLC stage	18.17	0.96 (0.94–0.98)	<0.0001
7 days after vaccination	Intercept	16.25	0.0006 (<0.0001–0.028)	0.0001
	Platelet	10.63	1.01 (1.003–1.01)	0.0011
	NSCLC stage	8.15	0.97 (0.95–0.99)	0.0043
	ELISA IgG [mg/L]	16.63	1.04 (1.02–1.06)	<0.0001
	Lymphocyte	2.78	1.42 (0.94–2.14)	0.095
	Hemoglobin	16.61	1.46 (1.22–1.74)	<0.0001
30 days after vaccination	Intercept	42.00	<0.0001	<0.0001
	Lymphocyte	4.78	0.42 (0.20–0.92)	0.029
	ELISA IgG [mg/L]	9.12	1.02 (1.01–1.04)	0.003
	Monocytes	10.26	0.12 (0.032–0.43)	<0.0001
	Platelet	4.05	1.01 (1.00–1.013)	0.044
	Hemoglobin	28.66	2.53 (1.80–3.55)	<0.0001
	Leukocytes	14.37	1.36 (1.16–1.59)	<0.0001

Due to the recorded percentage of increased mortality in patients with lung cancer diagnosed in stages III and IV, we decided to analyze whether the post-vaccination response of NSCLC patients can correlate with the stage of cancer. The obtained results are presented in Table 5. The post-vaccination response of NSCLC patients shows a significant negative correlation between the level of anti-pneumococcal antibodies, the level of IgG2 and IgG3, as well as the percentage of peripheral blood plasmablasts, and the tumor stage (Table 7). The recorded negative correlation means that with the increase in the stage of cancer, the post-vaccination response of the examined patients decreases in each of the analyzed aspects. In addition, we performed a detailed analysis of the correlation between the level of anti-pneumococcal antibodies, the level of IgG2 and IgG3, and the percentage of peripheral blood plasmablasts in the context of patients who survived and died during the study (Table 7). Vaccinated patients diagnosed with NSCLC who survived the 5 years of the study characterized by a high positive correlation between the level of anti-pneumococcal antibodies and the level of IgG2 ($R = 0.698$) and IgG3 ($R = 0.641$), as well as the percentage of total CD19+ peripheral blood plasmablasts ($R = 0.627$) and IgD -CD19+CD27+++ in CD19+ ($R = 0.614$), which was maintained throughout the study. In the case of unvaccinated patients who survived the experiment period, a significant low positive correlation was noted between the level of anti-pneumococcal antibodies and the percentage of peripheral blood plasmablasts IgD-CD19+CD27+++ in CD19+ ($R = 0.243$), which was most likely due to the natural immune response of this group of patients. Low positive correlations were also observed in vaccinated patients who did not survive the 5-year follow-up. These relationships were statistically significant for the level of anti-pneumococcal antibodies and the level of IgG2 (R = 0.211), as well as the total percentage of peripheral blood CD19+ plasmablasts (R = 0.237). In contrast, among unvaccinated patients who died during the study period, a negative correlation was found between the level of anti-pneumococcal antibodies and the total percentage of peripheral blood plasmablasts (R = −0.309). In addition, as the concentration of anti-pneumococcal antibodies increased, the annual incidence of upper and lower respiratory tract infections decreased in vaccinated NSCLC patients, which was not observed in unvaccinated patients.

Table 7. Correlation analysis of the post-vaccination response of NSCLC patients about the tumor stage at the 7th and 30th days after vaccination.

Period	Tumor Stage vs. Parameter	Spearman R	p-Value
Before vaccination	Anti-pneumococcal IgG antibodies [mg/L]	−0.035	0.56
	Level of IgG2 [g/L]	−0.035	0.55
	Level of IgG3 [g/L]	−0.034	0.56
	Frequency of total plasmablasts CD19+ in peripheral blood [%]	−0.026	0.66
	Frequency of IgD-CD19+CD27+++ plasmablasts in CD19+ [%]	0.031	0.61
	Prevalence of IgD-CD19+CD27+++ plasmablasts in peripheral blood [%]	0.082	0.17
7 days after vaccination	Anti-pneumococcal IgG antibodies [mg/L]	−0.37	<0.0001
	Level of IgG2 [g/L]	−0.19	0.0013
	Level of IgG3 [g/L]	−0.20	0.0018
	Frequency of total plasmablasts CD19+ in peripheral blood [%]	−0.17	0.004
	Frequency of IgD-CD19+CD27+++ plasmablasts in CD19+ [%]	−0.13	0.033
	Prevalence of IgD-CD19+CD27+++ plasmablasts in peripheral blood [%]	−0.038	0.517
30 days after vaccination	Anti-pneumococcal IgG antibodies [mg/L]	−0.45	<0.0001
	Level of IgG2 [g/L]	−0.37	<0.0001
	Level of IgG3 [g/L]	−0.41	<0.0001
	Frequency of total plasmablasts CD19+ in peripheral blood [%]	−0.26	0.0001
	Frequency of IgD-CD19+CD27+++ plasmablasts in CD19+ [%]	−0.25	0.0001
	Prevalence of IgD-CD19+CD27+++ plasmablasts in peripheral blood [%]	−0.33	0.0001

4. Discussion

This study is one of the first evaluations of comprehensive immunological responses in the case of NSCLC patients after anti-pneumococcal vaccination in a 5-year follow-up period. Previous studies, such as those by Mohr et al., indicate that among patients with lung cancer, compliance with recommendations regarding pneumococcal vaccinations, as well as other vaccinations, is low [24]. Therefore, in this context, the analyses conducted by our team, focusing on the immune response, enable arguments about the benefits resulting from the use of protective vaccinations and their impact on patients with NSCLC. The PCV13 vaccine is a preparation widely distributed within many healthcare systems in Poland and around the world. According to the manufacturer's information, each vaccine dose contains pneumococcal polysaccharides of serotypes 1, 3, 4, 5, 6A, 6B, 7F, 9V, 14, 18C, 19A, 19F, and 23F, which, according to epidemiological data, corresponds to coverage of 50–76% of all cases of invasive pneumococcal disease in adults [25]. Oncological patients are a special group of patients who very often suffer from pneumonia requiring hospitalization, caused not only by *S. pneumoniae* but also by infection with *Staphylococcus aureus* or *Haemophilus influenzae* [11,26]. All these pathogens are characterized by high resistance to commonly used antibiotics and contribute not only to a significant burden on the body's wealth but also to increased mortality of patients [12,27].

Bacteraemia caused by *S. pneumoniae* in patients with lung cancer can occur in more than 60% of cases [15]. Pneumonia is one of the most common complications diagnosed among cancer patients, especially those with lung cancer. Our findings concerning high levels of monocytes in patients with high risk of NSCLC-associated mortality are similar to those described by Mao et al. [28], who found, among others, higher infiltration of monocytes in the high-risk group of lung squamous cell carcinoma. Moreover, according to Ke et al. [29], high amounts of monocytes were associated with a significantly higher risk of all-cause mortality in asthma patients. It was also proven by Georgakis et al. [30] that the higher circulating monocyte chemoattractant protein-1 (MCP-1) levels were associated with higher long-term cardiovascular mortality in community-dwelling individuals free of overt cardiovascular disease.

The conducted research showed a significant increase in the percentage of both plasmablasts and specific anti-pneumococcal antibodies in voluntarily vaccinated NSCLC patients compared to unvaccinated patients. However, the post-vaccination response of NSCLC patients was significantly lower than that of healthy volunteers who were enrolled as controls, demonstrating the immune burden of NSCLC. Due to the length of the follow-up and the high mortality rate, our study also showed that patients vaccinated with NSCLC who survived for 5 years had significantly higher post-vaccination responses than patients who died, as well as reduced rates of respiratory infections, which may indicate the protective function of the vaccination used. Chiou et al. [31] noted that for elderly lung cancer patients aged $\geq$75 years, the 23-valent polysaccharide pneumococcal vaccine (PPSV23) inoculated during an anti-cancer treatment period could reduce community-acquired pneumonia hospitalizations and improve survival.

The International Agency for Research on Cancer (IARC) states that lung cancer remains the leading cause of cancer death, with an estimated 1.8 million deaths (18%) in 2020 [32]. In the case of our NSCLC patients, a total of 65.6% died during the 5-year follow-up. Even though there were significant differences in patients' immune responses about survival states, such differences were not significant about vaccination reception (p = 0.46, RR 1.1, 95%CI 0.87–1.37).

Data from the lung cancer report [33] published in 2021, presented by Polish experts, show that by 2040, the ratio of morbidity to mortality in lung cancer patients will reverse, which is associated with the implementation of effective treatment, including molecularly targeted treatment and personalized immunotherapy within the first line of treatment. However, even the best and most advanced therapies will have no chance of success if there are recurrent and severe *S. pneumoniae* infections among cancer patients. Both global and national public health institutions recommend the use of the PCV13 vaccine for specific groups of patients (age > 65 years and suffering from chronic heart and lung diseases, diabetes, alcoholism, nephrotic syndrome, congenital or acquired immunodeficiency, asplenia or post-splenectomy or Hodgkin's lymphoma), which was proven important based on results presented in this publication, to include oncological patients in said recommendations, especially those diagnosed with lung cancer. Considering that anti-cancer treatment (based on chemo- and/or radiotherapy) significantly affects the functioning of the patient's immune system, and the aggravating state of its dysfunction contributes to the increased incidence of oncological patients for life-threatening infections, both local (lung infections bronchitis) and generalized (bacteremia). As a consequence of difficult diagnostics or multi-resistance to antibiotics, such infections may, in many cases, lead to premature death of patients [34–36].

Potential synergistic effects of PCV vaccination in combination with other immunotherapies or treatments used in NSCLC should also be investigated. The case report by Huang et al. [37] reported that radiotherapy in combination with PCV could specifically stimulate immune response and remodel the tumor–immune microenvironment in tyrosine kinase inhibitor-resistant NSCLC, which may provide a new perspective for future immunotherapy in this challenging clinical situation. Combinations may enhance the overall immune response and lead to better clinical outcomes. It also seems important to develop and validate biomarkers to predict the response of NSCLC patients to PCV vaccination. Immune system monitoring can help to identify patients most likely to benefit from vaccination and guide treatment decisions. However, Mauro et al. [37] reported that patients with chronic lymphocytic leukemia previously treated with chemoimmunotherapy did not respond to pneumococcal vaccination. Moreover, age $\geq$ 60 years, IgG levels < 400 mg/L, prior treatment, and signs of disease progression were associated with a lower response rate in these patients [38].

Evaluation of the cost-effectiveness of PCV vaccination in patients with lung cancer should also be considered. Considering the economic impact of vaccination is critical to understanding its benefits and justifying its inclusion in routine clinical practice. Promoting awareness among healthcare professionals and patients of the importance of PCV vaccination in NSCLC turns out crucial. Increasing knowledge and understanding could lead to higher vaccination rates in this vulnerable population.

This may require long-term observational studies or randomized controlled trials comparing outcomes in vaccinated and unvaccinated NSCLC patients. The results by Mustafa et al. [39] showed that vaccination with PCV13 of patients with multiple myeloma produces a similar immunologic response as compared to normal controls, but the duration of response to vaccination may wane at 180 days compared to the control group. In this study, the response of NSCLC patients with fatal outcomes was statistically lower from the very beginning (7 days after vaccination).

Despite the above conclusions from our study, there are some limitations, such as the fact that due to the diversity of NSCLC and the different therapies used in patients, the correlation between survival and vaccine uptake may be limited to some extent. However, when designing our study, we tried to match patients by gender, age, vaccination status, and smoking status to mitigate these confounding factors as much as possible. Another issue related to the above limitation is heterogeneity in terms of disease stage—this variability is significant because different stages of NSCLC may respond differently to both vaccination and disease progression. Therefore, we performed a statistical analysis comparing the response between early-stage (0–II) and advanced-stage (III–IV) NSCLC groups to address this issue. However, it is important to remember that heterogeneity within these groups may still influence the observed correlation between survival and vaccine uptake. Therefore, further research in this direction is necessary.

These limitations highlight the complexity of interpreting the impact of pneumococcal vaccination on the survival of patients with NSCLC, given the variability in disease progression, response to treatment, and immune system interactions. Despite these challenges, we believe that our findings provide valuable information about the potential benefits of pneumococcal vaccination in patients with NSCLC, warranting further research.

5. Conclusions

In this study, we analyzed the comprehensive immunological response in the case of NSCLC patients after anti-pneumococcal vaccination in a 5-year follow-up period. It seemed that the PCV13 vaccination did not increase the overall survival rate in NSCLC patients in this period, and we observed a lack of vaccine response in patients with fatal outcomes, which was definitively correlated with the advanced stage of disease at the time of recruitment. This finding will be elaborated upon much more deeply by our team. The recognized factors associated with survival state were higher anti-pneumococcal IgG concentration and less progressive disease. We hope that the presented long-term research will increase patients' and physicians' awareness of the importance of including pneumococcal vaccinations in the standard oncological treatment, which will extend the survival time of lung cancer patients. However, we are aware that NSCLC patients may, therefore, remain at risk of pneumococcal infection despite vaccination, and it remains to be alert about additional strategies to prevent infectious complications in this high-risk population. First, there seems to be a need for more detailed studies to determine whether PCV vaccination positively affects NSCLC progression and treatment response.

Supplementary Materials: The following supporting information can be downloaded at https://www.mdpi.com/article/10.3390/jcm13051520/s1, Table S1 Analysis of selected parameters of peripheral blood and CRP levels in NSCLC patients and healthy volunteers 7 and 30 days after receiving the PCV13 vaccine in relation to unvaccinated patients and Table S2 Analysis of selected parameters of peripheral blood and CRP levels in NSCLC patients divided regarding stage of the disease in 7 and 30 days after receiving the PCV13 vaccine in relation to unvaccinated patients.

Author Contributions: Conceptualization, J.S.-K., P.M., E.G. and I.K.-G.; methodology, J.S.-K., P.M., E.G., S.M., K.G., J.S., Z.G., P.N-R., D.B. and I.K.-G.; software, S.M., A.S., K.G., J.S., Z.G., S.G. and I.K.-G.; validation, J.S.-K., P.M., I.K.-G., S.M., E.G., A.S., S.G., P.N.-R. and J.R.; formal analysis, J.S.-K., P.M., J.R. and I.K.-G.; investigation, J.S.-K., P.M., I.K.-G., S.M., E.G., A.S., S.G. and J.R.; resources, J.S.-K., P.M., I.K.-G., S.M., E.G., A.S., S.G. and J.R.; data curation, J.S.-K., P.M., I.K.-G., S.M., E.G., K.G., J.S., Z.G., A.S., S.G., P.N.-R., D.B. and J.R.; writing—original draft preparation, J.S.-K., P.M., I.K.-G., S.M., E.G., P.N-R. and D.B.; writing—review and editing, A.S., S.G. and J.R.; visualization, J.S.-K., P.M., I.K.-G., S.M., E.G., A.S., S.G., P.N.-R., D.B. and J.R.; supervision, S.G., A.S. and J.R.; project administration, J.S.-K., P.M., I.K.-G., S.M., E.G., A.S., S.G., P.N.-R. and J.R.; funding acquisition, S.G. and E.G. All authors have read and agreed to the published version of the manuscript.

Funding: This research was supported by the Medical University of Lublin grant no. DS640.

Institutional Review Board Statement: The study was conducted by the Declaration of Helsinki and approved by the Bioethics Committee of the Regional Chamber of Physicians in Kielce (No. KB7/2012 approved on 18 December 2012). The study protocol also received the necessary approval from the Bioethics Committee at the Medical University of Lublin under reference number KE-0254/283/2015 (approved on 15 January 2015).

Informed Consent Statement: Informed consent was obtained from all subjects involved in the study.

Data Availability Statement: The data presented in this study are available upon request from the first author.

Conflicts of Interest: The authors declare no conflicts of interest.

References

1. Lung Cancer Statistics | How Common Is Lung Cancer? | American Cancer Society. Available online: https://www.cancer.org/cancer/types/lung-cancer/about/key-statistics.html (accessed on 10 September 2023).
2. Ganti, A.K.; Klein, A.B.; Cotarla, I.; Seal, B.; Chou, E. Update of Incidence, Prevalence, Survival, and Initial Treatment in Patients with Non-Small Cell Lung Cancer in the US. *JAMA Oncol.* **2021**, *7*, 1824–1832. [CrossRef] [PubMed]
3. Zhu, T.; Bao, X.; Chen, M.; Lin, R.; Zhuyan, J.; Zhen, T.; Xing, K.; Zhou, W.; Zhu, S. Mechanisms and Future of Non-Small Cell Lung Cancer Metastasis. *Front. Oncol.* **2020**, *10*, 585284. [CrossRef]
4. Cooper, W.A.; Lam, D.C.L.; O'Toole, S.A.; Minna, J.D. Molecular Biology of Lung Cancer. *J. Thorac. Dis.* **2013**, *5* (Suppl. 5), S479–S490. [CrossRef] [PubMed]
5. Wu, J.; Lin, Z. Non-Small Cell Lung Cancer Targeted Therapy: Drugs and Mechanisms of Drug Resistance. *Int. J. Mol. Sci.* **2022**, *23*, 15056. [CrossRef]
6. Zhao, Y.; Liu, Y.; Li, S.; Peng, Z.; Liu, X.; Chen, J.; Zheng, X. Role of Lung and Gut Microbiota on Lung Cancer Pathogenesis. *J. Cancer Res. Clin. Oncol.* **2021**, *147*, 2177–2186. [CrossRef]
7. McLean, A.E.B.; Kao, S.C.; Barnes, D.J.; Wong, K.K.H.; Scolyer, R.A.; Cooper, W.A.; Kohonen-Corish, M.R.J. The Emerging Role of the Lung Microbiome and Its Importance in Non-Small Cell Lung Cancer Diagnosis and Treatment. *Lung Cancer* **2022**, *165*, 124–132. [CrossRef] [PubMed]
8. Ramírez-Labrada, A.G.; Isla, D.; Artal, A.; Arias, M.; Rezusta, A.; Pardo, J.; Gálvez, E.M. The Influence of Lung Microbiota on Lung Carcinogenesis, Immunity, and Immunotherapy. *Trends Cancer* **2020**, *6*, 86–97. [CrossRef]
9. Peters, B.A.; Pass, H.I.; Burk, R.D.; Xue, X.; Goparaju, C.; Sollecito, C.C.; Grassi, E.; Segal, L.N.; Tsay, J.-C.J.; Hayes, R.B.; et al. The Lung Microbiome, Peripheral Gene Expression, and Recurrence-Free Survival after Resection of Stage II Non-Small Cell Lung Cancer. *Genome Med.* **2022**, *14*, 121. [CrossRef]
10. Belluomini, L.; Caldart, A.; Avancini, A.; Dodi, A.; Trestini, I.; Kadrija, D.; Sposito, M.; Tregnago, D.; Casali, M.; Riva, S.T.; et al. Infections and Immunotherapy in Lung Cancer: A Bad Relationship? *Int. J. Mol. Sci.* **2020**, *22*, 42. [CrossRef]
11. Budisan, L.; Zanoaga, O.; Braicu, C.; Pirlog, R.; Covaliu, B.; Esanu, V.; Korban, S.S.; Berindan-Neagoe, I. Links between Infections, Lung Cancer, and the Immune System. *Int. J. Mol. Sci.* **2021**, *22*, 9394. [CrossRef]
12. Patel, A.J.; Nightingale, P.; Naidu, B.; Drayson, M.T.; Middleton, G.W.; Richter, A. Characterising the Impact of Pneumonia on Outcome in Non-Small Cell Lung Cancer: Identifying Preventative Strategies. *J. Thorac. Dis.* **2020**, *12*, 2236–2246. [CrossRef]
13. Song, X.; Liu, B.; Zhao, G.; Pu, X.; Liu, B.; Ding, M.; Xue, Y. Streptococcus Pneumoniae Promotes Migration and Invasion of A549 Cells in Vitro by Activating mTORC2/AKT through up-Regulation of DDIT4 Expression. *Front. Microbiol.* **2022**, *13*, 1046226. [CrossRef] [PubMed]
14. Li, N.; Zhou, H.; Holden, V.K.; Deepak, J.; Dhilipkannah, P.; Todd, N.W.; Stass, S.A.; Jiang, F. Streptococcus Pneumoniae Promotes Lung Cancer Development and Progression. *iScience* **2023**, *26*, 105923. [CrossRef]

15. Zhou, S.; Zhao, Q. Colonization of Streptococcus Pneumoniae in Pneumonia Patients with Lung Cancer. *Jundishapur. J. Microbiol.* **2018**, *11*, e57300. [CrossRef]
16. Streptococcus Pneumoniae: Information for Clinicians | CDC. Available online: https://www.cdc.gov/pneumococcal/clinicians/streptococcus-pneumoniae.html (accessed on 10 September 2023).
17. Mousavi, S.F.; Nobari, S.; Rahmati Ghezelgeh, F.; Lyriai, H.; Jalali, P.; Shahcheraghi, F.; Oskoui, M. Serotyping of Streptococcus Pneumoniae Isolated from Tehran by Multiplex PCR: Are Serotypes of Clinical and Carrier Isolates Identical? *Iran. J. Microbiol.* **2013**, *5*, 220–226.
18. Cleary, D.W.; Jones, J.; Gladstone, R.A.; Osman, K.L.; Devine, V.T.; Jefferies, J.M.; Bentley, S.D.; Faust, S.N.; Clarke, S.C. Changes in Serotype Prevalence of Streptococcus Pneumoniae in Southampton, UK between 2006 and 2018. *Sci. Rep.* **2022**, *12*, 13332. [CrossRef]
19. Shildt, R.A.; Boyd, J.F.; McCracken, J.D.; Schiffman, G.; Giolma, J.P. Antibody response to pneumococcal vaccine in patients with solid tumors and lymphomas. *Med. Pediatr. Oncol.* **1983**, *11*, 305–309. [CrossRef] [PubMed]
20. Nordøy, T.; Aaberge, I.S.; Husebekk, A.; Samdal, H.H.; Steinert, S.; Melby, H.; Kolstad, A. Cancer patients undergoing chemotherapy show adequate serological response to vaccinations against influenza virus and Streptococcus pneumoniae. *Med. Oncol.* **2002**, *19*, 71–78. [CrossRef]
21. HHung, T.Y.; Kotecha, R.S.; Blyth, C.C.; Steed, S.K.; Thornton, R.B.; Ryan, A.L.; Cole, C.H.; Richmond, P.C. Immunogenicity and safety of single-dose, 13-valent pneumococcal conjugate vaccine in pediatric and adolescent oncology patients. *Cancer* **2017**, *123*, 4215–4223. [CrossRef]
22. Abrahamian, F.; Agrawal, S.; Gupta, S. Immunological and Clinical Profile of Adult Patients with Selective Immunoglobulin Subclass Deficiency: Response to Intravenous Immunoglobulin Therapy. *Clin. Exp. Immunol.* **2010**, *159*, 344–350. [CrossRef]
23. de la Torre, M.C.; Torán, P.; Serra-Prat, M.; Palomera, E.; Güell, E.; Vendrell, E.; Yébenes, J.C.; Torres, A.; Almirall, J. Serum Levels of Immunoglobulins and Severity of Community-Acquired Pneumonia. *BMJ Open Respir. Res.* **2016**, *3*, e000152. [CrossRef] [PubMed]
24. Mohr, A.; Kloos, M.; Schulz, C.; Pfeifer, M.; Salzberger, B.; Bauernfeind, S.; Hitzenbichler, F.; Plentz, A.; Loew, T.; Koch, M. Low Adherence to Pneumococcal Vaccination in Lung Cancer Patients in a Tertiary Care University Hospital in Southern Germany. *Vaccines* **2022**, *10*, 311. [CrossRef] [PubMed]
25. Prevenar 13 | European Medicines Agency. Available online: https://www.ema.europa.eu/en/medicines/human/EPAR/prevenar-13 (accessed on 2 March 2024).
26. Wong, J.L.; Evans, S.E. Bacterial Pneumonia in Patients with Cancer: Novel Risk Factors and Management. *Clin. Chest Med.* **2017**, *38*, 263–277. [CrossRef] [PubMed]
27. Valvani, A.; Martin, A.; Devarajan, A.; Chandy, D. Postobstructive Pneumonia in Lung Cancer. *Ann. Transl. Med.* **2019**, *7*, 357. [CrossRef] [PubMed]
28. Mao, G.; Yang, D.; Liu, B.; Zhang, Y.; Ma, S.; Dai, S.; Wang, G.; Tang, W.; Lu, H.; Cai, S.; et al. Deciphering a Cell Death-Associated Signature for Predicting Prognosis and Response to Immunotherapy in Lung Squamous Cell Carcinoma. *Respir. Res.* **2023**, *24*, 176. [CrossRef] [PubMed]
29. Ke, J.; Qiu, F.; Fan, W.; Wei, S. Associations of Complete Blood Cell Count-Derived Inflammatory Biomarkers with Asthma and Mortality in Adults: A Population-Based Study. *Front. Immunol.* **2023**, *14*, 1205687. [CrossRef]
30. Georgakis, M.K.; de Lemos, J.A.; Ayers, C.; Wang, B.; Björkbacka, H.; Pana, T.A.; Thorand, B.; Sun, C.; Fani, L.; Malik, R.; et al. Association of Circulating Monocyte Chemoattractant Protein–1 Levels with Cardiovascular Mortality. *JAMA Cardiol.* **2021**, *6*, 587–592. [CrossRef]
31. Chiou, W.Y.; Hung, S.K.; Lai, C.L.; Lin, H.Y.; Su, Y.C.; Chen, Y.C.; Shen, B.J.; Chen, L.C.; Tsai, S.J.; Lee, M.S.; et al. Effect of 23-Valent Pneumococcal Polysaccharide Vaccine Inoculated During Anti-Cancer Treatment Period in Elderly Lung Cancer Patients on Community-Acquired Pneumonia Hospitalization: A Nationwide Population-Based Cohort Study. *Medicine* **2015**, *94*, e1022. [CrossRef]
32. World Health Organization. Cancer Mortality and Morbidity. 2023. Available online: https://www.who.int/news-room/fact-sheets/detail/lung-cancer (accessed on 18 November 2023).
33. Polska Koalicja Pacjentów Onkologicznych. 2021. Available online: https://immuno-onkologia.pl/wp-content/uploads/2021/06/rak-pluca-2021-Raport.pdf (accessed on 10 September 2023).
34. van Meir, H.; Nout, R.A.; Welters, M.J.P.; Loof, N.M.; de Kam, M.L.; van Ham, J.J.; Samuels, S.; Kenter, G.G.; Cohen, A.F.; Melief, C.J.M.; et al. Impact of (Chemo)Radiotherapy on Immune Cell Composition and Function in Cervical Cancer Patients. *Oncoimmunology* **2017**, *6*, e1267095. [CrossRef]
35. Karthikeyan, G.; Jumnani, D.; Prabhu, R.; Manoor, U.K.; Supe, S.S. Prevalence of Fatigue among Cancer Patients Receiving Various Anticancer Therapies and Its Impact on Quality of Life: A Cross-Sectional Study. *Indian J. Palliat. Care* **2012**, *18*, 165–175. [CrossRef]
36. Wargo, J.A.; Reuben, A.; Cooper, Z.A.; Oh, K.S.; Sullivan, R.J. Immune Effects of Chemotherapy, Radiation, and Targeted Therapy and Opportunities for Combination with Immunotherapy. *Semin. Oncol.* **2015**, *42*, 601–616. [CrossRef] [PubMed]
37. Huang, Y.S.; Li, Z.; Xiao, Z.F.; Li, D.; Liu, W.Y. Case report: Radiotherapy plus pneumococcal conjugate vaccine stimulates abscopal immune response in a patient with ALK+ NSCLC. *Front. Immunol.* **2022**, *13*, 950252. [CrossRef] [PubMed]

38. Mauro, F.R.; Giannarelli, D.; Galluzzo, C.M.; Vitale, C.; Visentin, A.; Riemma, C.; Rosati, S.; Porrazzo, M.; Pepe, S.; Coscia, M.; et al. Response to the conjugate pneumococcal vaccine (PCV13) in patients with chronic lymphocytic leukemia (CLL). *Leukemia* **2021**, *35*, 737–746. [CrossRef] [PubMed]
39. Mustafa, S.S.; Shah, D.; Bress, J.; Jamshed, S. Response to PCV13 vaccination in patients with multiple myeloma versus healthy controls. *Hum. Vaccines Immunother.* **2019**, *15*, 452–454. [CrossRef]

Disclaimer/Publisher's Note: The statements, opinions and data contained in all publications are solely those of the individual author(s) and contributor(s) and not of MDPI and/or the editor(s). MDPI and/or the editor(s) disclaim responsibility for any injury to people or property resulting from any ideas, methods, instructions or products referred to in the content.

Article

Analysis of Selected Toll-like Receptors in the Pathogenesis and Advancement of Non-Small-Cell Lung Cancer

Jolanta Smok-Kalwat [1], Paulina Mertowska [2,*], Sebastian Mertowski [2], Stanisław Góźdź [1,3], Izabela Korona-Głowniak [4], Wojciech Kwaśniewski [5] and Ewelina Grywalska [2]

1. Department of Clinical Oncology, Holy Cross Cancer Centre, 3 Artwinskiego Street, 25-734 Kielce, Poland; jolantasm@onkol.kielce.pl (J.S.-K.); stanislawgo@onkol.kielce.pl (S.G.)
2. Department of Experimental Immunology, Medical University of Lublin, 4a Chodzki Street, 20-093 Lublin, Poland; sebastianmertowski@umlub.pl (S.M.); ewelina.grywalska@umlub.pl (E.G.)
3. Institute of Medical Science, Collegium Medicum, Jan Kochanowski University of Kielce, IX Wieków Kielc 19A, 25-317 Kielce, Poland
4. Department of Pharmaceutical Microbiology, Medical University of Lublin, 20-093 Lublin, Poland; izabela.korona-glowniak@umlub.pl
5. Department of Gynecologic Oncology and Gynecology, Medical University of Lublin, Staszica 16 Street, 20-081 Lublin, Poland; wojciech.kwasniewski@umlub.pl
* Correspondence: paulinamertowska@umlub.pl

Abstract: (1) **Background:** Non-small-cell lung cancer (NSCLC) represents a significant global health challenge, contributing to numerous cancer deaths. Despite advances in diagnostics and therapy, identifying reliable biomarkers for prognosis and therapeutic stratification remains difficult. Toll-like receptors (TLRs), crucial for innate immunity, now show potential as contributors to cancer development and progression. This study aims to investigate the role of TLR expression as potential biomarkers in the development and progression of NSCLC. (2) **Materials and Methods:** The study was conducted on 89 patients diagnosed with NSCLC and 40 healthy volunteers, for whom the prevalence of TLR2, TLR3, TLR4, TLR7, TLR8, and TLR9 was assessed on selected subpopulations of T and B lymphocytes in the peripheral blood of recruited patients along with the assessment of their serum concentration. (3) **Result:** Our study showed several significant changes in NSCLC patients at the beginning of the study. This resulted in a 5-year follow-up of changes in selected TLRs in recruited patients. Due to the high mortality rate of NSCLC patients, only 16 patients survived the 5 years. (4) **Conclusions:** The results suggest that TLRs may constitute real biomarker molecules that may be used for future prognostic purposes in NSCLC. However, further validation through prospective clinical and functional studies is necessary to confirm their clinical utility. These conclusions may lead to better risk stratification and tailored interventions, benefiting NSCLC patients and bringing medicine closer to precision.

Keywords: toll-like receptors; non-small-cell lung cancer; biomarkers; tumor progression; innate immune system; clinicopathological characteristics

1. Introduction

Non-small-cell lung cancer (NSCLC) remains a significant global health burden, representing a substantial portion of cancer-related mortalities worldwide [1–3]. Despite advancements in early detection and treatment strategies, the prognosis for NSCLC patients remains diverse, necessitating the identification of robust predictive biomarkers to improve clinical management and patient outcomes [4,5]. Toll-like receptors (TLRs), as key components of the innate immune system, have recently emerged as potential contributors to the complex interplay between the tumor microenvironment and cancer progression [6–9].

The innate immune system plays a fundamental role in recognizing and responding to various pathogens, and danger signals through pattern recognition receptors (PRRs), among which TLRs are prominent members [10,11]. Aside from their role in infection control, TLRs have gained considerable attention due to their involvement in tumorigenesis and tumor progression [12]. Preclinical studies have revealed that aberrant TLR signaling can promote tumor cell proliferation, metastasis, and immune evasion, implicating TLRs as potential players in the intricate network of tumorigenic processes [13–16]. TLRs play a key role in the development and treatment of lung cancer, although their functions may be opposing (Figure 1). These receptors are widely expressed on various cell types, including those in the lung epithelium as well as immune cells such as myeloid and lymphoid cells. Studies indicate that TLR3 can promote the formation of metastases but also participate in the induction of apoptosis and the reactivation of local innate reactions. Another example is the role of TLR9, the increased expression of which in tissue supported the progression and metastasis of lung cancer, and on the other hand, its activation by CpG-ODN induced anticancer effects. Activation of TLR receptors may influence the development of the immune response and the balance in the tumor microenvironment (TME), which ultimately determines its progression or regression [17–21].

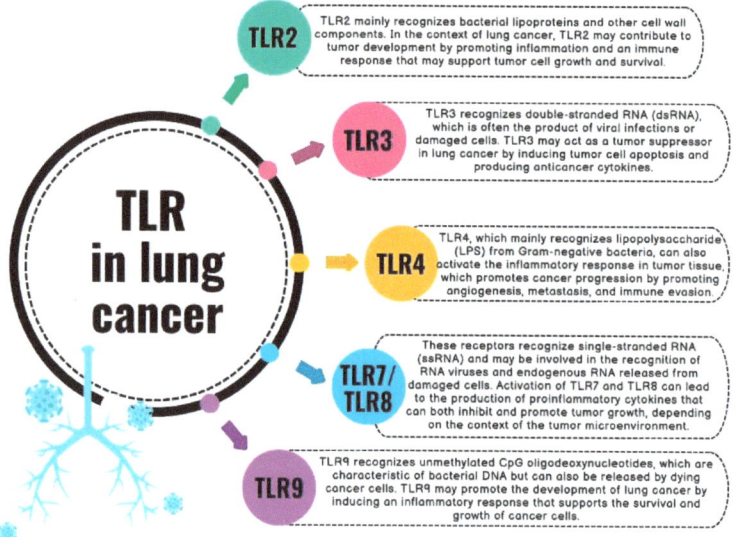

Figure 1. Description of the role of some TLRs in the context of lung cancer (based on [10–21]).

In recent years, investigations exploring TLRs' expression and functional significance in NSCLC have intensified. These studies have reported diverse TLR expression patterns across different NSCLC subtypes, prompting the question of whether TLRs could serve as valuable biomarkers for this heterogeneous disease [22–25]. Understanding the potential of TLR expression as an independent prognostic biomarker is crucial, as it could contribute to refining risk stratification and guiding personalized treatment approaches.

In light of the information and observations of our research team presented in the introduction, the publication aimed to determine the expression level of selected TLR receptors (TLR2, TLR3, TLR4, TLR7, TLR8, and TLR9) in subpopulations of peripheral blood lymphocytes in patients diagnosed with NSCLC. Additionally, we would like to check whether the percentage of lymphocytes positively expressing the tested TLRs and their soluble forms in serum can correlate with the patient's survival rate.

2. Materials and Methods

2.1. Characteristics of Patients and Research Material

Eighty-nine patients diagnosed with NSCLC and 40 healthy volunteers were analyzed. Patients were subject to several inclusion and exclusion criteria. The inclusion criteria for patients in the study included: histopathological confirmation of NSCLC; expressing the patient's informed consent to participate in the study; and lack of treatment before starting the study. The patients had not been previously treated for lung cancer and had not received any chemotherapy, radiotherapy, and/or immunotherapy. Blood samples were obtained from previously untreated patients with suspected lung cancer one day before surgery. Only patients who had NSCLC confirmed intraoperatively and in the histopathological examination following the surgery were included in the study. The control group consisted of healthy individuals matched in terms of gender and age to the study group. The health status of patients with NSCLC was confirmed by routine diagnostic tests performed during follow-up visits (at least 2 follow-up visits per year) with an internal medicine specialist and a pulmonologist. Samples for testing were collected each time during a follow-up visit. Smoking was not considered an exclusion criterion for patients in the study. The exclusion criteria for both groups were as follows: taking medications affecting the immune system, hormonal therapy, infection during the last three months before the study, any prior history of blood transfusion, autoimmune disease, cancer, allergies, and pregnancy or lactation within one year before this study. In addition, patients in each group became good in terms of age. Patients were recruited from January 2014 to January 2015, and the status—whether they are alive or not after five years, i.e., from January 2019 to January. Detailed information on the characteristics of the patients included in this study is presented in Table 1).

Table 1. Characteristics of patients included in the study.

Parameter		Patient with NSCLC (n = 89)		Healthy Volunteers (n = 40)	
		Mean ± SD	Median (Range)	Mean ± SD	Median (Range)
General information	Age	72.12 ± 8.0	73.0 (64.5–82)	74.5 ± 8.4	73.0 (70.5–83.0)
	Gender, male/female (%)	75/15 (83.33%/16.67%)		34/6 (85.0%/15.0%)	
	Smoking (%)	88 (97.77%)		14 (35.0%)	
Stages	IA	4 (4.49%)		NA	
	IB	14 (15.73%)			
	IIA	5 (5.62%)			
	IIB	9 (10.11%)			
	IIIA	11 (12.36%)			
	IIIB	18 (20.23%)			
	IIIC	3 (3.37%)			
	IV	25 (28.09%)			
Symptoms	Cough (lasting for weeks)	67 (74.44%)		NA	
	Shortness of breath	36 (40.00%)			
	Swallowing disorders	27 (30.00%)			
	Hoarseness	58 (64.44%)			
	Pain in the chest	68 (75.5%)			
	Weakness	72 (80.00%)			
	Weight loss	27 (30.00%)			
	Infections of the upper and lower respiratory tract requiring antibiotic therapy in the last year preceding diagnosis	63 (70.00%)		5 (12.5%)	
Therapy	Brachytherapy (%)	53 (58.88%)		NA	
	Chemotherapy (%)	48 (53.33%)		NA	
	Radiotherapy (%)	22 (24.44%)		NA	

NA—not applicable.

The research material consisted of 5 mL of peripheral blood collected in EDTA tubes (allowing for the assessment of the immunophenotype) and 5 mL of serum (allowing for the assessment of the concentration of soluble forms of the TLRs tested). The tests were each performed in two technical repetitions. The study protocol received the necessary approval from the Bioethics Committee at the esteemed Medical University of Lublin under reference number KE-0254/283/2015.

2.2. Immunophenotyping

The analysis of lymphocyte immunophenotype in peripheral blood was performed through the use of flow cytometry, a precise and accurate approach to cell analysis. A whole blood sample was collected and treated with a set of monoclonal human anti-bodies consisting of anti-CD45 AF700, anti-CD3 PerCp, anti-CD4 BV421, anti-CD8 BV605, anti-CD19 FITC, anti-CD56 BV650, and anti-CD16 BV650, as well as anti-TLR2 APC, anti-TLR3 PE, anti-TLR4 PE, anti-TLR7 PE, anti-TLR8 APC, and anti-TLR9 APC antibodies (BioLegend, San Diego, CA 92121, USA). Subsequently, a lysing buffer was utilized to remove any red blood cells, and the remaining cells were thoroughly washed and assessed through the use of a CytoFLEX LX instrument, which is a sophisticated flow cytometer (Beckman Coulter, Indianapolis, IN, USA). The resulting data were analyzed using the Kaluza Analysis program, as demonstrated in Figure 2. The CytoFLEX LX flow cytometer was subjected to daily quality control using CytoFLEX Ready to Use Daily QC Fluorospheres reagents (Beckman Coulter, Indianapolis, IN, USA).

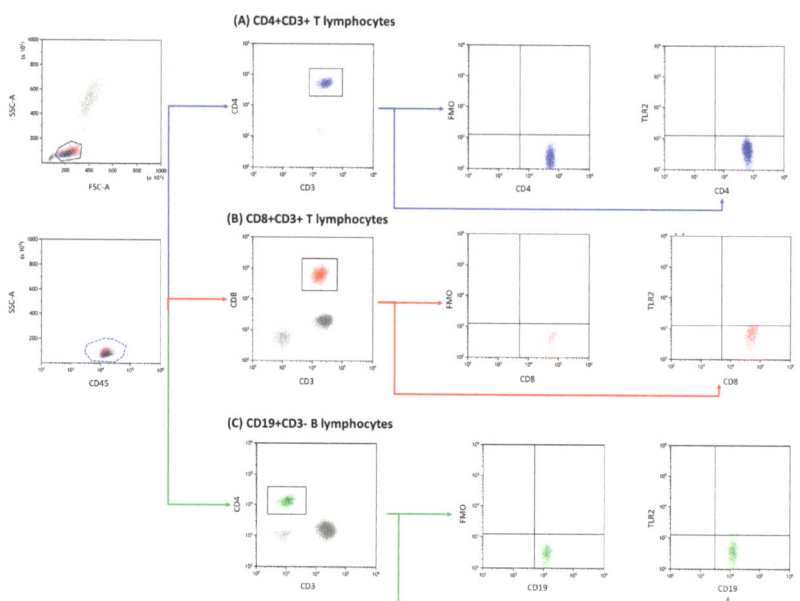

Figure 2. Exemplary analysis of the cells' immunophenotype and the determination of the percentage of positive TLR expression on the example of TLRCD4+CD3+ subpopulation marked in blue, CD8+CD3+ subpopulation in red, and CD19+CD3− subpopulation in green. Points (**A**–**C**) indicate the method of reading TLR2 using the FMO control.

2.3. Quantification of Soluble Forms of TLR Forms

Enzyme immunoassays (ELISA) were utilized to assess the concentration of soluble forms of TLR in serum samples collected from all patients participating in our study. Commercially available kits were employed, with particular use of the Human TLR2 ELISA Kit (range: 109.4–7000 pg/mL; sensitivity 17 pg/mL), Human TLR3 ELISA Kit (range: 156–10,000 pg/mL; sensitivity 10 pg/mL), Human TLR4 ELISA Kit (range: 0.41–100 ng/mL; sensitivity 0.4 ng/well), (Abcam in Cambridge, UK,) and the Human Toll-Like Receptor 7 (TLR7) ELISA Kit (range: 10–3500 ng/L; sensitivity 5.32 ng/mL), Human Toll-Like Receptor 8 (TLR-8) ELISA Kit (range: 20–0.312 ng/mL; sensitivity 0.06 ng/mL), and Human Toll-Like Receptor 9 (TLR-9) ELISA Kit (range: 20–0.312 ng/mL; sensitivity 0.06 ng/mL) from MyBiosource in San Diego, CA, USA. The manufacturer's instructions were followed diligently. For measurement, the VictorTM3 reader from PerkinElmer (Waltham, MA, USA).

2.4. Statistical Analysis

The data generated from this study were analyzed using Tibco Statistica 13.3 software, a highly regarded platform in data analytics and visualization, based in Palo Alto, California. The normality of the data distribution was assessed using the Shapiro–Wilk test, a widely used tool for testing the normality of data. The Kruskal–Wallis test was employed to examine differences between the groups, with Dunn's post hoc test being applied as a follow-up analysis. To account for multiple comparisons, the p-values for Dunn's test were adjusted using the Bonferroni method. The study also explored the relationships between pairs of variables using Spearman's correlation coefficients. Finally, ROC curves were utilized to evaluate the diagnostic performance of the laboratory test for patient-related parameters. To present the data clearly and concisely, GraphPad Prism, an industry-standard software platform for scientific graphing and analysis, was employed (GraphPad Prism Software v. 9.4.1, San Diego, CA, USA).

3. Results

3.1. Characteristics of Patients Included in the Study with Particular Emphasis on the Occurrence of TLR

The study recruited 89 newly diagnosed patients with a diagnosis confirmed histopathological as NSCLC. Detailed patient inclusion and exclusion criteria are described in the Materials and Methods section. The control group consisted of 40 healthy volunteers matched according to age to the study group. All collected information regarding patients recruited for the study and their results of peripheral blood morphology, biochemistry, and immunophenotype are summarized in Figure 3 and Table 2.

Table 2. Characteristics of the morphology and immunophenotype of peripheral blood of patients included in the study.

Parameter	Patient with NSCLC		Healthy Volunteers		p-Value
	Mean ± SD	Median (Range)	Mean ± SD	Median (Range)	
WBC [10^3/mm^3]	6.59 ± 2.05	6.19 (3.58–16.82)	6.29 ± 0.9	6.22 (5.6–6.8)	0.874
LYM [10^3/mm^3]	1.27 ± 0.54	1.15 (0.30–3.13)	1.86 ± 0.4	1.85 (1.6–2.0)	0.000 *
MON [10^3/mm^3]	0.55 ± 0.19	0.50 (0.23–1.18)	0.82 ± 0.3	0.77 (0.6–0.98)	0.000 *
NEU [10^3/mm^3]	4.59 ± 1.86	4.28 (2.18–14.76)	6.79 ± 2.9	6.55 (5.2–7.9)	0.000 *
RBC [10^6/mm^3]	3.12 ± 0.32	3.16 (2.24–3.74)	4.54 ± 0.3	4.55 (4.4–4.7)	0.000 *
HGB [g/gl]	9.06 ± 1.14	9.21 (6.26–12.04)	13.14 ± 1.65	13.7 (12.1–14.9)	0.000 *
PLT [10^3/mm^3]	228.94 ± 81.10	217.94 (84.32–540.60)	313.4 ± 93.1	312.0 (224.5–390.5)	0.000 *
CRP [mg/L]	17.54 ± 19.76	11.75 (0.50–107.63)	0.29 ± 0.4	0.16 (0.1–0.3)	0.000 *
CD3+ T lymphocytes [%]	47.47 ± 8.28	47.61 (13.87–62.55)	72.83 ± 6.4	71.94 (68.8–75.4)	0.000 *
CD3+CD8+ T lymphocytes [%]	20.38 ± 7.40	20.23 (6.09–39.93)	26.39 ± 3.0	26.91 (24.7–28.0)	0.000 *
CD3+CD4+ T lymphocytes [%]	26.63 ± 6.45	26.82 (7.05–38.76)	47.53 ± 4.8	46.76 (44.7–48.6)	0.000 *
Ratio CD3+CD4+/CD3+CD8	1.13 ± 0.96	0.92 (0.31–8.37)	1.82 ± 0.2	1.78 (1.6–2.1)	0.000 *
CD19+ B lymphocytes [%]	5.44 ± 3.07	4.91 (1.13–14.56)	12.59 ± 2.3	12.46 (11.6–13.7)	0.000 *

The symbol * denotes statistically significant results. Abbreviations: WBC—white blood cells; LYM- lymphocytes; MON—monocytes; NEU—neutrophils; RBC—red blood cells; HGB—hemoglobin; PLT—pellets; CRP—C-reactive protein; CD—cluster of differentiation.

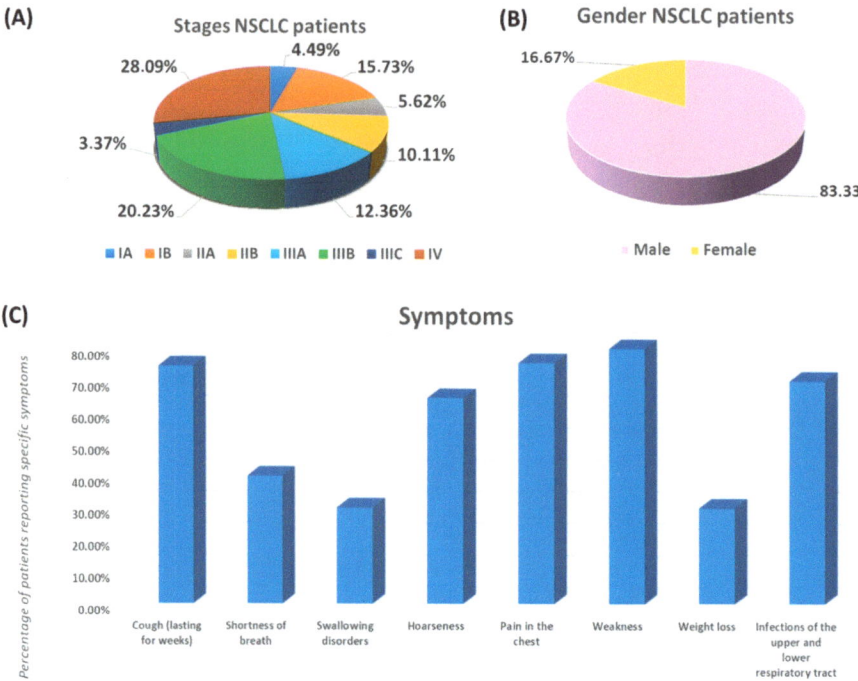

Figure 3. Characteristics of patients with NSCLC included in the study. (**A**) Stages of NSCLC patients; (**B**) Gender of NSCLC patients; (**C**) Most common symptoms reported by NSCLC patients.

The average age of patients included in the study was 72 years, which corresponds to the statistical data presented by the National Health Fund for patients from Poland, for whom the average age ranges between 70 and 75 years. Of the recruited patients, the majority of patients diagnosed with NSCLC were men. Analysis of the stage of patients included in the study showed a significant percentage of patients with advanced lung cancer: 32 people in stage III, 25 people in stage IV, 14 people in stage II, 18 people in stage I. This shows the need for deeper diagnostics of this group of diseases to increase the speed and effectiveness of detection, diagnosis, and implementation of treatment for these patients. Analysis of the symptoms of patients included in the study showed that they suffered from persistent cough, hoarseness, chest pain, and general weakness. Moreover, 70% of recruited patients struggled with upper and lower respiratory tract infections requiring antibiotic therapy in the last year before diagnosis. A detailed analysis of this aspect showed that 30 people struggled with 2–3 infections during the year; 10 people had one infection during the year; no infection was recorded in another 10 people; 8 people with 4–5 infections; and 3 people reported more than 6 infections in a year. Over 97% of recruited NSCLC patients admitted to smoking cigarettes (none of the patients used electronic cigarettes). The average number of pack-years was 35.66 ± 10.03, with a median of 37.5 (minimum: 15; maximum: 60).

As we can observe in Table 2, between patients recruited for the NSCLC study and the control group, there are several statistically significant differences in the analyzed parameters of morphology, biochemistry, and immunophenotype of peripheral blood.

However, the most important thing in our study was to determine the percentage of TLR2, TLR3, TLR4, TLR7, TLR8, and TLR9 occurrence on individual subpopulations of peripheral blood lymphocytes, the results of which are presented in Table 3.

Table 3. Peripheral blood immunophenotype analysis and serum concentration of sTLRs of NSCLC patients and healthy volunteers.

Lymphocyte Subset	Patient with NSCLC		Healthy Volunteers		p-Value
	Mean ± SD	Median (Range)	Mean ± SD	Median (Range)	
T CD4+TLR2+ [%]	4.08 ± 2.80	3.29 (0.91–14.29)	0.92 ± 0.6	0.83 (0.5–1.3)	<0.0001 *
T CD8+TLR2+ [%]	5.65 ± 3.03	4.79 (1.50–14.91)	0.88 ± 0.8	0.56 (0.3–1.2)	<0.0001 *
B CD19+TLR2+ [%]	5.78 ± 3.03	4.42 (0.90–12.29)	1.35 ± 0.5	1.32 (1.1–1.7)	<0.0001 *
T CD4+TLR3+ [%]	1.89 ± 0.61	1.79 (0.73–3.34)	0.94 ± 0.6	1.06 (0.3–1.3)	<0.0001 *
T CD8+TLR3+ [%]	1.71 ± 0.50	1.74 (0.54–2.71)	0.81 ± 0.5	0.67 (0.4–1.3)	<0.0001 *
B CD19+TLR3+ [%]	1.93 ± 0.56	1.92 (0.69–3.00)	0.49 ± 0.2	0.52 (0.3–0.6)	<0.0001 *
T CD4+TLR4+ [%]	5.06 ± 2.39	4.41 (1.67–11.83)	1.0 ± 0.5	1.08 (0.5–1.3)	<0.0001 *
T CD8+TLR4+ [%]	5.85 ± 2.76	5.24 (1.47–12.78)	0.98 ± 0.6	0.99 (0.5–1.5)	<0.0001 *
B CD19+TLR4+ [%]	5.46 ± 2.99	4.56 (2.45–17.09)	0.77 ± 0.4	0.79 (0.5–1.0)	<0.0001 *
T CD4+TLR7+ [%]	1.36 ± 0.37	1.34 (0.70–2.37)	0.49 ± 0.3	0.55 (0.2–0.7)	<0.0001 *
T CD8+TLR7+ [%]	1.76 ± 0.52	1.76 (0.72–3.04)	0.46 ± 0.3	0.32 (0.2–0.7)	<0.0001 *
B CD19+TLR7+ [%]	1.97 ± 0.41	1.94 (0.93–2.73)	0.43 ± 0.2	0.44 (0.3–0.6)	<0.0001 *
T CD4+TLR8+ [%]	2.83 ± 0.76	2.85 (1.52–4.37)	0.79 ± 0.5	0.76 (0.3–1.3)	<0.0001 *
T CD8+TLR8+ [%]	1.49 ± 0.65	1.43 (0.10–2.77)	0.42 ± 0.3	0.33 (0.3–0.7)	<0.0001 *
B CD19+TLR8+ [%]	1.66 ± 0.64	1.63 (0.69–2.91)	0.55 ± 0.3	0.56 (0.4–0.8)	<0.0001 *
T CD4+TLR9+ [%]	5.08 ± 3.10	4.31 (1.37–14.48)	0.97 ± 0.6	0.87 (0.5–1.3)	<0.0001 *
T CD8+TLR9+ [%]	5.85 ± 2.74	5.16 (0.80–14.00)	1.34 ± 0.6	1.41 (0.9–1.8)	<0.0001 *
B CD19+TLR-9+ [%]	8.25 ± 5.56	6.33 (1.18–25.96)	1.76 ± 0.7	1.59 (1.2–2.1)	<0.0001 *
sTLR2 [ng/mL]	6.78 ± 4.74	5.11 (0.80–19.35)	2.5 ± 1.0	2.63 (1.7–3.3)	<0.0001 *
sTLR3 [ng/mL]	6.25 ± 1.66	5.59 (4.79–11.89)	1.57 ± 0.8	1.47 (1.0–2.1)	<0.0001 *
sTLR4 [ng/mL]	6.34 ± 3.23	5.28 (2.14–16.02)	3.03 ± 0.7	3.26 (2.6–3.5)	<0.0001 *
sTLR7 [ng/mL]	4.92 ± 1.52	4.65 (3.47–10.10)	1.07 ± 0.6	1.07 (0.6–1.5)	<0.0001 *
sTLR8 [ng/mL]	6.22 ± 1.61	6.17 (3.49–12.14)	0.97 ± 0.6	1.01 (0.4–1.5)	<0.0001 *
sTLR9 [ng/mL]	8.82 ± 5.28	8.58 (0.88–21.56)	3.1 ± 0.6	3.21 (2.7–3.6)	<0.0001 *

The symbol * denotes statistically significant results. Abbreviations: CD—cluster of differentiation; TLR—Toll-like receptors; sTLR—soluble form of Toll-like receptors.

The obtained results confirm that patients with NSCLC have a higher percentage of all TLRs tested on the tested lymphocyte subpopulations compared to healthy volunteers. We additionally confirmed this study by analyzing the level of a soluble form of TLRs (sTLRs) in the serum of all patients, and the obtained results are also presented in Table 3.

Due to the extremely interesting research data obtained, our team decided to include these patients in further studies aimed at observing changes in the levels and concentrations of TLRs over time.

3.2. Changes in the Percentage of TLRs and Their Concentrations in Patients with NSCLC over Time

Our goal was to monitor the same parameters for 5 years in all patients diagnosed with NSCLC. Examinations were performed routinely during follow-up visits at least once a year. Due to the extremely high compliance rate observed among lung cancer patients, our study decreased the number of patients each year. From the initial pool of 89 diagnosed patients, 25 patients died in the first year (all in stage IV); in the second year, another 18 patients (15 patients in stage IIIB and 3 patients in stage IIIC); in the third year, another 19 patients (10 stage IIIA patients and 9 stage IIB patients); in the fourth year, 3 patients (all in stage IIA). In the fifth year of our observation, 8 more patients died (4 in stage IB, 4 in stage IA). This means that of all the patients recruited for this study, only 16 patients survived the 5-year follow-up period. Detailed causes of death of patients diagnosed with NSCLC included infection in 37 people (50.00%); multi-organ failure in 20 people (27.03%); cancer cachexia (13.51%); and thromboembolic complications in 7 people (9.46%).

Each year, we compiled the results of peripheral blood morphology and biochemistry tests along with its immunophenotyping, with particular emphasis on the percentage of the tested TLRs and their serum concentration. These lists have been presented in tables and included as supplementary materials marked as Supplementary Materials Tables S1–S8). All tables take into account the division of patients into living and dead patients in a given period in which the research was carried out.

In the main part of the manuscript, we would like to focus on the last 5 years of our observations, which may highlight the importance of the role of selected TLRs as potential biomarker molecules.

We observed much more statistically significant changes when analyzing the percentage of occurrence of individual subpopulations of T and B lymphocytes positive for the tested TLR receptors (Figures 4–6 and Table 4). Of course, the level of expression of the tested TLRs was significantly higher in NSCLC patients compared to healthy volunteers, but their analysis between NSCLC alive patients and NSCLC death deserves special attention. Except for CD19+TLR4+, all median values in NSCLC death patients were higher than in NSCLC alive patients. The ratio of the recorded values ranged from 1.39-fold for CD19+TLR7+ to 2.81-fold for CD19+TLR9+, which highlights the significant range of changes in the percentage of occurrence of individual subpopulations of lymphocytes, especially B-positive for the expression of the tested TLRs.

This is also emphasized by the analyses concerning the assessment of the concentration of soluble TLRs in the serum of all tested groups of patients (Table 5). As with the immunophenotypic analyses, all observed changes between NSCLC patients and controls were statistically significant. The highest differences were observed for sTLR-9 (2.80-fold), followed by sTLR-2 (2.02-fold), sTLR-4 (1.75-fold), sTLR-8 (1.55-fold), sTLR-7 (1.36-fold), and sTLR-3 (1.20-fold) in NSCLC dead versus NSCLC alive.

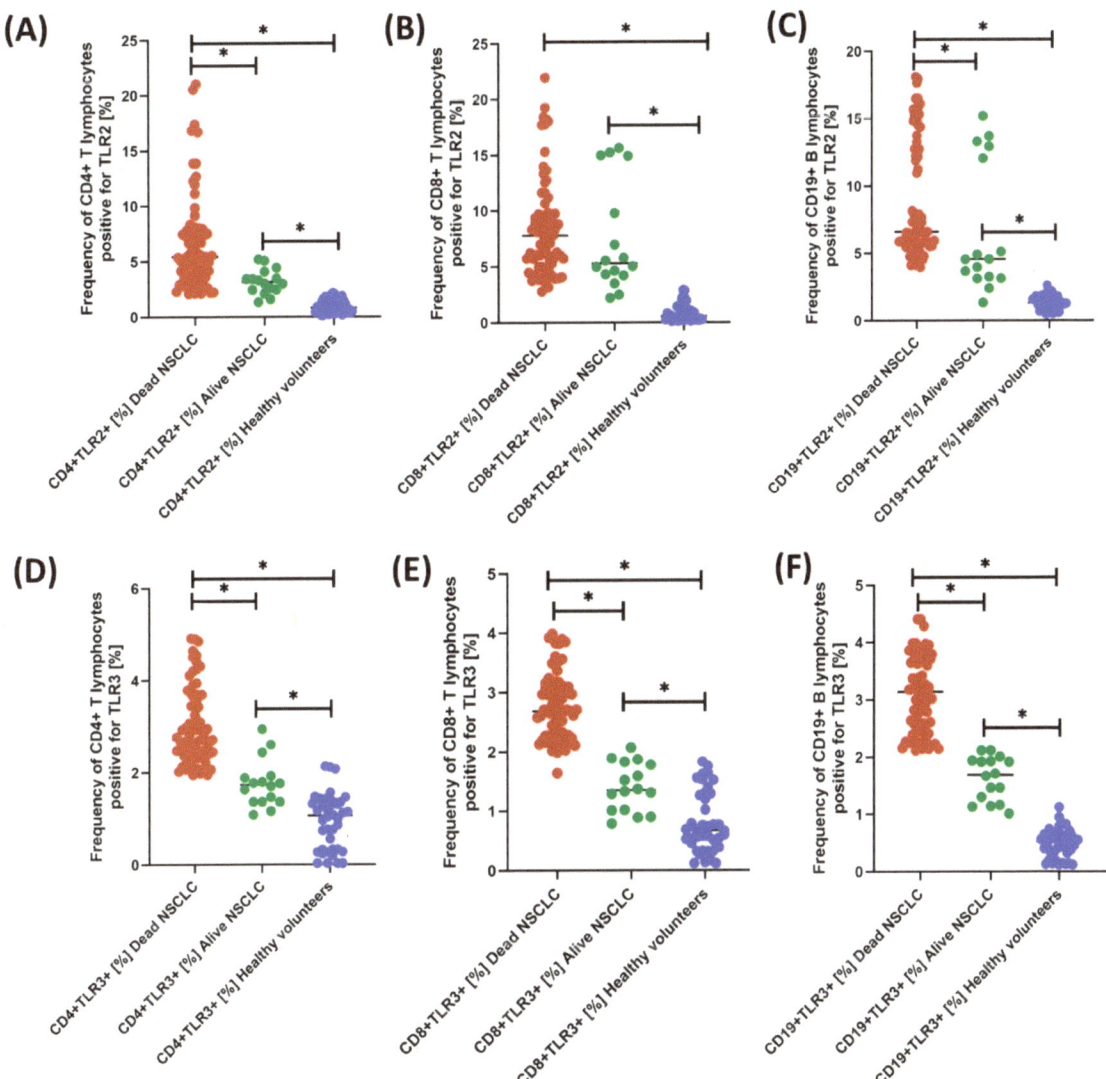

Figure 4. Graphical representation of the results regarding the evaluation of the percentage of TLR2- and TLR3-positive peripheral blood lymphocyte populations tested. (**A**) Percentage of CD4+TLR2+ lymphocytes; (**B**) Percentage of CD8+TLR2+ lymphocytes; (**C**) Percentage of CD19+TLR2+ lymphocytes; (**D**) Percentage of CD4+TLR3+ lymphocytes; (**E**) Percentage of CD8+TLR3+ lymphocytes; (**F**) Percentage of CD19+TLR3+ lymphocytes; * Statistically significant results are marked.

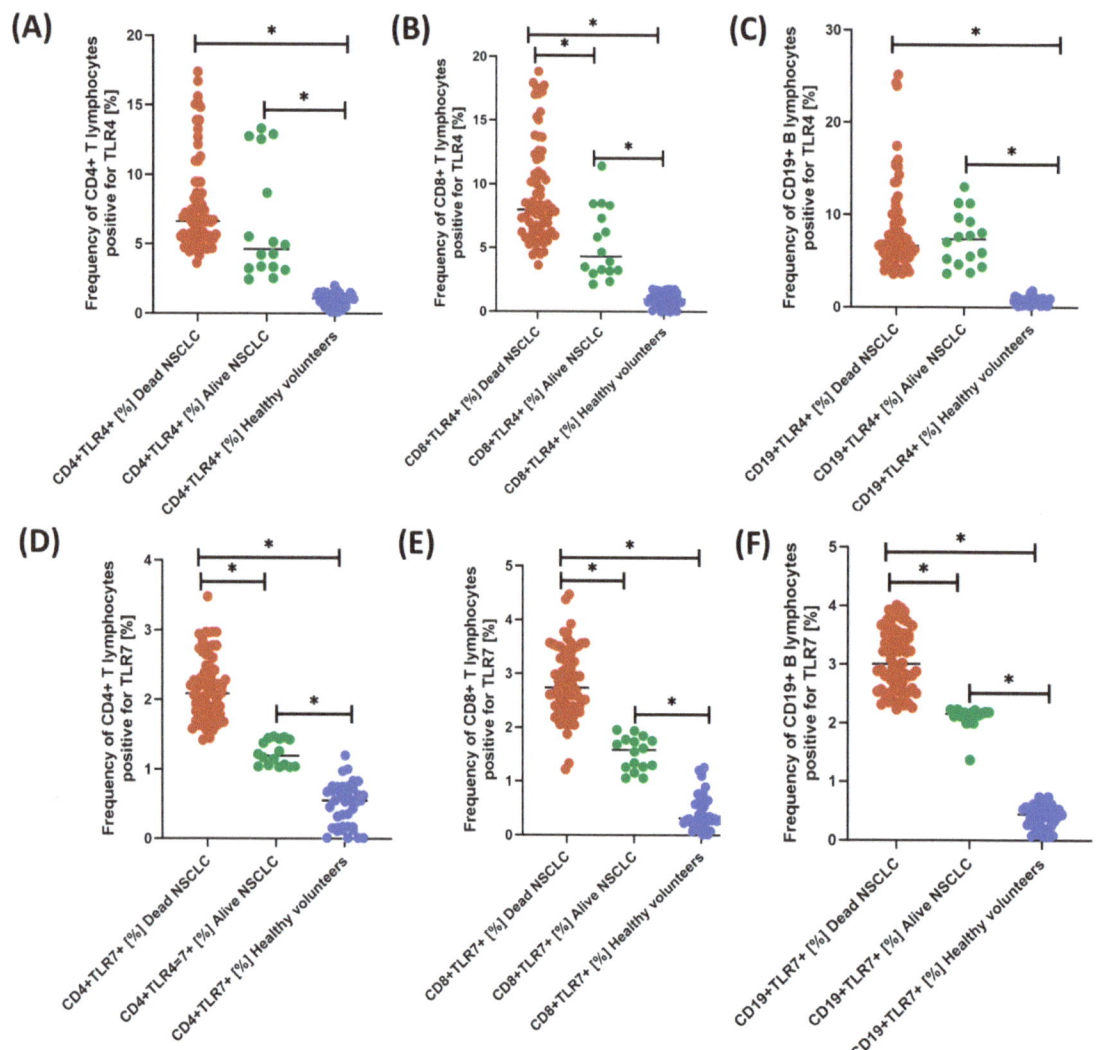

Figure 5. Graphical representation of the results regarding the evaluation of the percentage of TLR4- and TLR7-positive peripheral blood lymphocyte populations tested. (**A**) Percentage of CD4+TLR4+ lymphocytes; (**B**) Percentage of CD8+TLR4+ lymphocytes; (**C**) Percentage of CD19+TLR4+ lymphocytes; (**D**) Percentage of CD4+TLR7+ lymphocytes; (**E**) Percentage of CD8+TLR7+ lymphocytes; (**F**) Percentage of CD19+TLR7+ lymphocytes; * Statistically significant results are marked.

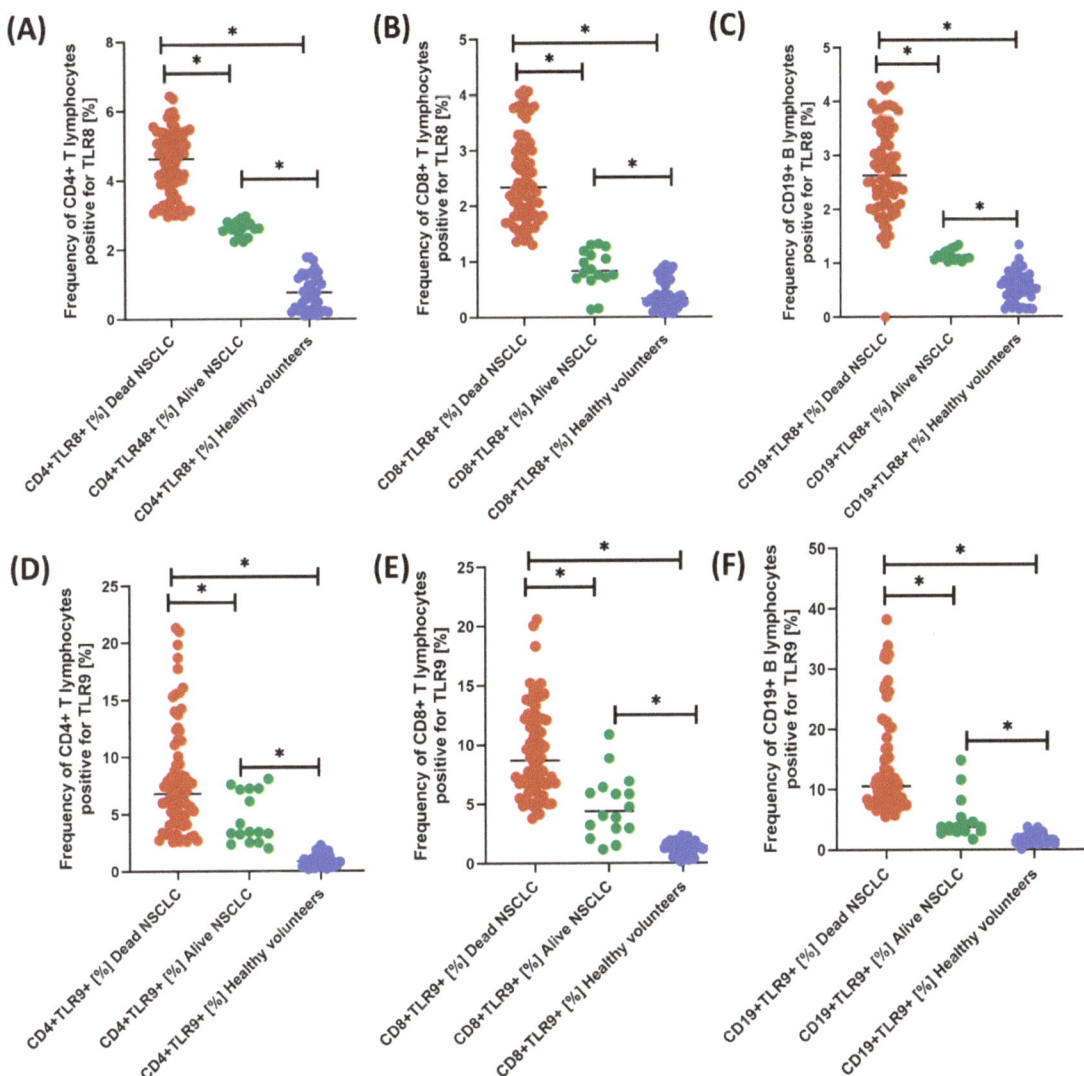

Figure 6. Graphical representation of the results regarding the evaluation of the percentage of TLR8- and TLR9-positive peripheral blood lymphocyte populations tested. (**A**) Percentage of CD4+TLR8+ lymphocytes; (**B**) Percentage of CD8+TLR8+ lymphocytes; (**C**) Percentage of CD19+TLR8+ lymphocytes; (**D**) Percentage of CD4+TLR9+ lymphocytes; (**E**) Percentage of CD8+TLR9+ lymphocytes; (**F**) Percentage of CD19+TLR9+ lymphocytes; * Statistically significant results are marked.

Table 4. Analysis of the percentage of TLR occurrence on selected subpopulations of peripheral blood lymphocytes in patients with NSCLC compared to healthy volunteers, with particular emphasis on survival status.

Parameter	Patient with NSCLC Alive (n = 16)		Patient with NSCLC Dead (n = 73)		p-Value	Healthy Volunteers (n = 40)		p-Value	NSCLC Alive vs. Dead	NSCLC Alive vs. Healthy Volunteers	NSCLC Dead vs. Healthy Volunteers
	Mean ± SD	Median (Range)	Mean ± SD	Median (Range)		Mean ± SD	Median (Range)				
T CD4+TLR2+ [%]	3.18 ± 1.1	3.16 (2.4–3.8)	7.11 ± 4.32	5.66 (2.10–21.02)	<0.0001 *	0.92 ± 0.6	0.83 (0.5–1.3)	<0.0001 *	<0.0001 *	<0.0001 *	<0.0001 *
T CD8+TLR2+ [%]	7.52 ± 4.9	5.30 (4.3–12.4)	9.02 ± 4.38	8.33 (3.17–21.93)	<0.0001 *	0.88 ± 0.8	0.56 (0.3–1.2)	<0.0001 *	0.21	<0.0001 *	<0.0001 *
B CD19+TLR2+ [%]	6.69 ± 4.8	4.55 (3.2–12.5)	9.16 ± 4.46	7.01 (3.99–18.08)	<0.0001 *	1.35 ± 0.5	1.32 (1.1–1.7)	<0.0001 *	0.0035 *	<0.0001 *	<0.0001 *
T CD4+TLR3+ [%]	1.76 ± 0.5	1.73 (1.4–1.9)	3.08 ± 0.83	2.81 (1.95–4.91)	<0.0001 *	0.94 ± 0.6	1.06 (0.3–1.3)	<0.0001 *	<0.0001 *	<0.0001 *	<0.0001 *
T CD8+TLR3+ [%]	1.40 ± 0.4	1.35 (1.0–1.8)	2.70 ± 0.54	2.77 (1.64–3.98)	<0.0001 *	0.81 ± 0.5	0.67 (0.4–1.3)	<0.0001 *	<0.0001 *	0.00016 *	<0.0001 *
B CD19+TLR3+ [%]	1.63 ± 0.4	1.69 (1.2–1.9)	3.21 ± 0.60	3.19 (2.12–4.41)	<0.0001 *	0.49 ± 0.2	0.52 (0.3–0.6)	<0.0001 *	<0.0001 *	<0.0001 *	<0.0001 *
T CD4+TLR4+ [%]	6.40 ± 4.1	4.62 (3.3–10.6)	7.91 ± 3.50	6.72 (3.62–17.39)	<0.0001 *	1.0 ± 0.5	1.08 (0.5–1.3)	<0.0001 *	0.020	<0.0001 *	<0.0001 *
T CD8+TLR4+ [%]	5.34 ± 2.8	4.30 (3.2–7.8)	9.54 ± 4.15	8.06 (3.63–18.80)	<0.0001 *	0.98 ± 0.6	0.99 (0.5–1.5)	<0.0001 *	0.0003 *	<0.0001 *	<0.0001 *
B CD19+TLR4+ [%]	7.37 ± 2.9	7.33 (4.9–9.5)	8.62 ± 4.79	6.82 (3.79–25.13)	<0.0001 *	0.77 ± 0.4	0.79 (0.5–1.0)	<0.0001 *	0.86	<0.0001 *	<0.0001 *
T CD4+TLR7+ [%]	1.23 ± 0.2	1.20 (1.1–1.4)	2.24 ± 0.44	2.19 (1.42–3.48)	<0.0001 *	0.49 ± 0.3	0.55 (0.2–0.7)	<0.0001 *	<0.0001 *	<0.0001 *	<0.0001 *
T CD8+TLR7+ [%]	1.52 ± 0.3	1.59 (1.3–1.8)	2.90 ± 0.61	2.79 (1.22–4.47)	<0.0001 *	0.46 ± 0.3	0.32 (0.2–0.7)	<0.0001 *	<0.0001 *	<0.0001 *	<0.0001 *
B CD19+TLR7+ [%]	2.09 ± 0.2	2.16 (2.1–2.2)	3.16 ± 0.48	3.22 (2.24–4.01)	<0.0001 *	0.43 ± 0.2	0.44 (0.3–0.6)	<0.0001 *	<0.0001 *	<0.0001 *	<0.0001 *
T CD4+TLR8+ [%]	2.61 ± 0.2	2.61 (2.5–2.8)	4.66 ± 0.86	4.76 (2.96–6.43)	<0.0001 *	0.79 ± 0.5	0.76 (0.3–1.3)	<0.0001 *	<0.0001 *	<0.0001 *	<0.0001 *
T CD8+TLR8+ [%]	0.86 ± 0.4	0.83 (0.7–1.2)	2.60 ± 0.75	2.40 (1.30–4.08)	<0.0001 *	0.42 ± 0.3	0.33 (0.3–0.7)	<0.0001 *	<0.0001 *	0.0004 *	<0.0001 *
B CD19+TLR8+ [%]	1.14 ± 0.1	1.11 (1.1–1.2)	2.85 ± 0.75	4.28 (2.83–1.20)	<0.0001 *	0.55 ± 0.3	0.56 (0.4–0.8)	<0.0001 *	<0.0001 *	<0.0001 *	<0.0001 *
T CD4+TLR9+ [%]	4.62 ± 2.2	3.45 (2.9–7.2)	8.16 ± 4.84	7.16 (2.60–21.30)	<0.0001 *	0.97 ± 0.6	0.87 (0.5–1.3)	<0.0001 *	0.0032 *	<0.0001 *	<0.0001 *
T CD8+TLR9+ [%]	4.82 ± 2.7	4.38 (2.9–6.2)	9.48 ± 4.04	8.44 (3.79–20.59)	<0.0001 *	1.34 ± 0.6	1.41 (0.9–1.8)	<0.0001 *	<0.0001 *	<0.0001 *	<0.0001 *
B CD19+TLR9+ [%]	5.04 ± 3.5	3.74 (3.1–5.0)	14.18 ± 8.37	11.15 (5.52–38.17)	<0.0001 *	1.76 ± 0.7	1.59 (1.2–2.1)	<0.0001 *	<0.0001 *	<0.0001 *	<0.0001 *

The symbol * denotes statistically significant results. Abbreviations: CD—cluster of differentiation; TLR—Toll-like receptors; denotes statistically significant results.

Table 5. The concentration of soluble forms of TLRs in the serum of NSCLC patients among healthy volunteers.

Serum Concentration [ng/mL]	Patient with NSCLC Alive (n = 16)		Patient with NSCLC Dead (n = 74)		Healthy Volunteers (n = 40)		p-Value	p-Value	p-Value
	Mean ± SD	Median (Range)	Mean ± SD	Median (Range)	Mean ± SD	Median (Range)	NSCLC Alive vs. Dead	NSCLC Alive vs. Healthy Volunteers	NSCLC Dead vs. Healthy Volunteers
sTLR2 [ng/mL]	5.27 ± 4.0	4.28 (3.1–6.0)	10.98 ± 7.47	8.67 (1.17–28.46)	2.5 ± 1.0	2.63 (1.7–3.3)	<0.0001 *	<0.0001 *	<0.0001 *
sTLR3 [ng/mL]	7.21 ± 0.1	7.18 (7.1–7.3)	9.62 ± 2.56	8.65 (7.3–17.48)	1.57 ± 0.8	1.47 (1.0–2.1)	<0.0001 *	<0.0001 *	<0.0001 *
sTLR4 [ng/mL]	4.47 ± 0.6	4.68 (4.2–4.8)	10.37 ± 4.79	8.63 (4.03–23.57)	3.03 ± 0.7	3.26 (2.6–3.5)	<0.0001 *	<0.0001 *	<0.0001 *
sTLR7 [ng/mL]	5.32 ± 0.2	5.25 (5.2–5.4)	7.65 ± 2.31	7.14 (5.71–14.86)	1.07 ± 0.6	1.07 (0.6–1.5)	<0.0001 *	<0.0001 *	<0.0001 *
sTLR8 [ng/mL]	6.13 ± 0.7	6.09 (5.6–6.5)	9.97 ± 2.10	9.47 (5.99–17.86)	0.97 ± 0.6	1.01 (0.4–1.5)	<0.0001 *	<0.0001 *	<0.0001 *
sTLR9 [ng/mL]	5.41 ± 2.2	5.02 (3.8–6.5)	14.61 ± 7.5	14.07 (1.30–31.70)	3.1 ± 0.6	3.21 (2.7–3.6)	<0.0001 *	<0.0001 *	<0.0001 *

The symbol * denotes statistically significant results. Abbreviations: sTLR—soluble form of Toll-like receptors.

Due to the high mortality of patients included in the study and their diversity in terms of stage, we decided to analyze the data obtained regarding the percentage of TLRs tested on selected T and B lymphocyte subpopulations in the context of their changes at the time of recruitment and the death of patients. For this purpose, we selected only a small group of patients with stages IA, IIIB, IIIC, and IV, because all patients did not survive the 5-year follow-up period. In the case of the remaining groups analyzed at the stage, a small percentage of patients survived the observation period; therefore, the comparison of entire groups is significantly difficult because, due to changes in the number of individual groups of patients, the obtained results may have low statistical significance. In the case of the groups selected for this analysis, detailed data were collected and are presented in tabular form (Tables 6–9).

Table 6. Analysis of the TLR results obtained in patients with stage IA at the time of recruitment and death.

Parameters	Results of Tested TLRs for Patients with IA at Recruitment	Results of Tested TLRs for IA Patients Who Died	p-Value
	Median (Range)	Median (Range)	
T CD4+TLR2+ [%]	2.48 (1.43–5.11)	2.67 (2.30–4.64)	0.885
T CD8+TLR2+ [%]	4.44 (2.45–6.59)	5.28 (2.79–5.69)	0.685
B CD19+TLR2+ [%]	4.21 (3.92–7.45)	6.55 (5.20–12.72)	0.200
T CD4+TLR3+ [%]	2.27 (2.07–2.51)	2.55 (1.95–2.95)	0.485
T CD8+TLR3+ [%]	1.96 (1.50–2.16)	2.17 (1.99–2.62)	0.200
B CD19+TLR3+ [%]	2.49 (2.45–2.54)	2.20 (2.15–2.64)	0.342
T CD4+TLR4+ [%]	3.18 (3.16–9.45)	5.66 (5.44–6.76)	0.342
T CD8+TLR4+ [%]	4.42 (2.47–11.91)	7.81 (4.77–10.01)	0.485
B CD19+TLR4+ [%]	3.93 (3.18–10.59)	4.55 (3.61–5.39)	0.885
T CD4+TLR7+ [%]	1.63 (1.57–1.79)	1.65 (1.61–1.90)	0.685
T CD8+TLR7+ [%]	1.82 (1.78–1.90)	2.08 (2.04–3.26)	0.028 *
B CD19+TLR7+ [%]	2.37 (2.28–2.40)	2.37 (2.32–2.74)	0.685
T CD4+TLR8+ [%]	3.54 (3.47–3.66)	3.13 (3.06–3.99)	0.342
T CD8+TLR8+ [%]	1.91 (1.86–2.04)	1.54 (1.39–1.97)	0.200
B CD19+TLR8+ [%]	2.32 (2.10–2.43)	1.77 (1.55–2.31)	0.114
T CD4+TLR9+ [%]	4.08 (3.22–10.42)	6.36 (5.92–17.76)	0.200
T CD8+TLR9+ [%]	6.00 (4.77–8.55)	9.75 (7.72–11.34)	0.057
B CD19+TLR9+ [%]	7.77 (7.15–9.16)	8.29 (6.58–21.26)	0.685
sTLR2 [ng/mL]	4.02 (0.80–18.33)	9.41 (7.71–14.25)	0.342
sTLR3 [ng/mL]	6.56 (6.35–7.34)	7.64 (7.56–8.09)	0.028 *
sTLR4 [ng/mL]	4.32 (2.74–8.03)	7.97 (7.23–12.79)	0.200
sTLR7 [ng/mL]	5.09 (5.05–5.14)	5.88 (5.76–6.54)	0.028 *
sTLR8 [ng/mL]	6.49 (6.26–6.68)	8.36 (7.91–11.63)	0.028 *
sTLR9 [ng/mL]	9.25 (8.21–16.46)	15.49 (6.65–19.87)	0.485

The symbol * denotes statistically significant results. Abbreviations: CD—cluster of differentiation; TLR—Toll-like receptors; sTLR—soluble form of Toll-like receptors.

Table 7. Analysis of the TLR results obtained in patients with stage IIIB at the time of recruitment and death.

Parameters	Results of Tested TLRs for Patients with IIIB at Recruitment	Results of Tested TLRs for IIIB Patients Who Died	p-Value
	Median (Range)	Median (Range)	
T CD4+TLR2+ [%]	2.73 (1.51–13.97)	5.62 (2.15–12.70)	0.001 *
T CD8+TLR2+ [%]	3.90 (2.60–9.08)	8.47 (3.17–21.93)	0.000 *

Table 7. Cont.

Parameters	Results of Tested TLRs for Patients with IIIB at Recruitment	Results of Tested TLRs for IIIB Patients Who Died	p-Value
	Median (Range)	Median (Range)	
B CD19+TLR2+ [%]	4.04 (3.07–12.29)	5.87 (4.11–15.71)	0.001 *
T CD4+TLR3+ [%]	1.67 (1.33–3.34)	2.68 (2.06–4.31)	0.000 *
T CD8+TLR3+ [%]	1.71 (1.41–2.16)	2.74 (1.64–3.92)	0.000 *
B CD19+TLR3+ [%]	1.75 (1.46–3.00)	3.16 (2.12–3.93)	0.000 *
T CD4+TLR4+ [%]	3.95 (2.46–9.02)	6.55 (4.60–12.70)	0.000 *
T CD8+TLR4+ [%]	5.41 (3.02–11.59)	7.82 (5.46–17.73)	0.001 *
B CD19+TLR4+ [%]	4.04 (2.58–16.50)	6.81 (3.81–15.21)	0.000 *
T CD4+TLR7+ [%]	1.24 (0.99–2.37)	2.15 (1.42–2.88)	0.000 *
T CD8+TLR7+ [%]	1.80 (0.90–2.56)	2.85 (1.22–3.57)	0.000 *
B CD19+TLR7+ [%]	1.75 (1.54–2.70)	3.08 (2.24–3.77)	0.000 *
T CD4+TLR8+ [%]	2.55 (2.03–4.37)	4.71 (2.96–5.64)	0.000 *
T CD8+TLR8+ [%]	1.24 (0.92–2.56)	2.35 (1.30–3.79)	0.000 *
B CD19+TLR8+ [%]	1.43 (0.99–2.91)	2.64 (1.35–3.92)	0.000 *
T CD4+TLR9+ [%]	4.82 (1.77–14.26)	7.05 (2.60–14.03)	0.621
T CD8+TLR9+ [%]	5.05 (3.13–13.63)	6.91 (3.79–18.30)	0.087
B CD19+TLR9+ [%]	7.55 (4.42–22.99)	8.46 (6.54–32.35)	0.117
sTLR2 [ng/mL]	5.67 (2.60–17.69)	5.64 (2.48–25.20)	0.695
sTLR3 [ng/mL]	5.45 (5.09–11.65)	8.69 (7.48–13.49)	0.000 *
sTLR4 [ng/mL]	5.38 (3.43–12.35)	8.50 (4.21–21.46)	0.000 *
sTLR7 [ng/mL]	4.34 (3.91–10.10)	7.16 (5.71–10.56)	0.000 *
sTLR8 [ng/mL]	5.86 (4.07–10.46)	9.47 (8.41–11.92)	0.000 *
sTLR9 [ng/mL]	10.01 (3.45–19.60)	11.00 (3.33–27.83)	0.824

The symbol * denotes statistically significant results. Abbreviations: CD—cluster of differentiation; TLR—Toll-like receptors; sTLR—soluble form of Toll-like receptors.

Table 8. Analysis of the TLR results obtained in patients with stage IIIC at the time of recruitment and death.

Parameters	Results of Tested TLRs for Patients with IIIC at Recruitment	Results of Tested TLRs for IIIC Patients Who Died	p-Value
	Median (Range)	Median (Range)	
T CD4+TLR2+ [%]	3.18 (2.46–3.36)	8.35 (5.29–12.31)	0.041 *
T CD8+TLR2+ [%]	6.05 (3.39–6.38)	9.19 (8.09–11.21)	0.041 *
B CD19+TLR2+ [%]	4.10 (3.25–8.07)	14.36 (12.16–15.82)	0.021 *
T CD4+TLR3+ [%]	1.83 (1.51–1.84)	3.90 (3.09–4.25)	0.041 *
T CD8+TLR3+ [%]	1.84 (1.54–1.84)	3.09 (2.96–3.98)	0.041 *
B CD19+TLR3+ [%]	1.87 (1.64–1.90)	3.79 (2.92–3.92)	0.041 *
T CD4+TLR4+ [%]	4.91 (3.36–6.43)	8.29 (7.93–16.71)	0.041 *
T CD8+TLR4+ [%]	5.30 (4.72–9.38)	13.67 (12.58–17.27)	0.031 *
B CD19+TLR4+ [%]	4.35 (4.32–5.57)	4.26 (4.20–15.96)	0.041 *
T CD4+TLR7+ [%]	1.32 (1.22–1.35)	2.74 (2.04–2.84)	0.041 *
T CD8+TLR7+ [%]	2.23 (1.54–2.34)	3.22 (2.95–3.51)	0.041 *
B CD19+TLR7+ [%]	1.91 (1.73–1.92)	3.66 (2.88–3.76)	0.041 *
T CD4+TLR8+ [%]	2.75 (2.30–2.84)	5.43 (4.28–5.57)	0.041 *
T CD8+TLR8+ [%]	1.40 (1.18–1.41)	3.28 (2.19–3.79)	0.041 *
B CD19+TLR8+ [%]	1.60 (1.37–1.62)	3.65 (2.43–3.90)	0.041 *

Table 8. Cont.

Parameters	Results of Tested TLRs for Patients with IIIC at Recruitment	Results of Tested TLRs for IIIC Patients Who Died	p-Value
	Median (Range)	Median (Range)	
T CD4+TLR9+ [%]	2.78 (2.32–6.36)	12.62 (12.43–15.69)	0.020 *
T CD8+TLR9+ [%]	4.58 (3.42–8.30)	14.05 (12.27–15.19)	0.031 *
B CD19+TLR9+ [%]	5.03 (4.67–14.59)	31.62 (15.05–32.57)	0.001 *
sTLR2 [ng/mL]	2.65 (1.93–12.05)	22.96 (20.32–24.46)	0.001 *
sTLR3 [ng/mL]	5.54 (5.39–5.56)	11.44 (8.45–13.46)	0.041 *
sTLR4 [ng/mL]	5.51 (2.86–6.08)	17.76 (17.44–18.74)	0.031 *
sTLR7 [ng/mL]	4.49 (4.25–7.18)	7.59 (6.84–7.87)	0.041 *
sTLR8 [ng/mL]	5.81 (5.75–5.86)	8.82 (8.73–11.19)	0.041 *
sTLR9 [ng/mL]	3.57 (2.72–15.90)	23.06 (22.18–25.31)	0.020 *

The symbol * denotes statistically significant results. Abbreviations: CD—cluster of differentiation; TLR—Toll-like receptors; sTLR—soluble form of Toll-like receptors.

Table 9. Analysis of the TLR results obtained in patients with stage IV at the time of recruitment and death.

Parameters	Results of Tested TLRs for Patients with IV at Recruitment	Results of Tested TLRs for IV Patients Who Died	p-Value
	Median (Range)	Median (Range)	
T CD4+TLR2+ [%]	2.03 (1.09–3.53)	7.35 (2.10–21.02)	0.000 *
T CD8+TLR2+ [%]	3.41 (1.69–10.64)	8.35 (3.61–19.25)	0.000 *
B CD19+TLR2+ [%]	3.74 (0.90–10.32)	7.33 (3.96–17.63)	0.000 *
T CD4+TLR3+ [%]	1.31 (0.73–2.05)	2.81 (1.98–4.85)	0.000 *
T CD8+TLR3+ [%]	1.24 (0.61–1.78)	2.97 (2.02–3.83)	0.000 *
B CD19+TLR3+ [%]	1.37 (0.69–1.79)	3.39 (2.15–4.41)	0.000 *
T CD4+TLR4+ [%]	3.70 (1.67–9.06)	6.95 (4.16–17.39)	0.000 *
T CD8+TLR4+ [%]	4.58 (1.47–7.77)	7.62 (4.65–18.80)	0.000 *
B CD19+TLR4+ [%]	3.74 (2.45–8.86)	6.82 (4.07–25.13)	0.000 *
T CD4+TLR7+ [%]	0.99 (0.70–1.29)	2.28 (1.56–2.97)	0.000 *
T CD8+TLR7+ [%]	1.21 (0.72–2.22)	2.66 (1.33–4.47)	0.000 *
B CD19+TLR7+ [%]	1.51 (1.36–1.86)	3.35 (2.27–4.01)	0.000 *
T CD4+TLR8+ [%]	1.91 (1.52–2.71)	5.04 (2.98–5.99)	0.000 *
T CD8+TLR8+ [%]	0.86 (0.10–1.34)	2.67 (1.36–4.08)	0.000 *
B CD19+TLR8+ [%]	0.86 (0.69–1.57)	2.98 (0.00–4.21)	0.000 *
T CD4+TLR9+ [%]	4.13 (1.37–12.08)	6.41 (2.65–21.30)	0.000 *
T CD8+TLR9+ [%]	4.36 (0.80–7.71)	8.85 (4.17–20.59)	0.000 *
B CD19+TLR9+ [%]	4.47 (1.18–14.46)	11.59 (6.50–38.17)	0.000 *
sTLR2 [ng/mL]	4.33 (1.37–13.12)	8.98 (1.17–28.46)	0.000 *
sTLR3 [ng/mL]	5.02 (4.81–5.50)	9.16 (7.49–17.48)	0.000 *
sTLR4 [ng/mL]	3.29 (2.14–8.69)	8.26 (4.03–23.57)	0.000 *
sTLR7 [ng/mL]	3.79 (3.52–4.45)	7.41 (5.75–14.86)	0.000 *
sTLR8 [ng/mL]	4.45 (3.49–7.91)	9.96 (5.99–17.04)	0.000 *
sTLR9 [ng/mL]	4.52 (2.00–13.51)	14.04 (1.30–31.70)	0.000 *

The symbol * denotes statistically significant results. Abbreviations: CD—cluster of differentiation; TLR—Toll-like receptors; sTLR—soluble form of Toll-like receptors.

As we can see in Table 6, among patients with stage IA, statistically significant changes in the percentage of the tested TLRs concerned T CD8+ TLR7+ and serum concentrations of sTLR3, sTLR7, and sTLR8 between the moment of recruitment and the death of the patients. We noted much more significant correlations for stage IIIB patients, where almost all results, except the percentage of TLR9 on T and B lymphocytes and serum sTLR2 and sTLR9 concentrations, were significantly higher at the time of patients' death than at the time of recruitment (Table 7). In patients with stages IIIC and IV, all observed changes in TLRs tested on immune cells and their serum concentrations of soluble forms were significantly higher at the time of death than at the time of recruitment of NSCLC patients to this study (Tables 8 and 9). Due to the extremely small sample size in the relevant stages, these results should be replicated with a much larger sample size in the relevant stages. However, the results obtained from this analysis present interesting relationships that should be further explored and understood.

3.3. Correlation Analysis and ROC (Receiver Operating Characteristic) Curve of Dead NSCLC and Alive NSCLC Patients

Next, we performed a Spearman rank correlation analysis for dead NSCLC and alive NSCLC patients. Details are provided in Supplementary Materials Tables S9 and S10, and Figure 7A,B.

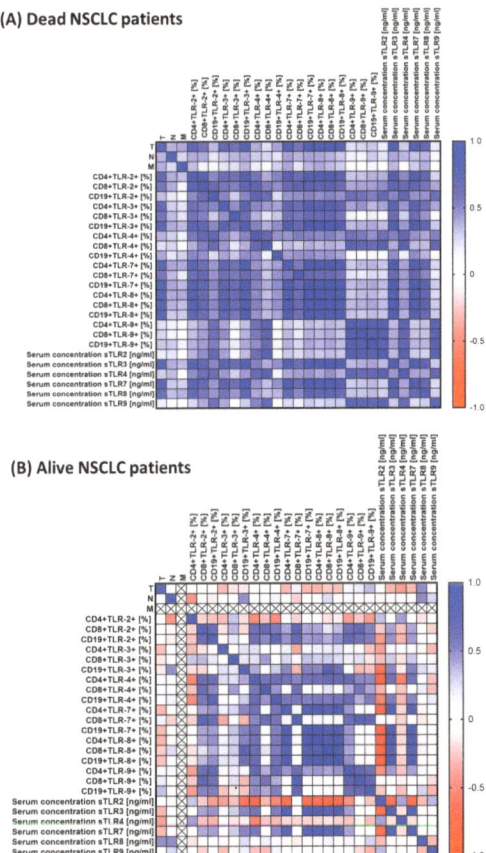

Figure 7. Graphical representation of Spearman rank correlations obtained for NSCLC dead (**A**) and NSCLC alive (**B**) patients. Positive correlations are marked in blue, while negative correlations are marked in red. The differentiation of shades of the mentioned colors is equivalent to the level of correlation. By positive correlations, we mean that as one parameter increases, the values of the other parameter increase, while by negative correlations we mean that as the value of one parameter increases, the values of the other parameter decrease. Abbreviations: CD—cluster of differentiation; TLR—Toll-like receptors; sTLR—soluble form of Toll-like receptors.

In dead NSCLC patients, we can observe nearly 170 positive correlations, of which 66 were moderate, 61 were high, and 43 very high. Among the NSCLC patients alive, we recorded 80 statistically significant correlations, of which 11 were negative (1 very high, 6 high, and 4 moderate) and 69 positive (24 very high, 26 high, and 19 moderate).

Due to such an important role of TLR disorders in the course of NSCLC, it seemed important to assess the prognostic value of the tested receptors in the context of mortality in NSCLC patients. The obtained test results are presented in Table 10 and Figures 7–9. The most sensitive markers of poor prognosis in NSCLC patients were: sTLR3, sTLR7, and CD4+TLR8+, as well as CD19+TLR7+.

Table 10. ROC prognostic analysis.

Factor	Parameter [%]	Prognostic Value	Youden Index	Area under the Curve (AUC)	95% CI	p-Value
Fatal prognosis of NSCLS patients	CD4+TLR2+ T cells [%]	5.27	0.55	0.814	0.72–0.91	<0.0001 *
	CD8+TLR2+ T cells [%]	6.03	0.3	0.60	0.43–0.77	0.26
	CD19+TLR2+ B cells [%]	5.18	0.54	0.734	0.56–0.91	0.0078 *
	CD4+TLR3+ T cells [%]	1.95	0.81	0.924	0.84–1.0	<0.0001 *
	CD8+TLR3+ T cells [%]	2.11	0.93	0.993	0.98–1.0	<0.0001 *
	CD19+TLR3+ B cells [%]	2.15	0.99	0.999	0.996–1.0	<0.0001 *
	CD4+TLR4+ T cells [%]	4.45	0.47	0.69	0.5–0.88	0.052
	CD8+TLR4+ T cells [%]	4.77	0.51	0.79	0.66–0.92	<0.0001 *
	CD19+TLR4+ B cells [%]	13.5	0.15	0.51	0.35–0.68	0.86
	CD4+TLR7+ T cells [%]	1.56	0.97	0.994	0.98–1.0	<0.0001 *
	CD8+TLR7+ T cells [%]	2.04	0.96	0.979	0.95–1.0	<0.0001 *
	CD19+TLR7+ B cells [%]	2.24	1.00	1.0	1.0	<0.0001 *
	CD4+TLR8+ T cells [%]	2.98	0.99	1.0	0.998–1.0	<0.0001 *
	CD8+TLR8+ T cells [%]	1.36	0.99	0.999	0.995–1.0	<0.0001 *
	CD19+TLR8+ B cells [%]	1.35	0.99	0.986	0.96–1.0	<0.0001 *
	CD4+TLR9+ T cells [%]	4.22	0.42	0.74	0.61–0.87	0.0003 *
	CD8+TLR9+ T cells [%]	6.69	0.57	0.85	0.74–0.95	<0.0001 *
	CD19+TLR9+ B cells [%]	5.52	0.81	0.90	0.79–1.0	<0.0001 *
	sTLR2 [ng/mL]	6.89	0.57	0.79	0.67–0.91	<0.0001 *
	sTLR3 [ng/mL]	7.48	1.00	1.0	1.0	<0.0001 *
	sTLR4 [ng/mL]	5.50	0.95	0.97	0.93–1.0	<0.0001 *
	sTLR7 [ng/mL]	5.71	1.0	1.0	1.0	<0.0001 *
	sTLR8 [ng/mL]	7.83	0.92	0.985	0.965–1.0	<0.0001 *
	sTLR9 [ng/mL]	11.46	0.69	0.87	0.80–0.95	<0.0001 *

The symbol * denotes statistically significant results.

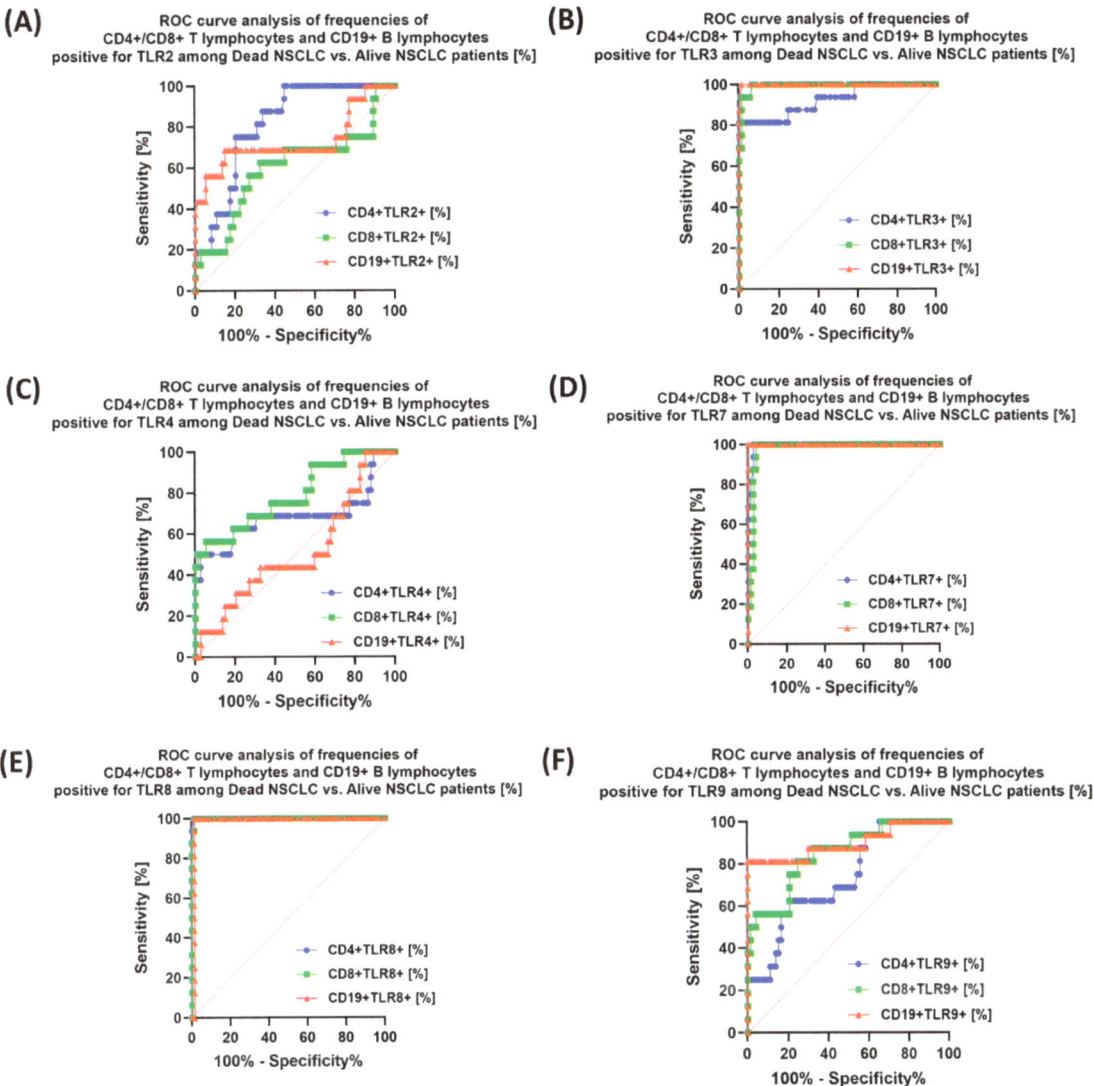

Figure 8. Graphical representation of the ROC analysis of selected immunophenotype parameters of dead NSCLC and alive NSCLC patients: (**A**) ROC curve for TLR2-positive lymphocyte percentage; (**B**) ROC curve for the percentage of TLR3-positive lymphocytes; (**C**) ROC curve for the percentage of TLR4-positive lymphocytes; (**D**) ROC curve for the percentage of TLR7-positive lymphocytes; (**E**) ROC curve for the percentage of TLR8-positive lymphocytes; (**F**) ROC curve for the percentage of TLR9-positive lymphocytes. Abbreviations: CD—cluster of differentiation; TLR—Toll-like receptors; ROC—Receiver Operating Characteristic.

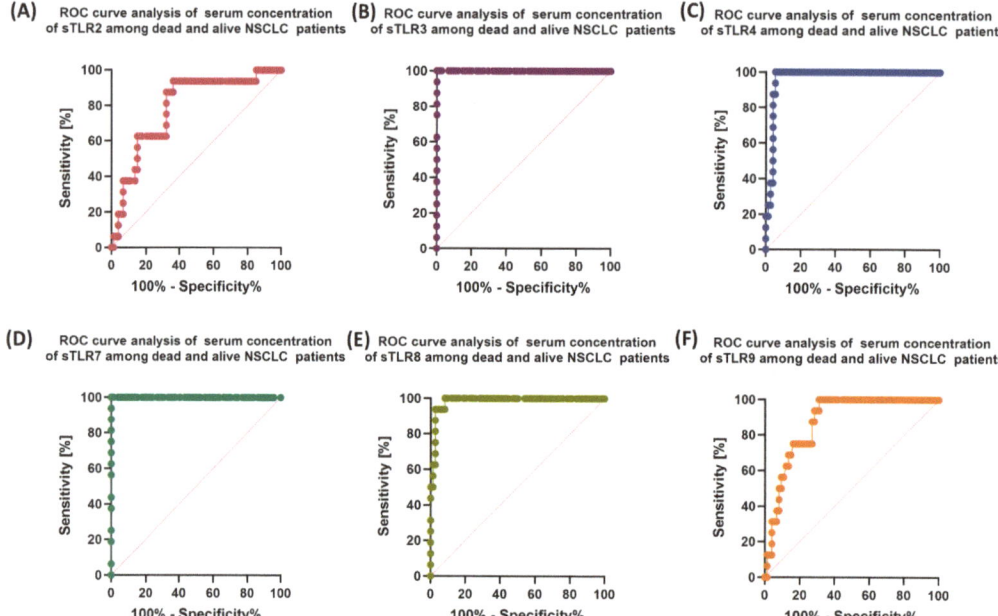

Figure 9. Graphical representation of ROC analysis of dissolved TLR concentrations for dead NSCLC and alive NSCLC patients: (**A**) ROC curve for sTLR2; (**B**) ROC curve for sTLR3; (**C**) ROC curve for sTLR4; (**D**) ROC curve for sTLR7; (**E**) ROC curve for sTLR8; (**F**) ROC curve for sTLR9. Abbreviations: sTLR—soluble form of Toll-like receptors; ROC—Receiver Operating Characteristic.

4. Discussion

The research results presented in this publication reflect, to some extent, the state of diagnostics and medical care not only in Poland but also around the world. The average age of patients participating in the study was 72 years, which correlates with statistical data on patients from Poland, for whom the average age is from 70 to 75 years. This indicates that the study is representative of the demographics of NSCLC patients in Poland but does not differ much from global data, where the average age of patients is over 65 years. The majority of NSCLC patients in our study were men, which is consistent with the generally higher risk of lung cancer in men. Moreover, a significant percentage of patients were in an advanced stage of the disease (32 people in stage III and 25 in stage IV), which emphasizes the need for deeper diagnostics and faster detection of this disease. Patients suffered symptoms such as chronic cough, hoarseness, chest pain, and general weakness. Additionally, 70% of patients had infections of the upper and lower respiratory tract requiring antibiotic therapy in the year preceding diagnosis, which may indicate negligence in earlier diagnosis. Virtually all patients (97%) admitted to smoking cigarettes, with an average number of pack-years of 35.66. This indicates a strong association between smoking and the development of NSCLC. Of course, this is in line with global trends, where the relationship between smoking and the development of NSCLC is well known. Moreover, studies indicate that mortality in patients who smoked was higher than mortality in never-smokers, and current smoking was an independent risk factor for worse prognosis. In our study, only three people declared that they did not smoke cigarettes (moreover, they were in IB). The expression of the tested TLRs in these patients was lower than in the remaining recruited people, but the sample size was too small to indicate statistically significant differences.

The study found that NSCLC patients had a higher prevalence of all tested TLRs (TLR2, TLR3, TLR4, TLR7, TLR8, TLR9) in peripheral blood lymphocyte subpopulations compared to healthy volunteers. This indicates a possible role of these receptors in the pathogenesis or immune response to NSCLC. Analysis of the levels of soluble forms of TLRs (sTLRs) in serum confirmed their higher concentrations in patients with NSCLC, which additionally suggests their potential importance in the dynamics of the disease.

Our results are consistent with the literature data that confirm the involvement of TLRs in the pathogenesis of lung cancer. Much of the literature consistently shows that TLRs are expressed in NSCLC tissues, and cell lines TLR expression levels were found to be higher in NSCLC compared to healthy lung tissues. This suggests that TLRs play a role in developing and maintaining NSCLC [26,27]. TLR signaling pathways are involved in promoting cancer cell proliferation, invasion, and metastasis [8,28,29]. Activation of TLRs in NSCLC cells leads to upregulation of pro-inflammatory cytokines and chemokines (TNF-α or CCL2), contributing to the immunosuppressive nature of the tumor microenvironment [30–36]. TLRs (especially TLR4) have been shown to influence immune evasion mechanisms in NSCLC. Cancer cells can use TLR signaling to suppress anticancer immune responses, leading to a reduced ability of the immune system to recognize and eliminate cancer cells [37,38]. Targeting TLR signaling pathways has emerged as a potential therapeutic strategy for NSCLC. Preclinical studies have explored the use of TLR agonists and antagonists to modulate the immune response and enhance the effectiveness of treatments such as chemotherapy and immunotherapy [39–42]. Studies have shown that TLR expression profiles can influence the response to specific therapies in NSCLC. For example, TLR activation has been linked to resistance to certain chemotherapeutic agents, while TLR modulation has been shown to make cancer cells more sensitive to immunotherapies [43].

High expression of TLR4 has been associated with resistance to cisplatin, a commonly used chemotherapy drug in NSCLC. TLR4 activation in cancer cells can promote the upregulation of anti-apoptotic proteins and DNA repair mechanisms. leading to reduced sensitivity to cisplatin-induced cell death [44,45]. TLR7 is similarly affected, which is responsible for promoting tumor progression, resistance to chemotherapy, and, as the study indicates, poor clinical results [46]. On the other hand, TLR3 expression has been linked to increased sensitivity to chemotherapy in NSCLC. TLR3 activation in cancer cells can enhance the production of pro-apoptotic proteins and increase the susceptibility of tumor cells to chemotherapeutic agents [29,47]. Combining TLR-targeted therapies with other treatments, such as checkpoint inhibitors, has shown promising results in preclinical models. This approach aims to harness the immunomodulatory effects of TLRs to enhance the anticancer immune response and improve treatment outcomes [27,48–50].

The research results we presented show how the expression of the tested TLRs changes over time in individual patients depending on the stage of disease advancement. The statistically significant differences demonstrated between the percentage of tested TLRs and the concentration of their soluble forms in patients who survived the 5-year observation period were significantly lower than in patients who died. In the case of immunophenotyping tests, these differences were: 2.23-fold (CD4+TLR2+); 1.20-fold (CD8+TLR2+) and 1.37-fold (CD19+TLR2+); 1.75-fold (CD4+TLR3+); 1.92-fold (CD8+TLR3+) and 1.97-fold (CD19+TLR3+); 1.23-fold (CD4+TLR4+); 1.79-fold (CD8+TLR4+) and 1.16-fold (CD19+TLR4+); 1.82-fold (CD4+TLR7+); 1.91-fold (CD8+TLR7+) and 1.51-fold (CD19+TLR7+); 1.78-fold (CD4+TLR8+); 3.02-fold (CD8+TLR8+) and 2.5-fold (CD19+TLR8+); 1.77-fold (CD4+TLR9+); 1.97-fold (CD8+TLR9+) and 2.81-fold (CD19+TLR9+). However, in the case of serum concentrations of the tested TLRs, these differences were higher by 2.08 times (sTLR2), respectively; 1.33-fold (sTLR3); 2.32-fold (sTLR4); 1.44-fold (sTLR7); 1.63-fold (sTLR8); 2.70 times (sTLR9). Despite the limitations of this study, TLR expression on different lymphocyte subpopulations (such as CD4+, CD8+, and CD19+) may influence the way the immune system recognizes and responds to cancer cells. TLRs may promote the formation of a tumor microenvironment by inducing proinflammatory cytokines, which may support tumor cell growth and survival. Our results suggest that higher TLR expressions are associated with poorer survival, which may reflect their role in promoting cancer progression. Moreover, some TLRs can also induce apoptosis of cancer cells. Reduced TLR expression in the group of patients with better survival may indicate that, in their case, the body's defense mechanisms were more effective in eliminating cancer cells. Additionally, as the literature data suggest, different TLRs may differentiate the immune response, e.g., by activating different types of T cells (CD4+, CD8+) and B cells (CD19+). In the case of our results, higher TLR expressions may be associated with a more aggressive or ineffective immune response, leading to worse survival outcomes. However, our studies also indicate the need for further research into the mechanisms regulating their expression and function in the context of lung cancer.

Our research is currently a pilot study and was conducted on a relatively small group of patients, which may significantly affect the aspects of TLR testing that are insufficient for clinical inclusion. However, among the obtained results, the analysis of ROC curves of NSCLC patients who did not survive the study period compared to living patients showed the highest sensitivity only for the expression of TLR7 and TLR8 on selected subpopulations of T and B lymphocytes, as well as TLR3 on B lymphocytes, in the remaining cases' sensitivity, and the specificity of the tested TLRs was not that promising. These observations were also confirmed in the analysis of soluble forms of TLRs, for which the highest sensitivity concerned TLR3, TLR7, and TLR8. The results, although interesting and perhaps too optimistic, are only a small selection of the analyses that need to be performed to be able to include TLRs in the diagnosis of NSCLC. We hope that this research will also inspire other researchers to consider more detailed studies that will allow the involvement of TLRs as biomarker molecules in the future.

In summary, studies on the role of TLRs in NSCLC have shown significant effects on tumor progression, immune evasion, and treatment response. The findings suggest that TLRs serve as potential prognostic markers and therapeutic targets in NSCLC, opening up new avenues for precision medicine and tailored interventions to improve patient outcomes. However further research and clinical trials are needed to confirm the clinical usefulness of TLR targeting in treating NSCLC.

5. Conclusions

In conclusion, this comprehensive study's findings highlight the critical role of TLR expression in NSCLC and its potential as an independent prognostic biomarker. The analysis of NSCLC patient cohorts and healthy volunteers revealed statistically significant differences in TLR expression, indicating the involvement of TLRs in the pathogenesis of the disease. The implications of these findings are substantial, as they provide valuable insights into the complex interplay between TLR expression and NSCLC progression. Identifying potential prognostic markers holds promise for enhancing risk stratification and guiding personalized treatment approaches, ultimately leading to improved clinical management and patient outcomes.

It is important to acknowledge some limitations of this study, including the small sample size and potential confounding factors that may impact TLR expression. Thus, further validation through larger prospective studies is warranted to solidify the clinical utility of these TLR markers in NSCLC management.

Nonetheless, the results presented pave the way for future research into the molecular mechanisms underlying TLR involvement in NSCLC and open new avenues for targeted therapeutic interventions. The elucidation of TLR-related pathways and their impact on immune response and tumor microenvironment may offer novel opportunities for developing tailored immunotherapies and combination treatments.

Overall, this study contributes valuable evidence to the growing knowledge surrounding TLR expression in NSCLC and highlights its potential significance as an independent prognostic biomarker. These findings serve as a foundation for advancing precision medicine in NSCLC, aiming to improve patient stratification and treatment efficacy while fostering the development of innovative therapeutic strategies to combat this devastating disease.

Supplementary Materials: The following supporting information can be downloaded at: https://www.mdpi.com/article/10.3390/jcm13102793/s1, Table S1. Selected parameters of morphology, biochemistry, and immunophenotype of NSCLC patients after one year of observation, taking into account their survival status. Table S2. Analysis of the percentage of TLRs tested on selected subpopulations of peripheral blood lymphocytes and their serum concentration in NSCLC patients after one year of observation, taking into account their survival status. Table S3. Selected parameters of morphology, biochemistry, and immunophenotype of NSCLC patients after two years of observation, taking into account their survival status. Table S4. Analysis of the percentage of TLRs tested on selected subpopulations of peripheral blood lymphocytes and their serum concentration in NSCLC patients after two years of observation, taking into account their survival status. Table S5. Selected parameters of morphology, biochemistry, and immunophenotype of NSCLC patients after three years of observation, taking into account their survival status. Table S6. Analysis of the percentage of TLRs tested on selected subpopulations of peripheral blood lymphocytes and their serum concentration in NSCLC patients after three years of observation, taking into account their survival status. Table S7. Selected parameters of morphology, biochemistry, and immunophenotype of NSCLC patients after four years of observation, taking into account their survival status. Table S8. Analysis of the percentage of TLRs tested on selected subpopulations of peripheral blood lymphocytes and their serum concentration in NSCLC patients after four years of observation, taking into account their survival status. Table S9. Spearman rank correlation analysis for dead NSCLC patients. Table S10. Spearman rank correlation analysis for alive NSCLC patients.

Author Contributions: Conceptualization, P.M., J.S.-K. and E.G.; methodology, P.M. and S.M.; software, P.M. and S.M.; validation, P.M. and S.M.; formal analysis, P.M. and I.K.-G.; investigation, P.M., S.M. and J.S.-K.; resources, J.S.-K. and S.G.; data curation, P.M. and S.M.; writing—original draft preparation, P.M. and S.M. writing—review and editing, J.S.-K., W.K., I.K.-G. and E.G.; visualization, P.M. and S.M.; supervision, E.G., J.S.-K. and S.G.; funding acquisition E.G. and W.K. All authors have read and agreed to the published version of the manuscript.

Funding: This research was supported by the Medical University of Lublin grant no. DS128 and DS127.

Institutional Review Board Statement: The study protocol was approved by the Bioethics Committee at the esteemed Medical University of Lublin under reference number KE-0254/283/2015 (approved on 15 January 2015).

Informed Consent Statement: Informed consent was obtained from all subjects involved in the study.

Data Availability Statement: All necessary information regarding the preparation of this work is available upon written request from the corresponding author.

Conflicts of Interest: The authors declare no conflicts of interest. The funders had no role in the study's design or collection, analyses, or interpretation of data; in the writing of the manuscript; or in the decision to publish the results.

References

1. Molina, J.R.; Yang, P.; Cassivi, S.D.; Schild, S.E.; Adjei, A.A. Non–Small Cell Lung Cancer: Epidemiology, Risk Factors, Treatment, and Survivorship. *Mayo Clin. Proc.* **2008**, *83*, 584–594. [CrossRef] [PubMed]
2. Schabath, M.B.; Cote, M.L. Cancer Progress and Priorities: Lung Cancer. *Cancer Epidemiol. Biomark. Prev.* **2019**, *28*, 1563–1579. [CrossRef] [PubMed]
3. Mithoowani, H.; Febbraro, M. Non-Small-Cell Lung Cancer in 2022: A Review for General Practitioners in Oncology. *Curr. Oncol.* **2022**, *29*, 1828–1839. [CrossRef] [PubMed]
4. Tang, Y.; Qiao, G.; Xu, E.; Xuan, Y.; Liao, M.; Yin, G. Biomarkers for Early Diagnosis, Prognosis, Prediction, and Recurrence Monitoring of Non-Small Cell Lung Cancer. *Onco Targets Ther.* **2017**, *10*, 4527–4534. [CrossRef] [PubMed]
5. Balata, H.; Fong, K.M.; Hendriks, L.E.; Lam, S.; Ostroff, J.S.; Peled, N.; Wu, N.; Aggarwal, C. Prevention and Early Detection for NSCLC: Advances in Thoracic Oncology 2018. *J. Thorac. Oncol.* **2019**, *14*, 1513–1527. [CrossRef] [PubMed]
6. Shcheblyakov, D.V.; Logunov, D.Y.; Tukhvatulin, A.I.; Shmarov, M.M.; Naroditsky, B.S.; Gintsburg, A.L. Toll-Like Receptors (TLRs): The Role in Tumor Progression. *Acta Naturae* **2010**, *2*, 21–29. [CrossRef]
7. Duan, T.; Du, Y.; Xing, C.; Wang, H.Y.; Wang, R.-F. Toll-Like Receptor Signaling and Its Role in Cell-Mediated Immunity. *Front. Immunol.* **2022**, *13*, 812774. [CrossRef] [PubMed]

8. Chen, X.; Zhang, Y.; Fu, Y. The Critical Role of Toll-like Receptor-Mediated Signaling in Cancer Immunotherapy. *Med. Drug Discov.* **2022**, *14*, 100122. [CrossRef]
9. Farooq, M.; Batool, M.; Kim, M.S.; Choi, S. Toll-Like Receptors as a Therapeutic Target in the Era of Immunotherapies. *Front. Cell Dev. Biol.* **2021**, *9*, 756315. [CrossRef] [PubMed]
10. Thompson, M.R.; Kaminski, J.J.; Kurt-Jones, E.A.; Fitzgerald, K.A. Pattern Recognition Receptors and the Innate Immune Response to Viral Infection. *Viruses* **2011**, *3*, 920–940. [CrossRef]
11. Akira, S.; Uematsu, S.; Takeuchi, O. Pathogen Recognition and Innate Immunity. *Cell* **2006**, *124*, 783–801. [CrossRef]
12. Liu, C.; Han, C.; Liu, J. The Role of Toll-Like Receptors in Oncotherapy. *Oncol. Res.* **2019**, *27*, 965–978. [CrossRef] [PubMed]
13. Yang, J.; Li, M.; Zheng, Q.C. Emerging Role of Toll-like Receptor 4 in Hepatocellular Carcinoma. *J. Hepatocell. Carcinoma* **2015**, *2*, 11–17. [CrossRef] [PubMed]
14. Giurini, E.F.; Madonna, M.B.; Zloza, A.; Gupta, K.H. Microbial-Derived Toll-like Receptor Agonism in Cancer Treatment and Progression. *Cancers* **2022**, *14*, 2923. [CrossRef] [PubMed]
15. Zhao, H.; Wu, L.; Yan, G.; Chen, Y.; Zhou, M.; Wu, Y.; Li, Y. Inflammation and Tumor Progression: Signaling Pathways and Targeted Intervention. *Signal Transduct. Target. Ther.* **2021**, *6*, 263. [CrossRef]
16. Du, B.; Jiang, Q.L.; Cleveland, J.; Liu, B.R.; Zhang, D. Targeting Toll-like Receptors against Cancer. *J. Cancer Metastasis Treat.* **2016**, *2*, 463–470. [CrossRef]
17. Liu, Y.; Gu, Y.; Han, Y.; Zhang, Q.; Jiang, Z.; Zhang, X.; Huang, B.; Xu, X.; Zheng, J.; Cao, X. Tumor Exosomal RNAs Promote Lung Pre-Metastatic Niche Formation by Activating Alveolar Epithelial TLR3 to Recruit Neutrophils. *Cancer Cell* **2016**, *30*, 243–256. [CrossRef]
18. Bianchi, F.; Alexiadis, S.; Camisaschi, C.; Truini, M.; Centonze, G.; Milione, M.; Balsari, A.; Tagliabue, E.; Sfondrini, L. TLR3 Expression Induces Apoptosis in Human Non-Small-Cell Lung Cancer. *Int. J. Mol. Sci.* **2020**, *21*, 1440. [CrossRef]
19. Zhang, Y.-B.; He, F.-L.; Fang, M.; Hua, T.-F.; Hu, B.-D.; Zhang, Z.-H.; Cao, Q.; Liu, R.-Y. Increased Expression of Toll-like Receptors 4 and 9 in Human Lung Cancer. *Mol. Biol. Rep.* **2009**, *36*, 1475–1481. [CrossRef]
20. Ren, T.; Xu, L.; Jiao, S.; Wang, Y.; Cai, Y.; Liang, Y.; Zhou, Y.; Zhou, H.; Wen, Z. TLR9 Signaling Promotes Tumor Progression of Human Lung Cancer Cell in Vivo. *Pathol. Oncol. Res.* **2009**, *15*, 623–630. [CrossRef]
21. Kell, S.A.; Kachura, M.A.; Renn, A.; Traquina, P.; Coffman, R.L.; Campbell, J.D. Preclinical Development of the TLR9 Agonist DV281 as an Inhaled Aerosolized Immunotherapeutic for Lung Cancer: Pharmacological Profile in Mice, Non-Human Primates, and Human Primary Cells. *Int. Immunopharmacol.* **2019**, *66*, 296–308. [CrossRef] [PubMed]
22. Wang, K.; Wang, J.; Wei, F.; Zhao, N.; Yang, F.; Ren, X. Expression of TLR4 in Non-Small Cell Lung Cancer Is Associated with PD-L1 and Poor Prognosis in Patients Receiving Pulmonectomy. *Front. Immunol.* **2017**, *8*, 456. [CrossRef]
23. Bauer, A.K.; Upham, B.L.; Rondini, E.A.; Tennis, M.A.; Velmuragan, K.; Wiese, D. Toll-like Receptor Expression in Human Non-Small Cell Lung Carcinoma: Potential Prognostic Indicators of Disease. *Oncotarget* **2017**, *8*, 91860–91875. [CrossRef]
24. Bianchi, F.; Milione, M.; Casalini, P.; Centonze, G.; Le Noci, V.M.; Storti, C.; Alexiadis, S.; Truini, M.; Sozzi, G.; Pastorino, U.; et al. Toll-like Receptor 3 as a New Marker to Detect High Risk Early Stage Non-Small-Cell Lung Cancer Patients. *Sci. Rep.* **2019**, *9*, 14288. [CrossRef]
25. Baranašić, J.; Šutić, M.; Catalano, C.; Drpa, G.; Huhn, S.; Majhen, D.; Nestić, D.; Kurtović, M.; Rumora, L.; Bosnar, M.; et al. TLR5 Variants Are Associated with the Risk for COPD and NSCLC Development, Better Overall Survival of the NSCLC Patients and Increased Chemosensitivity in the H1299 Cell Line. *Biomedicines* **2022**, *10*, 2240. [CrossRef] [PubMed]
26. Arora, S.; Ahmad, S.; Irshad, R.; Goyal, Y.; Rafat, S.; Siddiqui, N.; Dev, K.; Husain, M.; Ali, S.; Mohan, A.; et al. TLRs in Pulmonary Diseases. *Life Sci.* **2019**, *233*, 116671. [CrossRef] [PubMed]
27. Hoden, B.; DeRubeis, D.; Martinez-Moczygemba, M.; Ramos, K.S.; Zhang, D. Understanding the Role of Toll-like Receptors in Lung Cancer Immunity and Immunotherapy. *Front. Immunol.* **2022**, *13*, 1033483. [CrossRef] [PubMed]
28. Mokhtari, Y.; Pourbagheri-Sigaroodi, A.; Zafari, P.; Bagheri, N.; Ghaffari, S.H.; Bashash, D. Toll-like Receptors (TLRs): An Old Family of Immune Receptors with a New Face in Cancer Pathogenesis. *J. Cell. Mol. Med.* **2021**, *25*, 639–651. [CrossRef]
29. Haroun, R.; Naasri, S.; Oweida, A.J. Toll-Like Receptors and the Response to Radiotherapy in Solid Tumors: Challenges and Opportunities. *Vaccines* **2023**, *11*, 818. [CrossRef]
30. Li, J.; Yang, F.; Wei, F.; Ren, X. The Role of Toll-like Receptor 4 in Tumor Microenvironment. *Oncotarget* **2017**, *8*, 66656–66667. [CrossRef]
31. Sato, Y.; Goto, Y.; Narita, N.; Hoon, D.S.B. Cancer Cells Expressing Toll-like Receptors and the Tumor Microenvironment. *Cancer Microenviron.* **2009**, *2*, 205–214. [CrossRef] [PubMed]
32. Martín-Medina, A.; Cerón-Pisa, N.; Martinez-Font, E.; Shafiek, H.; Obrador-Hevia, A.; Sauleda, J.; Iglesias, A. TLR/WNT: A Novel Relationship in Immunomodulation of Lung Cancer. *Int. J. Mol. Sci.* **2022**, *23*, 6539. [CrossRef] [PubMed]
33. Di Lorenzo, A.; Bolli, E.; Tarone, L.; Cavallo, F.; Conti, L. Toll-Like Receptor 2 at the Crossroad between Cancer Cells, the Immune System, and the Microbiota. *Int. J. Mol. Sci.* **2020**, *21*, 9418. [CrossRef]
34. Oft, M. Immune Regulation and Cytotoxic T Cell Activation of IL-10 Agonists—Preclinical and Clinical Experience. *Semin. Immunol.* **2019**, *44*, 101325. [CrossRef]
35. Jin, J.; Lin, J.; Xu, A.; Lou, J.; Qian, C.; Li, X.; Wang, Y.; Yu, W.; Tao, H. CCL2: An Important Mediator Between Tumor Cells and Host Cells in Tumor Microenvironment. *Front. Oncol.* **2021**, *11*, 722916. [CrossRef]

36. Zhou, H.; Jiang, M.; Yuan, H.; Ni, W.; Tai, G. Dual Roles of Myeloid-Derived Suppressor Cells Induced by Toll-like Receptor Signaling in Cancer. *Oncol. Lett.* **2021**, *21*, 149. [CrossRef]
37. He, W.; Liu, Q.; Wang, L.; Chen, W.; Li, N.; Cao, X. TLR4 Signaling Promotes Immune Escape of Human Lung Cancer Cells by Inducing Immunosuppressive Cytokines and Apoptosis Resistance. *Mol. Immunol.* **2007**, *44*, 2850–2859. [CrossRef] [PubMed]
38. Li, K.; Qu, S.; Chen, X.; Wu, Q.; Shi, M. Promising Targets for Cancer Immunotherapy: TLRs, RLRs, and STING-Mediated Innate Immune Pathways. *Int. J. Mol. Sci.* **2017**, *18*, 404. [CrossRef] [PubMed]
39. Zhu, J.; Mohan, C. Toll-Like Receptor Signaling Pathways—Therapeutic Opportunities. *Mediat. Inflamm.* **2010**, *2010*, 781235. [CrossRef]
40. Espinosa-Sánchez, A.; Suárez-Martínez, E.; Sánchez-Díaz, L.; Carnero, A. Therapeutic Targeting of Signaling Pathways Related to Cancer Stemness. *Front. Oncol.* **2020**, *10*, 1533. [CrossRef]
41. Sun, H.; Li, Y.; Zhang, P.; Xing, H.; Zhao, S.; Song, Y.; Wan, D.; Yu, J. Targeting Toll-like Receptor 7/8 for Immunotherapy: Recent Advances and Prospectives. *Biomark. Res.* **2022**, *10*, 89. [CrossRef]
42. Gu, J.; Liu, Y.; Xie, B.; Ye, P.; Huang, J.; Lu, Z. Roles of Toll-like Receptors: From Inflammation to Lung Cancer Progression. *Biomed. Rep.* **2018**, *8*, 126–132. [CrossRef] [PubMed]
43. Horvath, L.; Thienpont, B.; Zhao, L.; Wolf, D.; Pircher, A. Overcoming Immunotherapy Resistance in Non-Small Cell Lung Cancer (NSCLC)—Novel Approaches and Future Outlook. *Mol. Cancer* **2020**, *19*, 141. [CrossRef]
44. Ran, S. The Role of TLR4 in Chemotherapy-Driven Metastasis. *Cancer Res.* **2015**, *75*, 2405–2410. [CrossRef] [PubMed]
45. Sun, Z.; Luo, Q.; Ye, D.; Chen, W.; Chen, F. Role of Toll-like Receptor 4 on the Immune Escape of Human Oral Squamous Cell Carcinoma and Resistance of Cisplatin-Induced Apoptosis. *Mol. Cancer* **2012**, *11*, 33. [CrossRef] [PubMed]
46. Chatterjee, S.; Crozet, L.; Damotte, D.; Iribarren, K.; Schramm, C.; Alifano, M.; Lupo, A.; Cherfils-Vicini, J.; Goc, J.; Katsahian, S.; et al. TLR7 Promotes Tumor Progression, Chemotherapy Resistance, and Poor Clinical Outcomes in Non–Small Cell Lung Cancer. *Cancer Res.* **2014**, *74*, 5008–5018. [CrossRef]
47. Muresan, X.M.; Bouchal, J.; Culig, Z.; Souček, K. Toll-Like Receptor 3 in Solid Cancer and Therapy Resistance. *Cancers* **2020**, *12*, 3227. [CrossRef] [PubMed]
48. Seliger, B. Combinatorial Approaches With Checkpoint Inhibitors to Enhance Anti-Tumor Immunity. *Front. Immunol.* **2019**, *10*, 999. [CrossRef]
49. Khair, D.O.; Bax, H.J.; Mele, S.; Crescioli, S.; Pellizzari, G.; Khiabany, A.; Nakamura, M.; Harris, R.J.; French, E.; Hoffmann, R.M.; et al. Combining Immune Checkpoint Inhibitors: Established and Emerging Targets and Strategies to Improve Outcomes in Melanoma. *Front. Immunol.* **2019**, *10*, 453. [CrossRef] [PubMed]
50. Sato-Kaneko, F.; Yao, S.; Ahmadi, A.; Zhang, S.S.; Hosoya, T.; Kaneda, M.M.; Varner, J.A.; Pu, M.; Messer, K.S.; Guiducci, C.; et al. Combination Immunotherapy with TLR Agonists and Checkpoint Inhibitors Suppresses Head and Neck Cancer. *JCI Insight* **2017**, *2*, e93397. [CrossRef]

Disclaimer/Publisher's Note: The statements, opinions and data contained in all publications are solely those of the individual author(s) and contributor(s) and not of MDPI and/or the editor(s). MDPI and/or the editor(s) disclaim responsibility for any injury to people or property resulting from any ideas, methods, instructions or products referred to in the content.

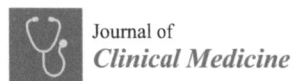

Review

Recent Advancements in Minimally Invasive Surgery for Early Stage Non-Small Cell Lung Cancer: A Narrative Review

Jibran Ahmad Khan [1], Ibrahem Albalkhi [1], Sarah Garatli [1] and Marcello Migliore [2,3,*]

[1] College of Medicine, Alfaisal University, Riyadh 11533, Saudi Arabia; jibrar@alfaisal.edu (J.A.K.); ialbalkhi@alfaisal.edu (I.A.); sarah@alfaisal.edu (S.G.)
[2] Thoracic Surgery & Lung Transplant, Lung Health Centre, Organ Transplant Center of Excellence (OTCoE), King Faisal Specialist Hospital & Research Center, Riyadh 12713, Saudi Arabia
[3] Department of Surgery & Medical Specialties, University of Catania, 96100 Catania, Italy
* Correspondence: mmiglior@hotmail.com

Abstract: Introduction: Lung cancer remains a global health concern, with non-small cell lung cancer (NSCLC) comprising the majority of cases. Early detection of lung cancer has led to an increased number of cases identified in the earlier stages of NSCLC. This required the revaluation of the NSCLC treatment approaches for early stage NSCLC. **Methods:** We conducted a comprehensive search using multiple databases to identify relevant studies on treatment modalities for early stage NSCLC. Inclusion criteria prioritized, but were not limited to, clinical trials and meta-analyses on surgical approaches to early stage NSCLC conducted from 2021 onwards. **Discussion:** Minimally invasive approaches, such as VATS and RATS, along with lung resection techniques, including sublobar resection, have emerged as treatments for early stage NSCLC. Ground-glass opacities (GGOs) have shown prognostic significance, especially when analyzing the consolidation/tumor ratio (CTR). There have also been updates on managing GGOs, including the non-surgical approaches, the extent of lung resection indicated, and the level of lymphadenectomy required. **Conclusions:** The management of early stage NSCLC requires a further assessment of treatment strategies. This includes understanding the required extent of surgical resection, interpreting the significance of GGOs (specifically GGOs with a high CTR), and evaluating the efficacy of alternative therapies. Customized treatment involving surgical and non-surgical interventions is essential for advancing patient care.

Keywords: non-small cell lung cancer; NSCLC; RATS; VATS; lobectomy; segmentectomy; ground-glass opacity

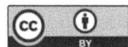

1. Introduction

Lung cancer is a global health burden that accounts for about 2 million deaths annually [1]. It can be histologically classified into two main types: small cell lung cancer (SCLC) and non-small cell lung cancer (NSCLC). Out of these two, NSCLC accounts for 85% of the cases. NSCLC is an aggressive disease and an early intervention has shown to decrease the 5-year mortality rate [2]. Unfortunately, most cases of NSCLC are detected at advanced stages, with only about 10% of cases identified in stage I [3]. This has a significant impact on the management strategy and prognosis of the disease [4]. It is further highlighted by the fact that the survival rates for stage I, stage II, stage III, and stage IV are 75–90%, 65%, 37%, and 9%, respectively [5,6]. Nevertheless, due to an increase in lung cancer screening, we see a rise in the prevalence of NSCLC in its earlier stages. Early stage NSCLC is typically defined as cancer at stage 2 or lower, providing an opportunity for intervention before the cancer has a chance to further metastasize.

Most thoracic cancer centers worldwide adopt standard treatment using surgery, radiation, chemotherapy, and palliative care. Surgical treatment plays a key role in managing early stage NSCLC, with an overall survival (OS) of 90% [7]. Surgical approaches for lung cancer may be divided based on the approaches to the surgery and how much lung is excised. Approaches to lung cancer surgery include video-assisted thoracoscopic surgery (VATS), robotic-assisted thoracoscopic surgery (RATS), or traditional open surgery. Resection of the lung is performed as either a wedge resection, segmentectomy, lobectomy, or pneumonectomy (Figure 1). Some specialized centers also utilize emerging treatments such as immunotherapy, targeted therapy, and radiofrequency ablation.

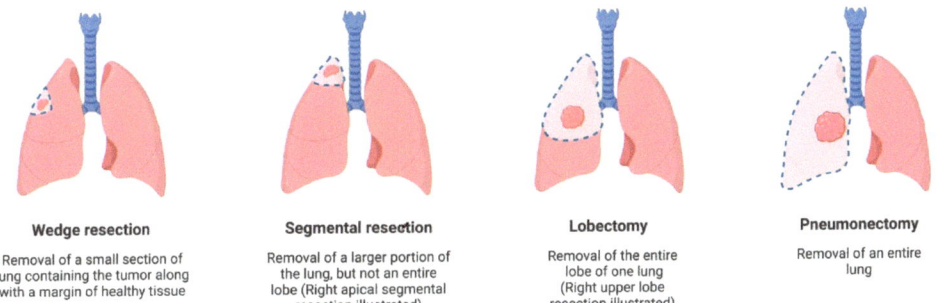

Figure 1. Different techniques of lung resection. Created with BioRender.com.

Despite all these treatment modalities, NSCLC exhibits recurrence rates between 30% and 55%, outlining the need for better treatment modalities [8]. Although the recent decade has witnessed multiple advancements in surgical techniques and approaches, unresolved questions remain in the management of early stage NSCLC:

1. How effective are the minimally invasive surgical approaches for NSCLC treatment?
2. Is sublobar resection superior to lobectomy for stage IA NSCLC treatment?
3. What is the prognostic value of ground-glass opacities (GGOs).
4. Is sublobar resection superior to lobectomy for GGOs?
5. What is the extent of the lymphadenectomy required for GGOs?

We aim to include a review of the literature on these four questions to update physicians on the most recent surgical advancements in the management of NSCLC. Additionally, we briefly alluded to recent updates in the non-surgical approaches to NSCLC.

2. Methods

To identify all studies evaluating the treatment modalities for early stage NSCLC, we performed a Boolean search using "non-small cell lung cancer", "NSCLC", "RATS", "VATS", "lobectomy", "segmentectomy", "lymphadenectomy", "lymph node dissection", "ground-glass opacity", "targeted therapy", "immunotherapy", "chemotherapy", and "radiotherapy" keywords. Two authors (J.K., I.A.) reviewed and included the relevant full-text articles in the English language using the PubMed/MEDLINE, Web of Science, Scopus, and Google Scholar databases. Afterward, the authors (J.K., I.A.) performed a more comprehensive review of the full manuscripts for inclusion. There was no year limit set. The inclusion criteria were prioritized but were not limited to clinical trials and meta-analyses on the surgical approaches of early stage NSCLC published from 2021 onwards.

3. Discussion

3.1. Surgical Approaches to NSCLC Treatment

3.1.1. How Effective Are the Minimally Invasive Surgical Approaches for NSCLC Treatment?

In the past, open lobectomy or pneumonectomy with mediastinal lymph node dissection was the primary surgical management approach. Nowadays, minimally invasive thoracoscopic techniques are becoming increasingly popular as they do not involve rib spreading or mechanical retractors, which are seen in traditional thoracotomy. These techniques have also developed over the years to include robot-assisted lobectomy, uniportal resection, and awake VATS [9]. Several studies have shown that VATS lobectomy is associated with reduced postoperative pain and preserved postoperative pulmonary function. For example, a retrospective analysis of 1079 patients at Duke University found that VATS lobectomy was associated with lower postoperative complications, including a decrease in prolonged air leak, atrial fibrillation, atelectasis, pneumonia, renal failure, blood transfusions, and death compared to thoracotomies [10]. Recent studies have also revealed that the conversion rate from VATS to thoracotomy can reach as low as 3 to 5% [11,12], which is considerably less than in the studies in the past, with an approximately 11% conversion in one trial [13]. Additionally, it was found that patients who undergo VATS have a decreased cytokine release and lower levels of C-reactive protein, which may result in decreased rates of atelectasis and relatively preserved postoperative lung function [14,15].

Robotic-assisted thoracoscopic surgery (RATS) is another option, with OS rates of 91% for stage IA cancer and 88% for stage IB cancer [16]. A meta-analysis by Singer et al. [17] demonstrated that RATS lobectomy costs more than VATS lobectomy. A nationwide comparative study published in 2014 by Paul et al. obtained similar results while further identifying an association of robotic lobectomy with increased rates of intraoperative injury and bleeding [18]. On the contrary, numerous recent studies revealed no significant difference in outcomes, while others exhibited better outcomes with robotic surgery. A 2019 meta-analysis demonstrated no significant difference in the short-term outcomes between VATS and RATS [19]. Another study conducted by the Society of Thoracic Surgeons (STS) saw no significant difference in OS between the two approaches [20]. Additional studies found improved 30-day mortality, number of conversions to open surgery [21,22], decreased postoperative complications, and reduced hospital stay [23]. The ROMAN trial recently published its findings on the perioperative outcomes of RATS and VATS for early stage NSCLC. Although there were inconclusive findings favoring RATS, it revealed notably improved lymph node sampling with RATS [24]. Another trial conducted by Catelli et al. found no difference in OS and disease-free survival (DFS), and instead found lower postoperative complications, such as pleural effusion, pain, and cardiovascular comorbidities, using RATS [25]. A recent meta-analysis, which included 25 studies, including 5 randomized controlled trials (RCTs), compared the postoperative quality of life (QoL) of RATS and robotic abdominal surgery with VATS and laparoscopic surgery (LS). They found no significant difference in global QoL with the robotic techniques compared to VATS [26].

Uniportal lobectomy is a minimally invasive technique that involves operating through a single access incision, removing the need to create an additional camera port [27,28]. A large European multicentric retrospective cohort comparing uniportal with multiportal surgery discovered no significant difference in the number of lymph nodes extracted and the conversion rate to open surgery [29]. Conversely, they found a statistically significant lower operative time and decreased hospital stay in the uniportal group. A randomized control trial conducted by Yao et al. saw no difference in operative time, lymph nodes harvested, chest tube duration, length of hospital stay, and pulmonary function; however, intraoperative blood loss and volume of total drainage were significantly decreased with uniportal VATS [30]. Similar outcomes between uniportal VATS and other VAT techniques were compared by Perna et al. in their prospective, randomized study. They concluded that uniportal VATS does not yield superior outcomes compared to other techniques of VATS [31]. A meta-analysis conducted in 2019, comparing open surgery, uniportal VATS, multiportal VATS, and RATS obtained equivalent findings. An emerging technique that is gaining popularity is uniportal subxiphoid VATS, known for its potential to reduce pain by avoiding intercostal nerve injury [32]. An added benefit of this approach is the possibility of performing bilateral procedures without the need for extra incisions or time spent repositioning the patient. A retrospective cohort saw comparable results to other techniques with uniportal subxiphoid VATS [33]. Nevertheless, clinical trials are required to compare the outcomes of uniportal subxiphoid VATS with other minimally invasive techniques.

3.1.2. Is Sublobar Resection Superior to Lobectomy for Stage Ia NSCLC Treatment?

While lobectomies have been the gold standard surgical resection in the treatment of early stage lung cancer since 1960, sublobar resection, comprising either segmentectomy or wedge resection, presents a notable difference in the surgical intensity. Segmentectomy is considered an alternative to lobectomy in terms of curative intensity in oncology, allowing for margin-positive or nodal metastasis to be assessed during surgery, while simultaneously being similar to wedge resection in terms of preservation of pulmonary parenchyma and postoperative respiratory function [34]. A recent clinical trial by Altorki et al. compared 362 individuals with peripheral cT1aN0 non-small cell lung cancer treated with either lobectomy, segmentectomy, or wedge resection. The outcomes they measured included DFS, OS, lung cancer-specific survival (LCSS), differences in surgical margins, locoregional recurrence rate, and expiratory flow rate at 6 months postoperatively. They found no significant difference in DFS, OS, LCSS, or pulmonary function between the three groups. Locoregional recurrence was numerically higher in wedge resection compared to segmentectomy but not statistically significant [35]. Another multicenter, noninferiority, phase 3 trial by Altorki and colleagues was conducted on a total of 697 patients with NSCLC clinically staged as T1aN0, who were randomly assigned to undergo sublobar resection or lobar resection after intraoperative confirmation of node-negative disease. The 5-year DFS rates after sublobar resection and lobectomy were 63.6% (95% CI, 57.9–68.8) and 64.1% (95% CI, 58.5–69.0), respectively. Hence, they concluded that sublobar resection was non-inferior to lobectomy in terms of DFS in patients with pathologically confirmed hilar and mediastinal lymph node-negative peripheral NSCLC [36]. A multicenter, open-label, phase 3 trial compared survival rates, mortality causes, and risk of recurrence between the two approaches in purely solid NSCLC less than or equal to 2cm. Their post hoc, supplemental analysis revealed a significantly improved 5-year OS with segmentectomy (86.1% [95% CI 81.4–89.7] with lobectomy vs. 92.4% [88.6-95.0] with segmentectomy). They further saw no statistically significant difference in the 5-year RFS (81.7% [95% CI 76.5–85.8] with lobectomy vs. 82.0% [76.9–86.0] with segmentectomy; HR 1.01 [95% CI 0.72–1.42]; $p = 0.94$). However, when considering demographics, better outcomes were observed with lobectomies in patients younger than 70 years ($p = 0.049$) and female patients ($p = 0.047$) [37]. Potter et al. aimed to compare these outcomes with the National Cancer Database in the United States in a propensity score-matched analysis. They found no significant difference in the 5-year OS between the two groups. Furthermore, subgroup analyses by histology and tumor grade exhibited no difference. Similar treatment patterns were also observed between the two approaches for second primary tumors [38]. A recent meta-analysis of randomized clinical trials comparing sublobar to lobar resection in stage IA NSCLC showed sublobar resection and lobectomy to have similar OS, DFS, and disease recurrence rates for stage IA NSCLC [39]. Another meta-analysis by Fong et al. also revealed similar outcomes, adding that sublobar resection ensures safer future treatments for patients experiencing recurrence or a second primary tumor [40]. A cross-sectional study by Brunelli et al. discussed dyspnea after segmentectomy versus lobectomy, comparing their Dyspnea Index Score. They found a reduced chance of perioperative dyspnea in the segmentectomy group.

These recent studies indicate that sublobar resection is a feasible alternative to lobectomy in NSCLC management. Numerous outcomes, including DFS, OS, and LCSS, show no significant difference between the two, particularly between segmentectomy and lobectomy. However, the data in terms of preservation of pulmonary function between sublobar resection and lobectomy also remain inconclusive. Therefore, more clinical trials may be required to determine any significant differences between the outcomes of these options.

3.1.3. What Is the Prognostic Value of Ground-Glass Opacities (GGOs)?

Ground-glass opacity (GGO) is defined as an area of hazy attenuation on CT scans with visible underlying blood vessels and bronchial structures [41]. GGOs are typically associated with adenocarcinomas, although they may be present in certain pulmonary conditions, such as COVID-19, potentially posing diagnostic challenges as the GGOs from such benign conditions mimic the ones observed in malignancy [42]. New imaging technologies are necessary to identify neoplastic or potential neoplastic GGOs which need operation. Pulmonary nodules possessing a GGO component are known as subsolid nodules (SSNs). SSNs are further divided into pure GGOs and part-solid GGOs [43]. The degree of GGO is measured using the consolidation-to-tumor ratio (CTR), defined as the solid portion size relative to the total size of the nodule [44]. The degree of malignancy has been associated with the proportion of GGO in each nodule, with the literature showing that nodules with large GGO components have a favorable prognosis [44–48]. Shigefuku et al. noted a positive impact of GGO on recurrence and 5-year survival after resection of adenocarcinoma [49]. Multifocal pure GGOs have exhibited a significantly higher 5-year OS (97.2%) compared to having a purely solid nodule (PSN) with additional GGOs (82.1%) or having only PSNs (41.3%) [50]. A recent cohort study by Choi et al. compared the metastatic potential of GGOs and PSNs with an increase in tumor size. Tumor size was observed as a significant predictor of outcomes in a multivariate analysis for the PSN, but not the GGO group. The GGO group also had a superior 5-year DFS [51]. Hence, while some studies found no association between CTR and tumor prognosis [52,53], the majority suggested the utilization of CTR to assess the T stage [40,45,54]. This prognosis may also differ based on the histologic characteristics of SSNs (Table 1) [40,55].

Table 1. Lepidic tumors presenting with GGO components.

Histologic Type	Size	Description
Atypical adenomatous hyperplasia (AAH)	Usually ≤0.5 cm	Solitary GGN usually smaller than 0.5 cm with no solid components
Adenocarcinoma in situ (AIS)	≤3 cm	Solitary GGN with purely lepidic growth, no stromal components, vascular, pleural and lymphatics invasion, or necrosis
Minimally invasive adenocarcinoma (MIA)	≤3 cm	Solitary GGN with mainly lepidic growth, ≤0.5 cm invasive foci, no stromal components, vascular, pleural, and lymphatics invasion, or necrosis
Lepidic predominant adenocarcinoma (LPA)	Any total size	Mainly lepidic growth, >0.5 cm invasive foci, or vascular, pleural, and lymphatics invasion, or necrosis

Due to their favorable prognostic value, possible alternative options to surgery for patients with GGOs have also been explored, particularly in patients who may be inoperable due to comorbidities, present with multiple lesions, or refuse surgery. Stereotactic body radiotherapy (SBRT) is one such option, proving to be a safe monotherapy with low toxicity for SSNs with a CTR ≤ 0.5 in a recent study [56]. Notably, in a retrospective study by Eriguchi et al., SBRT achieved a 3-year OS and cause-specific survival (CSS) of 100% for GGO tumors in operable patients [57]. Another study observed similar findings, with 3-year RFS and CSS rates of 96.0% and 100.0%, respectively. Furthermore, they noted no significant difference in the 3-year OS and RFS between operable and inoperable patients. Both these studies, therefore, explored the possibility of using stereotactic radiotherapy even in individuals who are deemed suitable for surgery. Carbon ion radiotherapy (CIRT) is another alternative, with one study revealing a Kaplan–Meier estimate of OS being significantly lower after CIRT than segmentectomy but with similar CSS [58]. Additionally, percutaneous radiofrequency ablation (RFA) could be used, with one study observing an OS and CSS of 96.4% and 100% at 3 years, and 96.4% and 100% at 5 years, respectively [59]. Lastly, another study by Iguchi et al. utilizing RFA found an OS and CSS of 93.3% and

100%, respectively, at 1 and 5 years [60]. Comparing the QoL of segmentectomy with SBRT has also been studied using the Short Form 8 (SF-8), for physical and mental health, and Functional Assessment of Cancer Therapy-Lung (FACT-L) surveys [61]. Patients reported better QoL immediately postop with SBRT but no significant difference between the two in long-term QoL. It is important to note that these studies are retrospective, with some having a small sample size; hence, a further evaluation with clinical trials is recommended before they can be routinely utilized for GGO management.

3.1.4. Is Sublobar Resection Superior to Lobectomy for GGOs?

The prevalence of GGOs has risen due to early detection from the application of lung cancer screening and CT scans. More GGOs are now being recognized in their early stages, thus increasing the feasibility of sublobar resection, such as wedge resection and segmentectomies, compared to lobectomies. A recent large cohort study included 1209 patients who either underwent wedge resection or segmentectomy. Wedge resection was found to have a significantly lower complication rate, shorter operating time, and shorter hospital stay. Along with that, they discovered statistically similar 5-year OS (98.8% vs. 99.6%, $p = 0.270$), 5-year RFS (98.8% vs. 99.5%, $p = 0.307$), and 5-year LCSS (99.9% vs. 99.6%, $p = 0.581$) with wedge resection and segmentectomy, respectively [62]. Another retrospective cohort by Zhang et al. included 424 patients with part-solid GGOs. They also discovered improved operative time, blood loss, and postoperative stay with sublobar resection. In addition, they saw similar postoperative complications and OS between the two for GGO-dominant lung adenocarcinomas ≤ 2 cm [63]. The Japan Clinical Oncology Group (JCOG) 1211 trial, a multicenter, single-arm, confirmatory phase 3 trial, confirmed these findings [64]. There is a need, however, for more clinical trials to better validate these findings. The ongoing GREAT trial is a prospective, open-label, randomized phase III trial across 19 hospitals in China, randomizing 1024 patients into segmentectomy and lobectomy. Their primary endpoint is 5-year RFS, and secondary endpoints include 5-year OS, perioperative outcomes, and pulmonary function preservation. They expect improved secondary endpoints and no statistical difference in the primary endpoint [65].

3.1.5. What Is the Extent of Lymphadenectomy Required for GGOs?

Lymphadenectomy, which includes lymph node sampling (LNS), and the more extensive lymph node dissection (LND), is an important component of NSCLC management. Due to the rise in the detection of early stage GGOs, the clinical significance of LND needs to be evaluated. A recent retrospective cohort study aimed to analyze the difference in clinical outcomes between LND and sampling for a CTR between 0.3 and 0.7. The Kaplan–Meier survival curves found similar outcomes for both approaches [66]. Another recent cohort concluded that complete exclusion of lymphadenectomy has a minimal impact on the curative management of GGOs for both sublobar and lobar resection [67]. A review by Kim et al. included numerous studies, including five clinical trials, discussing the extent of lymphadenectomy [68]. They discovered no significant difference in postoperative morbidities between lymph node sampling and dissection, with two studies noting an improved detection of occult N2 disease with dissection, and two other studies showing improved survival after dissection. However, they also noted methodologic uncertainties and a high risk of bias for all studies [68]. This was further highlighted in a meta-analysis of these studies. They saw a favorable OS but more complications with dissection. Nonetheless, they alluded to the limitations of the studies, particularly mentioning the asserted survival advantage not being backed up with reliable evidence [69]. Both reviews emphasized the need for larger randomized clinical trials that are more regulated. Another review by Deng et al. added that the studies they evaluated did not prove a survival benefit with dissection [70]. Moreover, five retrospective studies they referred to reported no or minimal lymph node involvement with pure GGOs and part-solid GGOs, respectively. With this, they suggested that lymph node dissection may not be required for pure GGOs and some part-solid GGOs. In contrast to the preceding two reviews, they also acknowledged that considering this excellent prognosis of GGOs, along with the intricacy of conducting RCTs, which demand excessive sampling and follow-up time, RCTs may not be imperative to determine the optimal lymphadenectomy strategy for GGOs, although studies are needed to understand lymphadenectomy for NSCLC in general [71]. Currently, two ongoing trials are assessing approaches to lymph node removal in GGOs. The LESSON trial is an ongoing, single-institutional, randomized, double-blind, and parallel-controlled trial in China aiming to assess lymph node dissection in clinically diagnosed stage IA NSCLC with GGO components $\geq 50\%$ (i.e., CTR ≤ 0.5) [71]. The MELDSIG trial is another ongoing multi-institutional randomized trial in China, analyzing the difference between dissection and sampling in stage Ia NSCLC with GGOs [72].

3.2. Non-Surgical Approaches to NSCLC

3.2.1. Radiotherapy and Adjuvant Chemotherapy

Patients who are medically unable to undergo surgery for early stage NSCLC are usually treated with radical radiotherapy. However, when standard fractionation is used, the outcomes are not as good as surgery, with 5-year OS rates of only 11% [73]. On the other hand, using stereotactic ablative radiotherapy (SABR) has shown similar local control rates and disease-specific survival rates to surgery [74]. Adjuvant cisplatin-based doublet chemotherapy has become the standard of care for completely resected stage II NSCLC based on the International Adjuvant Lung Cancer Trial in 2004 [75], but no significant innovations have been made since then. A phase II randomized TREAT study evaluated the role of cisplatin-pemetrexed versus cisplatin-vinorelbine, but a follow-up report showed no improvement in the 3-year survival period [76]. The addition of bevacizumab and erlotinib did not improve survival in the Eastern Cooperative Oncology Group 1505 study [77] nor the RADIANT study [78], respectively.

3.2.2. Immunotherapy

The mainstay for treating early stage NSCLC has traditionally been surgery alone. However, adjuvant immunotherapy has been proposed to reduce recurrence and facilitate cancer destruction. Surgery can cause immune dysfunction [79], which may allow unresected cancer cells to grow, but the use of adjuvant immunotherapy allows the timely treatment of subclinical micrometastatic disease [80]. Due to the groundbreaking outcomes of immune checkpoint inhibition (ICI) for metastatic (stage IV) NSCLC [81–83], investigating its potential in early stage NSCLC made sense. In addition, the success of durvalumab ICI in treating stage III unresectable NSCLC has increased interest in using ICI for non-metastatic early stage NSCLC [84].

Currently, four large randomized controlled phase III trials are investigating the use of ICI as an adjuvant treatment after surgical resection. These trials include PEARLS [85], Canadian Cancer Trials Group BR.31 [86], ANVIL [87], and IMpower010 [88]. All trials are conducted on patients with completely resected stage IB more than 4 cm, II, or IIIA, and allow adjuvant chemotherapy as per standard practice. Most allow resected tumors of any programmed death ligand 1(PD-L1) status, but the BR.31 trial will enrich the trial population with PD-L1-positive tumors after the enrollment of 600 patients. Two trials are placebo-controlled, whereas the ANVIL and IMpower010 are not. DFS is the primary endpoint in PEARLS. For the BR.31, this is DFS in PD-L1-positive tumors. IMpower010 has both endpoints, and ANVIL targets DFS and OS.

The IMpower010 trial showed a DFS benefit with atezolizumab, a PD-L1 inhibitor, versus best supportive care after adjuvant chemotherapy in patients with resected early stage NSCLC, with a pronounced benefit in the subgroup whose tumors expressed PD-L1 on 1% or more of tumor cells, and no new safety signals. However, there are certain disadvantages to neoadjuvant immunotherapy. First, it is unclear whether it will improve the patient's long-term survival. Second, it may jeopardize surgical feasibility by generating delays or raising the risk of complications. Furthermore, there are challenges in measuring the response and investigating biomarkers, which may limit its applicability and advancement.

3.2.3. Targeted Therapy

Targeted therapy using tyrosine kinase inhibitors (TKIs) has shown promise as an adjuvant treatment for *EGFR*-mutated NSCLC. The SELECT trial [89] found that adjuvant erlotinib improved 2-year DFS compared to historical controls. The CTONG1104/ADJUVANT trial [90] compared standard chemotherapy to gefitinib and found a superior DFS in the gefitinib arm. The ADAURA trial evaluated the impact of adjuvant osimertinib compared to a placebo and found an impressive DFS hazard ratio of 0.17 (95% CI 0.12–0.23, $p < 0.05$); however, controversy remains about whether these immature data should change practice. Additionally, neoadjuvant gefitinib has shown a 50% response rate among patients whose tumors harbored EGFR mutations, without a safety signal for increased surgical risk [91]. MET is a tyrosine kinase receptor for hepatocyte growth factor. *MET* gene amplification is observed in 2 to 4 percent of treatment-naïve NSCLC and in 5 to 20 percent of *EGFR*-mutated tumors that have acquired resistance to EGFR inhibitors. The literature suggests the use of MET inhibitors, such as capmatinib or crizotinib, in patients with a high-level MET amplification (>5-fold increase in gene copy number [GCN] or MET/CEP7 ratio >5) who have progressed despite being on chemotherapy or immunotherapy [92]. Hyperactivation mutations of the PI3K–AKT–mTOR signaling pathway are observed in many cancers, including NSCLC, where they have been heavily implicated in carcinogenesis and disease progression. Pilaralisib is a highly selective inhibitor of the class I PI3Ks and successfully inhibits tumor growth in vivo. Crizotinib is an ALK, MET, and ROS1 kinase inhibitor. The phase I study of Crizotinib in 50 patients who were positive for ROS1 rearrangement proved the antitumor activity of this drug in advanced NSCLC [93].

4. Future Directions and Conclusions

More research on early stage non-small cell lung cancer (NSCLC) is crucial to improve outcomes and find more effective treatments. With the increasing prevalence of early stage NSCLC, surgical techniques involving minimal resection of the lung parenchyma, i.e., sublobar resections, need to be explored, aiming to preserve function and minimize operative and postoperative complications. Moreover, while the prognostic significance of SSNs with major GGO components has been extensively studied, there is limited data regarding the relevance of GGOs with a CTR > 0.5. Studying the clinical progression of SSNs, such as lymph node involvement, will allow for the development of better treatment protocols, including the extent of lung resection, the extent of lymphadenectomy, and the utilization of non-surgical approaches. Lastly, as the range of treatment options expands, there is an increasing demand for a customized approach that incorporates a combination of surgical and non-surgical therapies and personalized medicine [94]. Potential selection biases in the reviewed studies, often from high-income countries, may limit generalizability. Additionally, many studies on surgical and non-surgical treatments like radiotherapy and ablation are retrospective, which can introduce biases, affecting their conclusions. More clinical trials are needed, and they are needed for a variety of populations to provide more generalizable conclusions.

Author Contributions: Conceptualization, M.M.; methodology, J.A.K., I.A. and M.M.; validation, M.M.; formal analysis, J.A.K. and I.A.; investigation, data curation, J.A.K. and I.A.; writing—original draft preparation, J.A.K.; writing—review and editing J.A.K., I.A., M.M. and S.G.; supervision, M.M. All authors have read and agreed to the published version of the manuscript.

Funding: This research received no external funding.

Acknowledgments: Figure 1: Adapted from "Lung Cancer Surgery with Description (Horizontal)". Created using BioRender.com (2024). Retrieved from https://app.biorender.com/biorender-templates.

Conflicts of Interest: The authors declare no conflicts of interest.

References

1. Bray, F.; Ferlay, J.; Soerjomataram, I.; Siegel, R.L.; Torre, L.A.; Jemal, A. Global cancer statistics 2018: GLOBOCAN estimates of incidence and mortality worldwide for 36 cancers in 185 countries. *CA. Cancer J. Clin.* **2018**, *68*, 394–424. [CrossRef] [PubMed]
2. Anggondowati, T.; Ganti, A.K.; Islam, K.M.M. Impact of time-to-treatment on overall survival of non-small cell lung cancer patients—An analysis of the national cancer database. *Transl. Lung Cancer Res.* **2020**, *9*, 1202–1211. [CrossRef] [PubMed]
3. Casal-Mouriño, A.; Ruano-Ravina, A.; Lorenzo-González, M.; Rodríguez-Martínez, Á.; Giraldo-Osorio, A.; Varela-Lema, L.; Pereiro-Brea, T.; Barros-Dios, J.M.; Valdés-Cuadrado, L.; Pérez-Ríos, M. Epidemiology of stage III lung cancer: Frequency, diagnostic characteristics, and survival. *Transl. Lung Cancer Res.* **2021**, *10*, 506–518. [CrossRef] [PubMed]
4. Krzakowski, M.; Jassem, J.; Antczak, A.; Chorostowska-Wynimko, J.; Dziadziuszko, R.; Głogowski, M.; Grodzki, T.; Kowalski, D.; Olszewski, W.; Orłowski, T.; et al. Cancer of the lung, pleura and mediastinum. *Oncol. Clin. Pract.* **2019**, *15*, 20–50. [CrossRef]
5. Surveillance, Epidemiology, and End Results Program. Available online: https://seer.cancer.gov/index.html (accessed on 2 April 2023).
6. Kay, F.U.; Kandathil, A.; Batra, K.; Saboo, S.S.; Abbara, S.; Rajiah, P. Revisions to the Tumor, Node, Metastasis staging of lung cancer (8th edition): Rationale, radiologic findings and clinical implications. *World J. Radiol.* **2017**, *9*, 269–279. [CrossRef] [PubMed]
7. Goldstraw, P.; Chansky, K.; Crowley, J.; Rami-Porta, R.; Asamura, H.; Eberhardt, W.E.E.; Nicholson, A.G.; Groome, P.; Mitchell, A.; Bolejack, V.; et al. The IASLC Lung Cancer Staging Project: Proposals for Revision of the TNM Stage Groupings in the Forthcoming (Eighth) Edition of the TNM Classification for Lung Cancer. *J. Thorac. Oncol.* **2016**, *11*, 39–51. [CrossRef] [PubMed]
8. Uramoto, H.; Tanaka, F. Recurrence after surgery in patients with NSCLC. *Transl. Lung Cancer Res.* **2014**, *3*, 242–249. [CrossRef]
9. Salfity, H.; Tong, B.C. VATS and Minimally Invasive Resection in Early-Stage NSCLC. *Semin. Respir. Crit. Care Med.* **2020**, *41*, 335–345. [CrossRef]
10. Villamizar, N.R.; Darrabie, M.D.; Burfeind, W.R.; Petersen, R.P.; Onaitis, M.W.; Toloza, E.; Harpole, D.H.; D'Amico, T.A. Thoracoscopic lobectomy is associated with lower morbidity compared with thoracotomy. *J. Thorac. Cardiovasc. Surg.* **2009**, *138*, 419–425. [CrossRef]
11. Villamizar, N.R.; Darrabie, M.; Hanna, J.; Onaitis, M.W.; Tong, B.C.; D'Amico, T.A.; Berry, M.F. Impact of T status and N status on perioperative outcomes after thoracoscopic lobectomy for lung cancer. *J. Thorac. Cardiovasc. Surg.* **2013**, *145*, 514–520; discussion 520–521. [CrossRef]
12. Byun, C.S.; Lee, S.; Kim, D.J.; Lee, J.G.; Lee, C.Y.; Jung, I.; Chung, K.Y. Analysis of Unexpected Conversion to Thoracotomy During Thoracoscopic Lobectomy in Lung Cancer. *Ann. Thorac. Surg.* **2015**, *100*, 968–973. [CrossRef]
13. Swanson, S.J.; Herndon, J.E.; D'Amico, T.A.; Demmy, T.L.; McKenna, R.J.; Green, M.R.; Sugarbaker, D.J. Video-assisted thoracic surgery lobectomy: Report of CALGB 39802—A prospective, multi-institution feasibility study. *J. Clin. Oncol. Off. J. Am. Soc. Clin. Oncol.* **2007**, *25*, 4993–4997. [CrossRef]
14. Leaver, H.A.; Craig, S.R.; Yap, P.L.; Walker, W.S. Lymphocyte responses following open and minimally invasive thoracic surgery. *Eur. J. Clin. Investig.* **2000**, *30*, 230–238. [CrossRef] [PubMed]
15. Kaseda, S.; Aoki, T.; Hangai, N.; Shimizu, K. Better pulmonary function and prognosis with video-assisted thoracic surgery than with thoracotomy. *Ann. Thorac. Surg.* **2000**, *70*, 1644–1646. [CrossRef] [PubMed]
16. Veronesi, G. Robotic lobectomy and segmentectomy for lung cancer: Results and operating technique. *J. Thorac. Dis.* **2015**, *7*, S122–S130. [CrossRef] [PubMed]
17. Singer, E.; Kneuertz, P.J.; D'Souza, D.M.; Moffatt-Bruce, S.D.; Merritt, R.E. Understanding the financial cost of robotic lobectomy: Calculating the value of innovation? *Ann. Cardiothorac. Surg.* **2019**, *8*, 194–201. [CrossRef] [PubMed]
18. Paul, S.; Jalbert, J.; Isaacs, A.J.; Altorki, N.K.; Isom, O.W.; Sedrakyan, A. Comparative effectiveness of robotic-assisted vs thoracoscopic lobectomy. *Chest* **2014**, *146*, 1505–1512. [CrossRef]
19. Guo, F.; Ma, D.; Li, S. Compare the prognosis of Da Vinci robot-assisted thoracic surgery (RATS) with video-assisted thoracic surgery (VATS) for non-small cell lung cancer: A Meta-analysis. *Medicine* **2019**, *98*, e17089. [CrossRef]
20. Louie, B.E.; Wilson, J.L.; Kim, S.; Cerfolio, R.J.; Park, B.J.; Farivar, A.S.; Vallières, E.; Aye, R.W.; Burfeind, W.R.; Block, M.I. Comparison of Video-Assisted Thoracoscopic Surgery and Robotic Approaches for Clinical Stage I and Stage II Non-Small Cell Lung Cancer Using The Society of Thoracic Surgeons Database. *Ann. Thorac. Surg.* **2016**, *102*, 917–924. [CrossRef]
21. Liang, H.; Liang, W.; Zhao, L.; Chen, D.; Zhang, J.; Zhang, Y.; Tang, S.; He, J. Robotic Versus Video-assisted Lobectomy/Segmentectomy for Lung Cancer: A Meta-analysis. *Ann. Surg.* **2018**, *268*, 254–259. [CrossRef]
22. Emmert, A.; Straube, C.; Buentzel, J.; Roever, C. Robotic versus thoracoscopic lung resection: A systematic review and meta-analysis. *Medicine* **2017**, *96*, e7633. [CrossRef] [PubMed]
23. Oh, D.S.; Reddy, R.M.; Gorrepati, M.L.; Mehendale, S.; Reed, M.F. Robotic-Assisted, Video-Assisted Thoracoscopic and Open Lobectomy: Propensity-Matched Analysis of Recent Premier Data. *Ann. Thorac. Surg.* **2017**, *104*, 1733–1740. [CrossRef] [PubMed]
24. Veronesi, G.; Abbas, A.E.-S.; Muriana, P.; Lembo, R.; Bottoni, E.; Perroni, G.; Testori, A.; Dieci, E.; Bakhos, C.T.; Car, S.; et al. Perioperative Outcome of Robotic Approach Versus Manual Videothoracoscopic Major Resection in Patients Affected by Early Lung Cancer: Results of a Randomized Multicentric Study (ROMAN Study). *Front. Oncol.* **2021**, *11*, 726408. [CrossRef] [PubMed]
25. Catelli, C.; Corzani, R.; Zanfrini, E.; Franchi, F.; Ghisalberti, M.; Ligabue, T.; Meniconi, F.; Monaci, N.; Galgano, A.; Mathieu, F.; et al. RoboticAssisted (RATS) versus Video-Assisted (VATS) lobectomy: A monocentric prospective randomized trial. *Eur. J. Surg. Oncol. J. Eur. Soc. Surg. Oncol. Br. Assoc. Surg. Oncol.* **2023**, *49*, 107256. [CrossRef] [PubMed]

26. Martins, R.S.; Fatimi, A.S.; Mahmud, O.; Mahar, M.U.; Jahangir, A.; Jawed, K.; Golani, S.; Siddiqui, A.; Aamir, S.R.; Ahmad, A. Quality of life after robotic versus conventional minimally invasive cancer surgery: A systematic review and meta-analysis. *J. Robot. Surg.* **2024**, *18*, 171. [CrossRef] [PubMed]
27. Migliore, M.; Calvo, D.; Criscione, A.; Borrata, F. Uniportal video assisted thoracic surgery: Summary of experience, mini-review and perspectives. *J. Thorac. Dis.* **2015**, *7*, E378–E380. [CrossRef] [PubMed]
28. Migliore, M.; Hirai, K. Uniportal VATS: Comment on the consensus report from the uniportal VATS interest group (UVIG) of the European Society of Thoracic Surgeons. *Eur. J. Cardio-Thorac. Surg.* **2020**, *57*, 612. [CrossRef] [PubMed]
29. Manolache, V.; Motas, N.; Bosinceanu, M.L.; de la Torre, M.; Gallego-Poveda, J.; Dunning, J.; Ismail, M.; Turna, A.; Paradela, M.; Decker, G.; et al. Comparison of uniportal robotic-assisted thoracic surgery pulmonary anatomic resections with multiport robotic-assisted thoracic surgery: A multicenter study of the European experience. *Ann. Cardiothorac. Surg.* **2023**, *12*, 102–109. [CrossRef] [PubMed]
30. Yao, J.; Chang, Z.; Zhu, L.; Fan, J. Uniportal versus multiportal thoracoscopic lobectomy: Ergonomic evaluation and perioperative outcomes from a randomized and controlled trial. *Medicine* **2020**, *99*, e22719. [CrossRef]
31. Perna, V.; Carvajal, A.F.; Torrecilla, J.A.; Gigirey, O. Uniportal video-assisted thoracoscopic lobectomy versus other video-assisted thoracoscopic lobectomy techniques: A randomized study. *Eur. J. Cardio-Thorac. Surg.* **2016**, *50*, 411–415. [CrossRef]
32. Chiu, C.-H.; Chao, Y.-K.; Liu, Y.-H. Subxiphoid approach for video-assisted thoracoscopic surgery: An update. *J. Thorac. Dis.* **2018**, *10*, S1662–S1665. [CrossRef] [PubMed]
33. Ali, J.; Haiyang, F.; Aresu, G.; Chenlu, Y.; Gening, J.; Gonzalez-Rivas, D.; Lei, J. Uniportal Subxiphoid Video-Assisted Thoracoscopic Anatomical Segmentectomy: Technique and Results. *Ann. Thorac. Surg.* **2018**, *106*, 1519–1524. [CrossRef]
34. Saji, H.; Okada, M.; Tsuboi, M.; Nakajima, R.; Suzuki, K.; Aokage, K.; Aoki, T.; Okami, J.; Yoshino, I.; Ito, H.; et al. Segmentectomy versus lobectomy in small-sized peripheral non-small-cell lung cancer (JCOG0802/WJOG4607L): A multicentre, open-label, phase 3, randomised, controlled, non-inferiority trial. *Lancet* **2022**, *399*, 1607–1617. [CrossRef] [PubMed]
35. Altorki, N.; Wang, X.; Damman, B.; Mentlick, J.; Landreneau, R.; Wigle, D.; Jones, D.R.; Conti, M.; Ashrafi, A.S.; Liberman, M.; et al. Lobectomy, segmentectomy, or wedge resection for peripheral clinical T1aN0 non-small cell lung cancer: A post hoc analysis of CALGB 140503 (Alliance). *J. Thorac. Cardiovasc. Surg.* **2024**, *167*, 338–347.e1. [CrossRef] [PubMed]
36. Altorki, N.; Wang, X.; Kozono, D.; Watt, C.; Landrenau, R.; Wigle, D.; Port, J.; Jones, D.R.; Conti, M.; Ashrafi, A.S.; et al. Lobar or Sublobar Resection for Peripheral Stage IA Non-Small-Cell Lung Cancer. *N. Engl. J. Med.* **2023**, *388*, 489–498. [CrossRef] [PubMed]
37. Hattori, A.; Suzuki, K.; Takamochi, K.; Wakabayashi, M.; Sekino, Y.; Tsutani, Y.; Nakajima, R.; Aokage, K.; Saji, H.; Tsuboi, M.; et al. Segmentectomy versus lobectomy in small-sized peripheral non-small-cell lung cancer with radiologically pure-solid appearance in Japan (JCOG0802/WJOG4607L): A post-hoc supplemental analysis of a multicentre, open-label, phase 3 trial. *Lancet Respir. Med.* **2024**, *12*, 105–116. [CrossRef] [PubMed]
38. Potter, A.L.; Kim, J.; McCarthy, M.L.; Senthil, P.; Mathey-Andrews, C.; Kumar, A.; Cao, C.; Lin, M.-W.; Lanuti, M.; Martin, L.W.; et al. Segmentectomy versus lobectomy in the United States: Outcomes after resection for first primary lung cancer and treatment patterns for second primary lung cancers. *J. Thorac. Cardiovasc. Surg.* **2024**, *167*, 350–364.e17. [CrossRef] [PubMed]
39. Meldola, P.F.; Toth, O.A.S.; Schnorrenberger, E.; Machado, P.G.; Chiarelli, G.F.C.; Kracik, J.L.S.; de Carvalho, C.C.; Lôbo, M.d.M.; Gross, J.L. Sublobar resection versus lobectomy for stage IA non-small-cell lung cancer: A systematic review and meta-analysis of randomized controlled trials. *Surg. Oncol.* **2023**, *51*, 101995. [CrossRef] [PubMed]
40. Fong, K.Y.; Chan, Y.H.; Chia, C.M.L.; Agasthian, T.; Lee, P. Sublobar resection versus lobectomy for stage IA non-small-cell lung cancer ≤ 2 cm: A systematic review and patient-level meta-analysis. *Updat. Surg.* **2023**, *75*, 2343–2354. [CrossRef]
41. Cardillo, G.; Petersen, R.H.; Ricciardi, S.; Patel, A.; Lodhia, J.V.; Gooseman, M.R.; Brunelli, A.; Dunning, J.; Fang, W.; Gossot, D.; et al. European guidelines for the surgical management of pure ground-glass opacities and part-solid nodules: Task Force of the European Association of Cardio-Thoracic Surgery and the European Society of Thoracic Surgeons. *Eur. J. Cardio-Thorac. Surg.* **2023**, *64*, ezad386. [CrossRef]
42. Migliore, M. Ground glass opacities of the lung before, during and post COVID-19 pandemic. *Ann. Transl. Med.* **2021**, *9*, 1042. [CrossRef] [PubMed]
43. Ettinger, D.S.; Wood, D.E.; Aisner, D.L.; Akerley, W.; Bauman, J.R.; Bharat, A.; Bruno, D.S.; Chang, J.Y.; Chirieac, L.R.; DeCamp, M.; et al. NCCN Guidelines® Insights: Non–Small Cell Lung Cancer, Version 2.2023: Featured Updates to the NCCN Guidelines. *J. Natl. Compr. Canc. Netw.* **2023**, *21*, 340–350. [CrossRef] [PubMed]
44. Hattori, A.; Matsunaga, T.; Hayashi, T.; Takamochi, K.; Oh, S.; Suzuki, K. Prognostic Impact of the Findings on Thin-Section Computed Tomography in Patients with Subcentimeter Non–Small Cell Lung Cancer. *J. Thorac. Oncol.* **2017**, *12*, 954–962. [CrossRef] [PubMed]
45. Sun, K.; You, A.; Wang, B.; Song, N.; Wan, Z.; Wu, F.; Zhao, W.; Zhou, F.; Li, W. Clinical T1aN0M0 lung cancer: Differences in clinicopathological patterns and oncological outcomes based on the findings on high-resolution computed tomography. *Eur. Radiol.* **2021**, *31*, 7353–7362. [CrossRef] [PubMed]
46. Ye, T.; Deng, L.; Wang, S.; Xiang, J.; Zhang, Y.; Hu, H.; Sun, Y.; Li, Y.; Shen, L.; Xie, L.; et al. Lung Adenocarcinomas Manifesting as Radiological Part-Solid Nodules Define a Special Clinical Subtype. *J. Thorac. Oncol.* **2019**, *14*, 617–627. [CrossRef] [PubMed]
47. Kamigaichi, A.; Tsutani, Y.; Mimae, T.; Miyata, Y.; Shimada, Y.; Ito, H.; Nakayama, H.; Ikeda, N.; Okada, M. The prognostic impact of the ground-glass opacity component in nearly pure-solid stage IA non-small-cell lung cancer. *Eur. J. Cardiothorac. Surg.* **2022**, *62*, ezac166. [CrossRef] [PubMed]

48. Migliore, M.; Fornito, M.; Palazzolo, M.; Criscione, A.; Gangemi, M.; Borrata, F.; Vigneri, P.; Nardini, M.; Dunning, J. Ground glass opacities management in the lung cancer screening era. *Ann. Transl. Med.* **2018**, *6*, 90. [CrossRef] [PubMed]
49. Shigefuku, S.; Shimada, Y.; Hagiwara, M.; Kakihana, M.; Kajiwara, N.; Ohira, T.; Ikeda, N. Prognostic Significance of Ground-Glass Opacity Components in 5-Year Survivors with Resected Lung Adenocarcinoma. *Ann. Surg. Oncol.* **2021**, *28*, 148–156. [CrossRef] [PubMed]
50. Hattori, A.; Takamochi, K.; Oh, S.; Suzuki, K. Prognostic Classification of Multiple Primary Lung Cancers Based on a Ground-Glass Opacity Component. *Ann. Thorac. Surg.* **2020**, *109*, 420–427. [CrossRef]
51. Choi, S.; Yoon, D.W.; Shin, S.; Kim, H.K.; Choi, Y.S.; Kim, J.; Shim, Y.M.; Cho, J.H. Importance of Lymph Node Evaluation in ≤2-cm Pure-Solid Non-Small Cell Lung Cancer. *Ann. Thorac. Surg.* **2024**, *117*, 586–593. [CrossRef]
52. Nakada, T.; Kuroda, H. Narrative review of optimal prognostic radiological tools using computed tomography for T1N0-staged non-small cell lung cancer. *J. Thorac. Dis.* **2021**, *13*, 3171–3181. [CrossRef] [PubMed]
53. Ye, T.; Deng, L.; Xiang, J.; Zhang, Y.; Hu, H.; Sun, Y.; Li, Y.; Shen, L.; Wang, S.; Xie, L.; et al. Predictors of Pathologic Tumor Invasion and Prognosis for Ground Glass Opacity Featured Lung Adenocarcinoma. *Ann. Thorac. Surg.* **2018**, *106*, 1682–1690. [CrossRef] [PubMed]
54. Zhai, W.Y.; Wong, W.S.; Duan, F.F.; Liang, D.C.; Gong, L.; Dai, S.Q.; Wang, J.Y. Distinct Prognostic Factors of Ground Glass Opacity and Pure-Solid Lesion in Pathological Stage I Invasive Lung Adenocarcinoma. *World J. Oncol.* **2022**, *13*, 259–271. [CrossRef] [PubMed]
55. Travis, W.D.; Brambilla, E.; Noguchi, M.; Nicholson, A.G.; Geisinger, K.; Yatabe, Y.; Powell, C.A.; Beer, D.; Riely, G.; Garg, K.; et al. International Association for the Study of Lung Cancer/American Thoracic Society/European Respiratory Society: International multidisciplinary classification of lung adenocarcinoma: Executive summary. *Proc. Am. Thorac. Soc.* **2011**, *8*, 381–385. [CrossRef] [PubMed]
56. Jang, J.Y.; Kim, S.S.; Song, S.Y.; Shin, Y.S.; Lee, S.W.; Ji, W.; Choi, C.-M.; Choi, E.K. Clinical Outcome of Stereotactic Body Radiotherapy in Patients with Early-Stage Lung Cancer with Ground-Glass Opacity Predominant Lesions: A Single Institution Experience. *Cancer Res. Treat.* **2023**, *55*, 1181–1189. [CrossRef] [PubMed]
57. Eriguchi, T.; Takeda, A.; Sanuki, N.; Tsurugai, Y.; Aoki, Y.; Oku, Y.; Hara, Y.; Akiba, T.; Shigematsu, N. Stereotactic body radiotherapy for operable early-stage non-small cell lung cancer. *Lung Cancer* **2017**, *109*, 62–67. [CrossRef]
58. Mizobuchi, T.; Nomoto, A.; Wada, H.; Yamamoto, N.; Nakajima, M.; Fujisawa, T.; Suzuki, H.; Yoshino, I. Outcomes of carbon ion radiotherapy compared with segmentectomy for ground glass opacity-dominant early-stage lung cancer. *Radiat. Oncol.* **2023**, *18*, 201. [CrossRef] [PubMed]
59. Kodama, H.; Yamakado, K.; Hasegawa, T.; Takao, M.; Taguchi, O.; Fukai, I.; Sakuma, H. Radiofrequency ablation for ground-glass opacity-dominant lung adenocarcinoma. *J. Vasc. Interv. Radiol. JVIR* **2014**, *25*, 333–339. [CrossRef] [PubMed]
60. Iguchi, T.; Hiraki, T.; Gobara, H.; Fujiwara, H.; Matsui, Y.; Soh, J.; Toyooka, S.; Kiura, K.; Kanazawa, S. Percutaneous Radiofrequency Ablation of Lung Cancer Presenting as Ground-Glass Opacity. *Cardiovasc. Interv. Radiol.* **2015**, *38*, 409–415. [CrossRef]
61. Wisnivesky, J.P.; Mudd, J.; Stone, K.; Slatore, C.G.; Flores, R.; Swanson, S.; Blackstock, W.; Smith, C.B.; Chidel, M.; Rosenzweig, K.; et al. Longitudinal quality of life after sublobar resection and stereotactic body radiation therapy for early-stage non-small cell lung cancer. *Cancer*, **2024**; ahead of print. [CrossRef]
62. Liu, C.; Yang, Z.; Li, Y.; Guo, C.; Xia, L.; Zhang, W.; Xiao, C.; Mei, J.; Liao, H.; Zhu, Y.; et al. Intentional wedge resection versus segmentectomy for ≤2 cm Ground-Glass-Opacity-Dominant Non-Small cell lung cancer: A Real-World study using inverse probability of treatment weighting. *Int. J. Surg.* **2024**. [CrossRef]
63. Zhang, C.; He, Z.; Cheng, J.; Cao, J.; Hu, J. Surgical Outcomes of Lobectomy Versus Limited Resection for Clinical Stage I Ground-Glass Opacity Lung Adenocarcinoma 2 Centimeters or Smaller. *Clin. Lung Cancer* **2021**, *22*, e160–e168. [CrossRef] [PubMed]
64. Aokage, K.; Suzuki, K.; Saji, H.; Wakabayashi, M.; Kataoka, T.; Sekino, Y.; Fukuda, H.; Endo, M.; Hattori, A.; Mimae, T.; et al. Segmentectomy for ground-glass-dominant lung cancer with a tumour diameter of 3 cm or less including ground-glass opacity (JCOG1211): A multicentre, single-arm, confirmatory, phase 3 trial. *Lancet Respir. Med.* **2023**, *11*, 540–549. [CrossRef] [PubMed]
65. Li, H.; Wang, Y.; Chen, Y.; Zhong, C.; Fang, W. Ground glass opacity resection extent assessment trial (GREAT): A study protocol of multi-institutional, prospective, open-label, randomized phase III trial of minimally invasive segmentectomy versus lobectomy for ground glass opacity (GGO)-containing early-stage invasive lung adenocarcinoma. *Front. Oncol.* **2023**, *13*, 1052796. [CrossRef] [PubMed]
66. Woo, W.; Cha, Y.J.; Lee, J.; Moon, D.H.; Lee, S. Impact of extended mediastinal lymph node dissection for stage I ground-glass opacity lesions. *J. Thorac. Dis.* **2023**, *15*, 6029–6039. [CrossRef] [PubMed]
67. Mimae, T.; Miyata, Y.; Tsubokawa, N.; Kudo, Y.; Nagashima, T.; Ito, H.; Ikeda, N.; Okada, M. Omitting lymph node dissection for small ground glass opacity-dominant tumors. *Ann. Thorac. Surg.* **2024**; ahead of print. [CrossRef] [PubMed]
68. Kim, H.K. What Should Thoracic Surgeons Consider during Surgery for Ground-Glass Nodules? Lymph Node Dissection. *J. Chest Surg.* **2021**, *54*, 342–347. [CrossRef] [PubMed]
69. Mokhles, S.; Macbeth, F.; Treasure, T.; Younes, R.N.; Rintoul, R.C.; Fiorentino, F.; Bogers, A.J.J.C.; Takkenberg, J.J.M. Systematic lymphadenectomy versus sampling of ipsilateral mediastinal lymph-nodes during lobectomy for non-small-cell lung cancer: A systematic review of randomized trials and a meta-analysis. *Eur. J. Cardiothorac. Surg.* **2017**, *51*, 1149–1156. [CrossRef] [PubMed]

70. Deng, C.; Zhang, Y.; Chen, H. Is it really necessary to perform mediastinal lymphadenectomy in surgery for ground glass opacity-featured lung adenocarcinoma? *AME Med. J.* **2022**, *7*, 24. [CrossRef]
71. Huang, W.; Deng, H.-Y.; Ren, Z.-Z.; Xu, K.; Wang, Y.-F.; Tang, X.; Zhu, D.-X.; Zhou, Q. LobE-Specific lymph node diSsectiON for clinical early-stage non-small cell lung cancer: Protocol for a randomised controlled trial (the LESSON trial). *BMJ Open* **2022**, *12*, e056043. [CrossRef]
72. Li, C.; Ni, Y.; Liu, C.; Liu, R.; Zhang, C.; Song, Z.; Liu, H.; Jiang, T.; Zhang, Z. Mediastinal lymph node dissection versus spared mediastinal lymph node dissection in stage IA non-small cell lung cancer presented as ground glass nodules: Study protocol of a phase III, randomised, multicentre trial (MELDSIG) in China. *BMJ Open* **2023**, *13*, e075242. [CrossRef]
73. Milano, M.T.; Zhang, H.; Usuki, K.Y.; Singh, D.P.; Chen, Y. Definitive radiotherapy for stage I nonsmall cell lung cancer. *Cancer* **2012**, *118*, 5572–5579. [CrossRef]
74. De Ruysscher, D.; Nakagawa, K.; Asamura, H. Surgical and nonsurgical approaches to small-size nonsmall cell lung cancer. *Eur. Respir. J.* **2014**, *44*, 483–494. [CrossRef] [PubMed]
75. Arriagada, R.; Bergman, B.; Dunant, A.; Le Chevalier, T.; Pignon, J.P.; Vansteenkiste, J.; International Adjuvant Lung Cancer Trial Collaborative Group. Cisplatin-based adjuvant chemotherapy in patients with completely resected non-small-cell lung cancer. *N. Engl. J. Med.* 2004; 350, 351–360. [CrossRef]
76. Kreuter, M.; Vansteenkiste, J.; Fischer, J.R.; Eberhardt, W.; Zabeck, H.; Kollmeier, J.; Serke, M.; Frickhofen, N.; Reck, M.; Engel-Riedel, W.; et al. Randomized phase 2 trial on refinement of early-stage NSCLC adjuvant chemotherapy with cisplatin and pemetrexed versus cisplatin and vinorelbine: The TREAT study. *Ann. Oncol. Off. J. Eur. Soc. Med. Oncol.* **2013**, *24*, 986–992. [CrossRef] [PubMed]
77. Wakelee, H.A.; E Dahlberg, S.; Keller, S.M.; Tester, W.J.; Gandara, D.R.; Graziano, S.L.; Adjei, A.; Leighl, N.B.; Aisner, S.C.; Rothman, J.M.; et al. Adjuvant chemotherapy with or without bevacizumab in patients with resected non-small-cell lung cancer (E1505): An open-label, multicentre, randomised, phase 3 trial. *Lancet Oncol.* **2017**, *18*, 1610–1623. [CrossRef] [PubMed]
78. Kelly, K.; Altorki, N.K.; Eberhardt, W.E.; O'Brien, M.E.; Spigel, D.R.; Crinò, L.; Tsai, C.-M.; Kim, J.-H.; Cho, E.K.; Hoffman, P.C.; et al. Adjuvant Erlotinib Versus Placebo in Patients with Stage IB-IIIA Non-Small-Cell Lung Cancer (RADIANT): A Randomized, Double-Blind, Phase III Trial. *J. Clin. Oncol.* **2015**, *33*, 4007–4014. [CrossRef] [PubMed]
79. Hogan, B.V.; Peter, M.B.; Shenoy, H.G.; Horgan, K.; Hughes, T.A. Surgery induced immunosuppression. *Surg. J. R. Coll. Surg. Edinb. Irel.* **2011**, *9*, 38–43. [CrossRef] [PubMed]
80. Ghysen, K.; Vansteenkiste, J. Immunotherapy in patients with early stage resectable nonsmall cell lung cancer. *Curr. Opin. Oncol.* **2019**, *31*, 13. [CrossRef]
81. Gandhi, L.; Rodríguez-Abreu, D.; Gadgeel, S.; Esteban, E.; Felip, E.; De Angelis, F.; Domine, M.; Clingan, P.; Hochmair, M.J.; Powell, S.F.; et al. Pembrolizumab plus Chemotherapy in Metastatic Non-Small-Cell Lung Cancer. *N. Engl. J. Med.* **2018**, *378*, 2078–2092. [CrossRef] [PubMed]
82. Reck, M.; Rodríguez–Abreu, D.; Robinson, A.G.; Hui, R.; Csőszi, T.; Fülöp, A.; Gottfried, M.; Peled, N.; Tafreshi, A.; Cuffe, S.; et al. Updated Analysis of KEYNOTE-024: Pembrolizumab Versus Platinum-Based Chemotherapy for Advanced Non–Small-Cell Lung Cancer With PD-L1 Tumor Proportion Score of 50% or Greater. *J. Clin. Oncol.* **2019**, *37*, 537–546. [CrossRef]
83. Paz-Ares, L.; Luft, A.; Vicente, D.; Tafreshi, A.; Gümüş, M.; Mazières, J.; Hermes, B.; Çay Şenler, F.; Csőszi, T.; Fülöp, A.; et al. Pembrolizumab plus Chemotherapy for Squamous Non–Small-Cell Lung Cancer. *N. Engl. J. Med.* **2018**, *379*, 2040–2051. [CrossRef]
84. Antonia, S.J.; Villegas, A.; Daniel, D.; Vicente, D.; Murakami, S.; Hui, R.; Kurata, T.; Chiappori, A.; Lee, K.H.; de Wit, M.; et al. Overall Survival with Durvalumab after Chemoradiotherapy in Stage III NSCLC. *N. Engl. J. Med.* **2018**, *379*, 2342–2350. [CrossRef]
85. Paz-Ares, L.; Hasan, B.; Dafni, U.; Menis, J.; Maio, M.E.D.; Oselin, K.; Albert, I.; Faehling, M.; Schil, P.V.; O'Brien, M.E.R. A randomized, phase 3 trial with anti-PD-1 monoclonal antibody pembrolizumab (MK-3475) versus placebo for patients with early stage NSCLC after resection and completion of standard adjuvant therapy (EORTC/ETOP 1416-PEARLS). *Ann. Oncol.* **2017**, *28*, ii23. [CrossRef]
86. Canadian Cancer Trials Group. A Phase III Prospective Double Blind Placebo Controlled Randomized Study of Adjuvant MEDI4736. In *Completely Resected Non-Small Cell Lung Cancer*; ClinicalTrials.gov: Bethesda, MD, USA, 2023.
87. Chaft, J.E.; Dahlberg, S.E.; Khullar, O.V.; Edelman, M.J.; Simone, C.B.; Heymach, J.; Rudin, C.M.; Ramalingam, S.S. EA5142 adjuvant nivolumab in resected lung cancers (ANVIL). *J. Clin. Oncol.* **2018**, *36*, TPS8581. [CrossRef]
88. Felip, E.; Altorki, N.; Zhou, C.; Csőszi, T.; Vynnychenko, I.; Goloborodko, O.; Luft, A.; Akopov, A.; Martinez-Marti, A.; Kenmotsu, H.; et al. Adjuvant atezolizumab after adjuvant chemotherapy in resected stage IB-IIIA non-small-cell lung cancer (IMpower010): A randomised, multicentre, open-label, phase 3 trial. *Lancet* **2021**, *398*, 1344–1357. [CrossRef] [PubMed]
89. Pennell, N.A.; Neal, J.W.; Chaft, J.E.; Azzoli, C.G.; Jänne, P.A.; Govindan, R.; Evans, T.L.; Costa, D.B.; Wakelee, H.A.; Heist, R.S.; et al. SELECT: A Phase II Trial of Adjuvant Erlotinib in Patients with Resected Epidermal Growth Factor Receptor-Mutant Non-Small-Cell Lung Cancer. *J. Clin. Oncol.* **2019**, *37*, 97–104. [CrossRef] [PubMed]
90. Wu, Y.-L.; Zhong, W.; Wang, Q.; Mao, W.; Xu, S.-T.; Wu, L.; Chen, C.; Cheng, Y.; Xu, L.; Wang, J.; et al. CTONG1104: Adjuvant gefitinib versus chemotherapy for resected N1-N2 NSCLC with EGFR mutation—Final overall survival analysis of the randomized phase III trial 1 analysis of the randomized phase III trial. *J. Clin. Oncol.* **2020**, *38*, 9005. [CrossRef]
91. Lara-Guerra, H.; Waddell, T.K.; Salvarrey, M.A.; Joshua, A.M.; Chung, C.T.; Paul, N.; Boerner, S.; Sakurada, A.; Ludkovski, O.; Ma, C.; et al. Phase II study of preoperative gefitinib in clinical stage I non-small-cell lung cancer. *J. Clin. Oncol.* **2009**, *27*, 6229–6236. [CrossRef] [PubMed]

92. Barlesi, F.; Mazieres, J.; Merlio, J.-P.; Debieuvre, D.; Mosser, J.; Lena, H.; Ouafik, L.; Besse, B.; Rouquette, I.; Westeel, V.; et al. Routine molecular profiling of patients with advanced non-small-cell lung cancer: Results of a 1-year nationwide programme of the French Cooperative Thoracic Intergroup (IFCT). *Lancet* **2016**, *387*, 1415–1426. [CrossRef] [PubMed]
93. Abbasian, M.H.; Ardekani, A.M.; Sobhani, N.; Roudi, R. The Role of Genomics and Proteomics in Lung Cancer Early Detection and Treatment. *Cancers* **2022**, *14*, 5144. [CrossRef]
94. Migliore, M.; Halezeroglu, S.; Mueller, M.R. Making precision surgical strategies a reality: Are we ready for a paradigm shift in thoracic surgical oncology? *Future Oncol.* **2020**, *16*, 1–5. [CrossRef]

Disclaimer/Publisher's Note: The statements, opinions and data contained in all publications are solely those of the individual author(s) and contributor(s) and not of MDPI and/or the editor(s). MDPI and/or the editor(s) disclaim responsibility for any injury to people or property resulting from any ideas, methods, instructions or products referred to in the content.

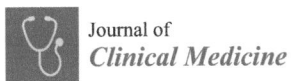

Article

Co-Occurring Driver Genomic Alterations in Advanced Non-Small-Cell Lung Cancer (NSCLC): A Retrospective Analysis

Ilaria Attili [1], Riccardo Asnaghi [2], Davide Vacirca [3], Riccardo Adorisio [3], Alessandra Rappa [3], Alberto Ranghiero [3], Mariano Lombardi [3], Carla Corvaja [1], Valeria Fuorivia [2], Ambra Carnevale Schianca [2], Pamela Trillo Aliaga [1], Gianluca Spitaleri [1], Ester Del Signore [1], Juliana Guarize [4], Lorenzo Spaggiari [2,5], Elena Guerini-Rocco [2,3], Nicola Fusco [2,3], Filippo de Marinis [1] and Antonio Passaro [1,*]

[1] Division of Thoracic Oncology, European Institute of Oncology IRCCS, 20141 Milan, Italy; ilaria.attili@ieo.it (I.A.)
[2] Department of Oncology and Hemato-Oncology, University of Milan, 20141 Milan, Italy
[3] Division of Pathology, IEO, European Institute of Oncology IRCCS, 20141 Milan, Italy
[4] Division of Interventional Pulmonology, IEO, European Institute of Oncology IRCCS, 20141 Milan, Italy
[5] Department of Thoracic Surgery, IEO, European Institute of Oncology IRCCS, 20141 Milan, Italy
* Correspondence: antonio.passaro@ieo.it

Abstract: Background: Actionable driver mutations account for 40–50% of NSCLC cases, and their identification clearly affects treatment choices and outcomes. Conversely, non-actionable mutations are genetic alterations that do not currently have established treatment implications. Among co-occurring alterations, the identification of concurrent actionable genomic alterations is a rare event, potentially impacting prognosis and treatment outcomes. **Methods:** We retrospectively evaluated the prevalence and patterns of concurrent driver genomic alterations in a large series of NSCLCs to investigate their association with clinicopathological characteristics, to assess the prognosis of patients whose tumor harbors concurrent alterations in the genes of interest and to explore their potential therapeutic implications. **Results:** Co-occurring driver alterations were identified in 26 out of 1520 patients with at least one gene alteration (1.7%). Within these cases, the incidence of concurrent actionable gene alterations was 39% (0.7% of the overall cohort). Among compound actionable gene mutations, *EGFR* was the most frequently involved gene (70%). The most frequent association was *EGFR* mutations with *ROS1* rearrangement. Front-line targeted treatments were the preferred approach in patients with compound actionable mutations, with dismal median PFS observed (6 months). **Conclusions:** Advances in genomic profiling technologies are facilitating the identification of concurrent mutations. In patients with concurrent actionable gene alterations, integrated molecular and clinical data should be used to guide treatment decisions, always considering rebiopsy at the moment of disease progression.

Keywords: molecular testing; next-generation sequencing; concurrent mutations; biopsy; tyrosine kinase inhibitors; treatments

Citation: Attili, I.; Asnaghi, R.; Vacirca, D.; Adorisio, R.; Rappa, A.; Ranghiero, A.; Lombardi, M.; Corvaja, C.; Fuorivia, V.; Carnevale Schianca, A.; et al. Co-Occurring Driver Genomic Alterations in Advanced Non-Small-Cell Lung Cancer (NSCLC): A Retrospective Analysis. *J. Clin. Med.* **2024**, *13*, 4476. https://doi.org/10.3390/jcm13154476

Academic Editors: Sukhwinder Singh Sohal and Milo Frattini

Received: 28 May 2024
Revised: 7 July 2024
Accepted: 16 July 2024
Published: 31 July 2024

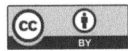

Copyright: © 2024 by the authors. Licensee MDPI, Basel, Switzerland. This article is an open access article distributed under the terms and conditions of the Creative Commons Attribution (CC BY) license (https://creativecommons.org/licenses/by/4.0/).

1. Introduction

Non-small-cell lung cancer (NSCLC) constitutes approximately 85% of all lung cancer cases, making it the most prevalent subtype worldwide [1]. The advent of precision medicine has illuminated the role of driver mutations in NSCLC pathogenesis. Within NSCLC, driver mutations play a significant role, with reported frequencies varying across populations, overall reaching up to 40–50% of NSCLC cases [2–4]. *EGFR*-activating mutations occur in about 10–15% of Caucasian and up to 50% of Asian NSCLC patients [5,6], while *ALK* and *ROS1* rearrangements are detected in 3–7% [7] and 2% of cases, respectively [8,9]. *KRAS* G12C mutations are overall the most frequent driver gene alteration (13%) [10]. Less common are *BRAF* V600 mutations (1–2%), *ERBB2* mutations (2–3%) and *RET* and *NTRK1,2,3* gene rearrangements (2% and 0.3%, respectively) [11–14].

These alterations are defined as actionable, representing key targets for tailored therapies, which can revolutionize treatment paradigms and improve patient outcomes. Indeed, tyrosine kinase inhibitors (TKIs) are currently the standard front-line treatment for *EGFR-*, *ALK-*, *ROS1-* and *BRAF*-positive patients, and targeted treatments are available in the pretreated setting or in clinical trials for *RET*, *ERBB2*, *KRAS* and *NTRK* actionable alterations [15].

On the other hand, non-actionable mutations are genetic alterations that do not currently have established targeted therapies or known treatment implications [16,17]. These mutations may still provide valuable information for understanding the biology of the tumor or predicting prognosis. Non-actionable mutations may include alterations in genes with unclear functional significance or those for which targeted therapies are still under investigation or development (i.e., *KRAS* non-G12C or *BRAF* non-V600 mutations). According to this definition, the use of comprehensive molecular profiling techniques, such as next-generation sequencing (NGS), may allow us to identify actionable and non-actionable mutations in most NSCLC samples [18].

Even more complex, the definition of concurrent mutations refers to the presence of multiple genomic alterations within the same tumor, often involving different driver genes [19]. These compound alterations can arise through various mechanisms, including clonal evolution, tumor heterogeneity and the selective pressure exerted by treatments [20–22]. The most frequent patterns of co-occurring alterations in NSCLC involve one actionable gene alteration and one alteration in genes involved in cell survival and proliferation (*TP53*, *STK11*, *PI3KCA* and DNA repair pathways), often defining a negative prognostic role compared with the non-co-mutated counterpart [18,19,23–26].

From a diagnostic standpoint, identifying and characterizing compound mutations requires comprehensive molecular profiling techniques. Additionally, interpreting the functional significance of these concurrent genomic alterations and predicting their impact on tumor behavior can be complex.

In clinical practice, the identification of concurrent actionable genomic alterations is a rare event (around 1%), described as anecdotical; however, these co-occurrences may influence treatment decisions [27–29]. Indeed, some combinations of mutations may confer resistance to specific targeted therapies, limiting their effectiveness. Conversely, certain compound mutations may offer opportunities for combination therapies targeting multiple pathways simultaneously, potentially enhancing treatment response. These aspects have been mainly investigated in the setting of acquired resistance to TKIs, but no data, besides case reports, are available for co-occurring actionable mutations present in treatment-naïve patients [30].

In the present study, we evaluate the prevalence and the pattern of concurrent driver genomic alterations in a large series of NSCLCs (i) to investigate their association with clinicopathological characteristics, (ii) to assess the prognosis of patients whose tumor harbors concurrent alterations in the gene of interest and (iii) to explore their potential therapeutic implications.

2. Materials and Methods

This retrospective analysis was conducted on a single institution's database (European Institute of Oncology—Milan, Italy) consisting of 1520 patients diagnosed with advanced NSCLC harboring at least one driver mutation between December 2016 and December 2022. Patients diagnosed with advanced/metastatic NSCLC, molecularly profiled at our institution, were screened for the presence of co-occurrent alterations in genes of interest. Medical records were reviewed to collect information on molecular classification, demographic features, disease characteristics, treatments administered, responses and follow-up. Information on rebiopsy at disease progression, when performed, was also collected.

We considered genes of interest: *EGFR*, *KRAS*, *BRAF*, *ALK*, *ROS1*, *RET*, *MET*, *ERBB2*, *NTRK* and *PIK3CA*. The population of the current work was defined including patients with at least 2 co-occurring alterations in NSCLC driver genes (*EGFR*, *KRAS*, *BRAF*, *ALK*, *ROS1*, *RET*, *MET*, *ERBB2* and *NTRK*).

The identified co-occurrent alterations were then grouped into 3 categories based on their actionability. The first group consisted of patients with two actionable alterations, defined as *EGFR*-activating mutations, *KRAS* p.G12C mutations, *BRAF* p.V600 mutations, *ALK*, *ROS1*, *RET* and *NTRK* gene rearrangements, *MET* exon skipping mutations and *ERBB2* exon 20 mutations. The second group included patients with one actionable and one non-actionable alteration, while patients with two non-actionable mutations on driver genes were categorized into the third group (Supplementary Figure S1). Testing methods used for molecular classification included DNA and/or RNA NGS assays and FISH.

NGS analysis was performed using the Oncomine Comprehensive Assay (OCA) v.3 (Thermo Fisher Scientific, Waltham, MA, USA) according to manufacturer instructions. Libraries were prepared by using an Ion AmpliSeq DL8 kit (Thermo Fisher Scientific, MA, USA) on an Ion Chef system (Thermo Fisher Scientific, MA, USA) following manufacturer instructions. After library reamplification and barcoding, libraries were diluted at 30 pM and newly loaded into the Ion Chef instrument for automatic template preparation and chip loading. Finally, libraries were automatically loaded on an Ion 540™ Chip and sequenced on an Ion S5™ System (Thermo Fisher Scientific, MA, USA). Data analysis was performed as follows: after alignment to the hg19 human reference genome, coverage analysis with custom bed-files was assessed using the coverage plug-in (v.5.0.2.0) from Torrent Suite (v.5.0.2) (Thermo Fisher Scientific, MA, USA); the variant caller plug-in was used with a dedicated workflow on Ion Reporter Torrent Suite 5.16 (Thermo Fisher Scientific, MA, USA). Criteria for annotating and classifying molecular alterations as pathogenic/likely pathogenic according to gene mutation databases (Catalogue of Somatic Mutations in Cancer (COSMIC), cBioPortal for Cancer Genomics, ClinVar–NCBI–NIH) were a minimum coverage depth of $500\times$, allele coverage and a quality score ≥ 20 and a minimum variant allele frequency (VAF) of 5%.

FISH analyses were performed using a dual-color probe (ALK, ROS1 and RET IQFISH Break Apart Probe and MET IQFISH Probe with CEP7, respectively; Agilent Technologies, Santa Clara, CA, USA).

All the study procedures were carried out with general authorization for the processing of personal data for scientific research purposes from "The Italian Data Protection Authority" (http://www.garanteprivacy.it/web/guest/home/docweb/-/docwebdisplay/export/2485392, accessed on 10 April 2024). All information regarding patients was managed adopting anonymous numerical codes, and all samples were handled in compliance with the Helsinki Declaration.

Variables were presented by using the median value for continuous variables and percentages (numbers) for categorical variables.

Overall survival (OS) was defined as the time from the diagnosis of advanced/metastatic disease to death. Progression-free survival (PFS) was defined as the time from treatment start to disease progression or death. OS and PFS were estimated by using Kaplan–Meier methods. Median follow-up was calculated with the reverse Kaplan–Meier method. The Cox regression model was used for subgroup analysis on survival outcomes, and data were evaluated as hazard ratios (HRs) and their 95% confidence interval (CI), as appropriate. Given the very small subset and heterogeneity of patients, no adjustments were considered and only univariate analyses were performed.

The statistical significance level was set at $p < 0.05$ for all tests. All statistical analyses were performed with RStudio (RStudio: Integrated Development for R. RStudio, Inc., Boston, MA, USA, v.4.1.2).

3. Results

3.1. Frequency and Distribution of Compound Driver Gene Alterations

Overall, 1520 cases of advanced NSCLC with at least one alteration in genes of interest were identified in the study period. Co-occurring alterations in genes of interest were observed in 36 cases (2.3% of the patients with at least one actionable mutation). Among them, we identified 26 patients with at least two co-occurring driver genomic alterations, representing the population of interest in the current work.

The most frequent testing method was the combined use of DNA/RNA NGS plus FISH (53%), followed by DNA NGS plus FISH (41%) (Table 1).

Table 1. Testing methods used for molecular assessment.

Testing Method	Baseline ($n = 26$)	Rebiopsy ($n = 8$)	Total ($n = 34$)
NGS DNA + FISH	12	2	14 (41%)
NGS DNA/RNA + FISH	14	4	18 (53%)
NGS DNA or DNA/RNA	0	1	1 (3%)
PCR alone	0	1	1 (3%)

The study population included $n = 10$ (39%) patients who had compound actionable alterations, $n = 12$ (46%) patients whose tumor harbored one actionable and at least one non-actionable alteration in driver genes and $n = 4$ (15%) patients with two or more non-actionable alterations in driver genes (Figure 1a; Table 2).

a.
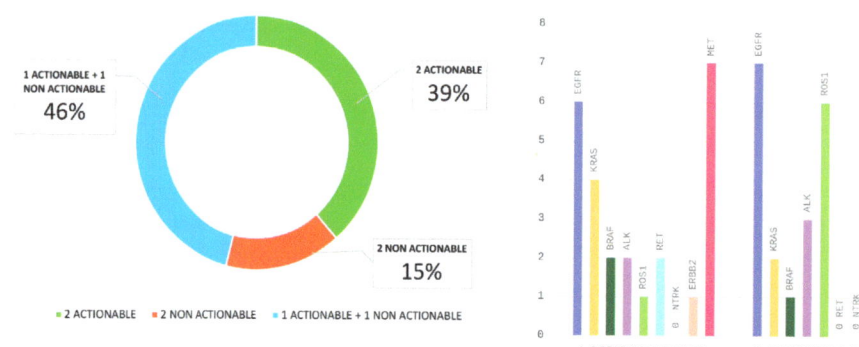

b.
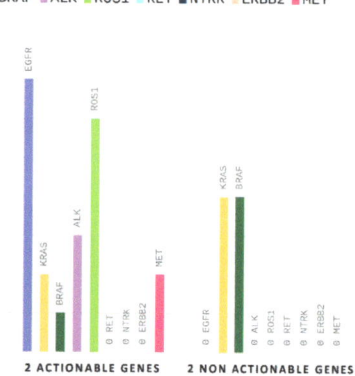

Figure 1. Distribution of concurrent driver genomic alterations. Distribution by actionability of compound driver genes (**a**) and distribution of compound mutations by involved genes (**b**).

Overall, the most frequent alterations involved in the compound group are fusion genes (seven *ROS1* rearrangements and five *ALK* rearrangements), followed by *EGFR* mutations ($n = 11$). Among the ten cases with concurrent actionable alterations, nine harbored gene rearrangements and seven *EGFR* mutations. The most frequent association was an *EGFR* mutation with *ROS1* gene rearrangement (Figure 1b).

KRAS and *BRAF* gene mutations were the most frequent compound non-actionable mutations in driver genes (Figure 1b).

Of note, rebiopsy was performed at the time of disease progression in eight cases (50% of those with concurrent actionable mutations). In 87.5% of cases, the site of rebiopsy was different from that of the baseline, including one case of liquid biopsy. Considering the presence of one driver mutation, the molecular results of the rebiopsy analysis were concordant with those of the baseline analysis. However, loss of one gene alteration was observed in four (50%) cases, and in three cases, one additional resistant mutation was detected (Table 2).

Table 2. Clinicopathological characteristics and molecular alteration at baseline and progression in the study population (n = 26 patients with at least 2 co-occurring driver genomic alterations).

| Patient # | Sex | Age [1] | Smoking Status | Baseline | | | | Progression | | | Baseline Tumor Cellularity | VAF§ | Rebiopsy Tumor Cellularity | Rebiopsy VAF |
				Baseline Biopsy Site	Collection Method	Baseline Testing Result	Rebiopsy Site (If Performed)	Collection Method	Rebiopsy Testing Result		Baseline VAF		
1	M	68	never	RSL	TISSUE-BLOCK	EGFR L858R KRAS Q61K	-	-	-	40–60%	69% 7%	-	-
2	M	76	former	RSL LIL	CITO-BLOCK	EGFR E906 KRAS G12C	-	-	-	60%	39% 50%	-	-
3	F	55	never	RPP LPP	CITO-BLOCK	EGFR L858R ERBB2 S310F	AL	TISSUE-BLOCK	EGFR L858R ERBB2 wt	20%	13% 9%	20–40%	6% -
4	F	78	never	RSL	TISSUE-BLOCK	EGFR L858R MET L1213F	RPP	TISSUE-BLOCK	EGFR L858R MET wt	60%	27% NA	40%	33% -
5	M	60	never	RSL	CITO-BLOCK	EGFR L858R MET: c.2942-15_2942-12del	RSL	TISSUE-BLOCK	EGFR L858R MET: c.2942-15_2942-12del	60%	57% NA	60%	62% NA
6	F	76	never	ML	CITO-BLOCK	EGFR V843I ALK rearrangement (2p23)	-	-	-	60%	5% NA	-	-
7	M	76	former	ML	CITO-BLOCK	KRAS Q61H BRAF G464V	-	-	-	40%	36% 23%	-	-
8	M	82	former	LIL	CITO-BLOCK	KRAS K117N BRAF G469V	-	-	-	20–40%	12% 12%	-	-
9	M	72	former	LIL	TISSUE-BLOCK	KRAS G13D BRAF G469V	-	-	-	60%	5% 17%	-	-
10	M	70	current	RIL	TISSUE-BLOCK	KRAS Q61R BRAF D594G PIK3CA E453K	-	-	-	20–40%	17% 10% 23%	-	-
11	F	52	never	RML	CITO-BLOCK	KRAS G12V BRAF D594N RET KIF5B	-	-	-	40%	11% 18% NA	-	-

Table 2. *Cont.*

Patient #	Sex	Age [1]	Smoking Status	Baseline			Progression				Baseline Tumor Cellularity	VAF §			
				Baseline Biopsy Site	Collection Method	Baseline Testing Result	Rebiopsy Site (If Performed)	Collection Method	Rebiopsy Testing Result			Baseline VAF	Rebiopsy Tumor Cellularity	Rebiopsy VAF	
12	M	62	never	LPP	TISSUE-BLOCK	EGFR L861Q ROS1 rearrangement (6q22)	LSL	TISSUE-BLOCK	EGFR L861Q ROS1 rearrangement (6q22)		20–40%	6% NA	40%	10% -	
13	M	75	never	PLEURAL LIQUID	CITO-BLOCK	EGFR L858R ALK rearrangement (2p23)	RPP	TISSUE-BLOCK	EGFR L858R EGFR T790M ALK rearrangement (2p23)		-	.	20%	25% NA	
14	F	71	never	T	TISSUE-BLOCK	EFGR E746_T751delinsA EGFR amplification (30.2) chr7 ALK rearrangement EML4 (ex 2)-ALK (ex 20	-	-	-		40%	82% NA	-	-	
15	F	62	current	T	TISSUE-BLOCK	EGFR L858R ROS1 rearrangement (6q22)	PLASMA TISSUE	LIQUID BIOPSY	EGFR L858R EGFR T790M ROS1 not estimated *		20%	12% NA	NA	NA	
16	F	84	never	RIL	CITO-BLOCK	EGFR L858R ROS1 rearrangement (6q22)	-	-	-		60%	95% NA	-	-	
17	F	48	current	LPP	TISSUE-BLOCK	EGFR E746_A750del ROS1 rearrangement (6q22)	LINGULA	TISSUE-BLOCK	EGFR E746_A750del EGFR T790M ROS1 wt		20–40%	26% NA	40%	58% 32% NA	

Table 2. Cont.

Patient #	Sex	Age [1]	Smoking Status	Baseline			Progression				VAF§			
				Baseline Biopsy Site	Collection Method	Baseline Testing Result	Rebiopsy Site (If Performed)	Collection Method	Rebiopsy Testing Result	Baseline Tumor Cellularity	Baseline VAF	Rebiopsy Tumor Cellularity	Rebiopsy VAF
18	F	70	never	T	TISSUE-BLOCK	EGFR L861Q ROS1 rearrangement (6q22)	-	-	-	60%	40% NA	-	-
19	M	67	never	ML	CITO-BLOCK	RET rearrangement (10q11) MET CNV (8.2) chr 7	-	-	-	60%	NA NA	-	-
20	F	27	never	RPP	TISSUE-BLOCK	ROS1 rearrangement (6q22) MET CNV (6.64) chr 7	LPP	TISSUE-BLOCK	ROS1 rearrangement (6q22) MET wt	20–40%	NA NA	20%	NA NA
21	M	49	former	RML	CITO-BLOCK	BRAF K601N MET ex14skipping	-	-	-	60%	42% NA	-	-
22	F	59	former	RIL	TISSUE-BLOCK	KRAS G12C ROS1 6q22 PIK3CA E545K	-	-	-	60%	7% NA 8%	-	-
23	F	69	current	RB	TISSUE-BLOCK	BRAFV600E ALK rearrangement EML4 ex 19-ALK ex 20	-	-	-	60%	18% NA	-	-
24	M	69	current	RSL	CITO-BLOCK	KRAS CNV (6) chr12 MET ex14skipping	-	-	-	20–40%	NA 52%	-	-

Table 2. Cont.

Patient #	Sex	Age [1]	Smoking Status	Baseline Biopsy Site	Baseline Collection Method	Baseline Testing Result	Rebiopsy Site (If Performed)	Progression Collection Method	Rebiopsy Testing Result	Baseline Tumor Cellularity	Baseline VAF	Rebiopsy Tumor Cellularity	Rebiopsy VAF
25	M	68	former	RPP	TISSUE-BLOCK	KRAS G12C MET ex14 skipping	-	-	-	20%	10% 6%	-	-
26	F	40	never	ML	CITO-BLOCK	ALK rearrangement EML4 ex 19-ALK ex 20 MET CNV (23.87) chr 7	-	-	-	60%	NA NA	-	-

Abbreviations: RSL = right superior lobe; RML = right middle lobe; RIL = right inferior lobe; LIL = left inferior lobe; LSL = left superior lobe; RPP = right parietal pleura; LPP = left parietal pleura; AL = axillar lymph node; ML = mediastinic lymph node; T = distal/carenal trachea; RB = right bronchus; NA = data not available § for concordant gene alterations. [1] Age at diagnosis of advanced/metastatic NSCLC. All patients were stage IV. * A different testing method from baseline was used in this case. # patient ID number.

3.2. Exploratory Evaluation of Therapeutic Approaches Used in Patients with Compound Actionable Gene Alterations

As expected, for patients with one actionable plus one non-actionable gene alteration, the therapeutic approach was chosen as per international guidelines.

In the group with compound actionable gene alterations ($n = 10$), the preferred treatment approach was an upfront targeted treatment (seven out of eight patients with available clinical follow-up), followed by an alternative driver-based targeted approach at disease progression in four cases. No subsequent treatment was possible in two patients due to worsening clinical conditions and death (Figure 2). The best responses to front-line targeted treatment were partial responses (4/7), stable disease (1/7) and progressive disease (2/7). Median PFS with front-line targeted treatment was 6 months (95% CI 3-NA), and median treatment duration was 8 months (95% CI 6-NA). Conversely, front-line chemotherapy was preferred only in one case, with 12-month lasting clinical benefit (Figure 2). Due to the unavailability of clinical trials in the setting, no patients were treated with dual TKIs.

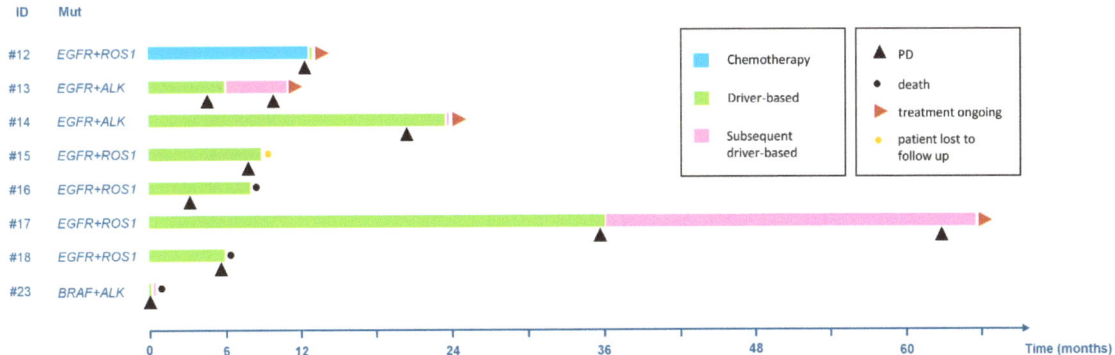

Figure 2. Swimmer plot of treatments in patients with co-occurring actionable gene alterations. The preferred treatment approach was the use of upfront targeted treatment (7 out of 8 patients), followed by an alternative driver-based targeted approach at disease progression in four cases. No subsequent treatment was possible in 2 patients due to worsening of clinical conditions and death.

3.3. Prognosis of Patients Harboring Compound Driver Gene Alterations

Follow-up data were available for eighteen out of twenty-six patients, including eight with concurrent actionable alterations, eight with compound actionable and non-actionable alterations and two in the concurrent non-actionable driver alteration group. The median follow-up was 28 months (IQR 22–70 months).

Overall, the median OS in the study population was 26 months (95% CI 22-NA).

Of note, the median OS was 25 months (95% CI 10-NA) in the compound actionable and 29 months (95% CI 22-NA) in the compound actionable plus non-actionable (HR 1.66, 95% CI 0.41–6.77) group.

In addition, no statistically significant differences in median survival were observed according to the presence or absence of the most represented genes.

4. Discussion

In NSCLC, concurrent molecular alterations pose both diagnostic and therapeutic challenges. We described a cohort of patients with NSCLC harboring concurrent alterations in driver genes ($n = 26$), including 10 patients with compound actionable alterations. We included in our study also $n = 4$ patients whose tumor harbored concurrent currently non-actionable *KRAS* and *BRAF* mutations, considering their potential future targetability with novel KRAS and BRAF inhibitors.

Overall, the incidence of co-occurring driver gene alterations in our cohort was 1.7%, with 50% of cases involving *EGFR* mutations. Within these cases, the incidence of concurrent actionable gene alterations was 39% (0.7% of the overall cohort). Among cases with compound actionable gene mutations, *EGFR* was the most frequently involved gene (70%).

Of note, a recently published retrospective study evaluated a total of 3077 patients with NSCLC who underwent molecular analysis by NGS, identifying 46 cases (1.5%) of co-occurring gene alterations, most (80%) involving EGFR mutations [28]. In this study, the incidence of compound driver actionable alterations was 41% (19 out of the 46 cases, 0.6%) [28]. However, the specific co-mutation patterns in this Asian population differed from our cohort. Indeed, in the Asian study, the most prevalent co-occurrence was represented by the association of *EGFR* and *ERBB2* actionable mutations (47%), whereas in our cohort, the most frequent association was *EGFR* mutations and *ROS1* gene rearrangements (50%). Of note, *ERBB2* actionable mutations were not observed in our compound study group, and *ROS1* rearrangements were not reported in the Asian compound population [28].

Due to the study period, testing methods were heterogeneous, and this might have represented a limitation of this study. Indeed, the time frame could affect the results due to the current modern molecular tools. First, we might have underestimated the real prevalence of co-occurring driver alterations; however, the incidence in our cohort was similar to those reported in the literature [28]. Second, we might have observed a higher rate of discordance at rebiopsy; however, this was only in one case, and different methods were used for baseline and progression analysis. Of note, the site of rebiopsy (progressive lesions) was different from that of the original diagnosis in all but one case, thus representing a good surrogate of tumor heterogeneity and clonal evolution under treatment-selective pressure.

Moreover, half of the rebiopsies were performed in patients with previously known co-occurring actionable mutations. Indeed, in the presence of concurrent actionable alterations, the need for molecular retesting at disease progression after any treatment is even stronger; this may allow for the identification of the persistence or disappearance of either clone, guiding subsequent treatment decisions [20].

In terms of treatment choice and outcomes, despite the very small numbers not powered to test for any difference nor to try valid estimations, we report a 6-month median PFS with front-line targeted treatments in patients with compound actionable mutations, which is quite low compared to the pivotal data of TKIs in *EGFR*-, *ALK*-, *ROS1*- and *BRAF*-mutated NSCLC patients. Of note, the population is highly heterogeneous (patients differ in age, driver mutation type and VAF), so these results are only exploratory. Another bias could indeed be due to the heterogeneity of the management protocols during the 6 years of the retrospective study.

In our opinion, the choice of a sequential targeted approach, which occurred in most (seven out of eight) patients, is a critical option. This choice might have been in part guided by the knowledge and treatments available at the time of treatment selection (the first approvals of front-line ALK TKIs and ROS1 TKIs in Italy occurred in 2017 and 2018, respectively). Such front-line choice may limit the considerations of the need for subsequent biopsy at disease progression because the focus was not on the presence of a dual driver. As such, assessing a subset of two patient cohorts before and after 2017 for ALK TKIs and before and after 2018 for ROS1 TKIs, respectively, could be an interesting continuation of this study.

Moreover, this approach does not consider the role of tumor heterogeneity and clone evolution during tumor progression. Therefore, we suggest a front-line agnostic treatment approach. Indeed, chemotherapy may exert cytotoxic effects on tumor cells and may be potentially effective across driver gene alterations, allowing the possibility to retest for actionable mutations to be targeted at disease progression. In our view, prospective clinical trials should be conducted to test this idea, not excluding the option of immunotherapy, looking at specific gene alterations and smoking status.

To this end, the combined use of tissue rebiopsy and plasma liquid biopsy might help to re-assess the presence of driver mutations and their VAF, which might guide the choice of subsequent selected targeted or agnostic treatment approaches (Figure 3).

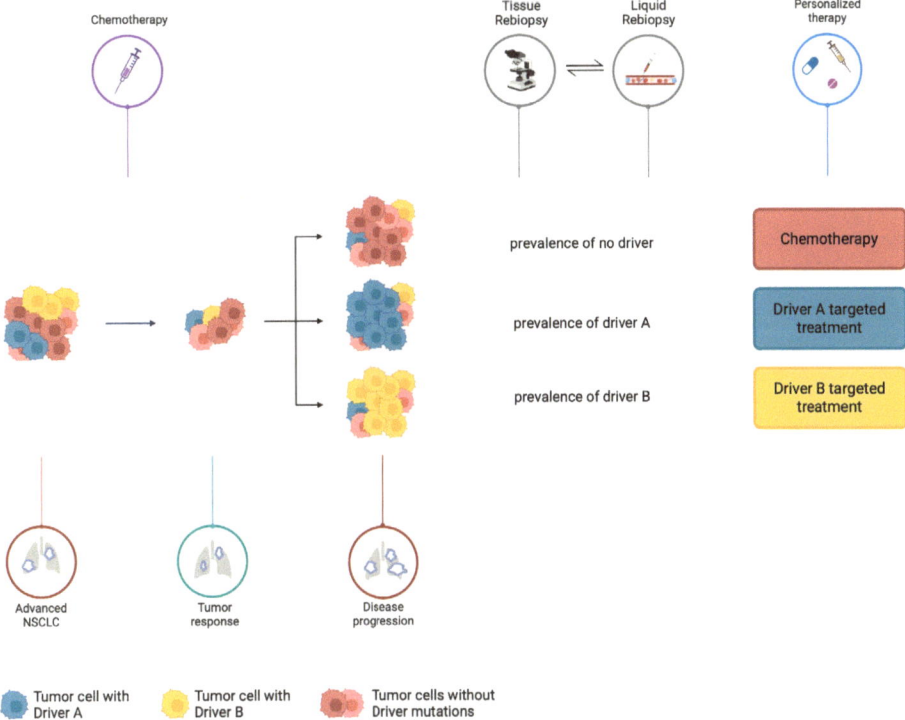

Figure 3. The proposed treatment approach to NSCLC with concurrent actionable genomic alterations. At diagnosis of advanced/metastatic NSCLC with compound driver actionable mutation, we propose front-line agnostic chemotherapy-based treatment. Indeed, chemotherapy exerts cytotoxic effects on tumor cells and is potentially active across driver gene alterations. At the time of disease progression, tumor rebiopsy, when feasible, should be performed to retest for residual driver mutations. To this end, the combined use of tissue rebiopsy and plasma liquid biopsy might investigate tumor heterogeneity more efficiently to detect the presence of residual or persistent mutations and their VAF, which might guide the choice of subsequent selected targeted treatments or subsequent agnostic approaches with chemotherapy-based regimens. Created with BioRender.com.

5. Conclusions

Despite the above-discussed limitations of a small, retrospectively evaluated population, our exploratory results point out the clinical needs for the rare but not absent population of patients with co-occurring actionable gene alterations.

Overall, understanding the landscape of co-occurring genomic alterations in NSCLC is essential for optimizing treatment strategies and improving patient outcomes. Advances in genomic profiling technologies and computational tools for analyzing complex mutational profiles are facilitating the identification and interpretation of concurrent mutation, driving personalized approaches to cancer therapy.

Supplementary Materials: The following supporting information can be downloaded at https://www.mdpi.com/article/10.3390/jcm13154476/s1. Figure S1 (Supplementary Figure S1): Study scheme. Diagram shows the study design and group categories defined.

Author Contributions: Conceptualization: I.A. and A.P.; methodology and data analysis: I.A. and R.A. (Riccardo Asnaghi); data collection: I.A., R.A. (Riccardo Asnaghi), D.V., R.A. (Riccardo Adorisio), A.R. (Alberto Ranghiero), V.F., A.C.S. and A.R. (Alessandra Rappa); patients: F.d.M., P.T.A., E.D.S., G.S., C.C., I.A., A.P., M.L., J.G., L.S., N.F. and E.G.-R.; writing—original draft preparation: I.A., R.A. (Riccardo Asnaghi) and A.P.; writing—review and editing: all authors; visualization: I.A. and R.A. (Riccardo Asnaghi); supervision: A.P., E.G.-R. and F.d.M. All authors have read and agreed to the published version of the manuscript.

Funding: This work was partially supported by the Italian Ministry of Health with "Ricerca Corrente", "5 × 1000".

Institutional Review Board Statement: All the study procedures were carried out with general authorization for the processing of personal data for scientific research purposes from "The Italian Data Protection Authority" (DSC.RE.7173.A, 13 July 2019) (http://www.garanteprivacy.it/web/guest/home/docweb/-/docwebdisplay/export/2485392, accessed on 10 April 2024). All information regarding patients was managed using anonymous numerical codes, and all samples were handled in compliance with the Helsinki Declaration.

Informed Consent Statement: According to the aforementioned national guidelines, the study did not require ethical committee approval since it did not affect the clinical management of the involved patients.

Data Availability Statement: The raw data supporting the conclusions of this article will be made available by the authors on request.

Conflicts of Interest: I. Attili received consulting fees from Bristol-Myers Squibb, outside the submitted work. F. de Marinis received honoraria or consulting fees from AstraZeneca, Boehringer Ingelheim, Bristol-Myers Squibb, Merck Sharp & Dohme, Pfizer, Novartis, Takeda, Xcovery and Roche, outside the submitted work. A. Passaro reports personal fees, as speaker bureau or advisor, for AstraZeneca, Agilent/Dako, Boehringer Ingelheim, Bristol-Myers Squibb, Eli-Lilly, Merck Sharp & Dohme, Janssen, Novartis, Pfizer and Roche Genentech, outside the submitted work. The authors have no other relevant affiliations or financial involvement with any organization or entity with a financial interest in or financial conflict with the subject matter or materials discussed in the manuscript apart from those disclosed.

References

1. Bray, F.; Laversanne, M.; Sung, H.; Ferlay, J.; Siegel, R.L.; Soerjomataram, I.; Jemal, A. Global cancer statistics 2022: GLOBOCAN estimates of incidence and mortality worldwide for 36 cancers in 185 countries. *CA Cancer J. Clin.* **2024**, *74*, 229–263. [CrossRef] [PubMed]
2. Tan, A.C.; Tan, D.S.W. Targeted Therapies for Lung Cancer Patients with Oncogenic Driver Molecular Alterations. *J. Clin. Oncol.* **2022**, *40*, 611–625. [CrossRef] [PubMed]
3. Chevallier, M.; Borgeaud, M.; Addeo, A.; Friedlaender, A. Oncogenic driver mutations in non-small cell lung cancer: Past, present and future. *World J. Clin. Oncol.* **2021**, *12*, 217–237. [CrossRef] [PubMed]
4. Grodzka, A.; Knopik-Skrocka, A.; Kowalska, K.; Kurzawa, P.; Krzyzaniak, M.; Stencel, K.; Bryl, M. Molecular alterations of driver genes in non-small cell lung cancer: From diagnostics to targeted therapy. *EXCLI J.* **2023**, *22*, 415–432. [CrossRef] [PubMed]
5. Melosky, B.; Kambartel, K.; Häntschel, M.; Bennetts, M.; Nickens, D.J.; Brinkmann, J.; Kayser, A.; Moran, M.; Cappuzzo, F. Worldwide Prevalence of Epidermal Growth Factor Receptor Mutations in Non-Small Cell Lung Cancer: A Meta-Analysis. *Mol. Diagn. Ther.* **2022**, *26*, 7–18. [CrossRef]
6. Zhang, Y.L.; Yuan, J.Q.; Wang, K.F.; Fu, X.H.; Han, X.R.; Threapleton, D.; Yang, Z.Y.; Mao, C.; Tang, J.L. The prevalence of EGFR mutation in patients with non-small cell lung cancer: A systematic review and meta-analysis. *Oncotarget* **2016**, *7*, 78985–78993. [CrossRef] [PubMed]
7. Blackhall, F.H.; Peters, S.; Bubendorf, L.; Dafni, U.; Kerr, K.M.; Hager, H.; Soltermann, A.; O'Byrne, K.J.; Dooms, C.; Sejda, A.; et al. Prevalence and clinical outcomes for patients with ALK-positive resected stage I to III adenocarcinoma: Results from the European Thoracic Oncology Platform Lungscape Project. *J. Clin. Oncol. Off. J. Am. Soc. Clin. Oncol.* **2014**, *32*, 2780–2787. [CrossRef] [PubMed]
8. Davies, K.D.; Doebele, R.C. Molecular pathways: ROS1 fusion proteins in cancer. *Clin. Cancer Res. An. Off. J. Am. Assoc. Cancer Res.* **2013**, *19*, 4040–4045. [CrossRef] [PubMed]
9. Kwak, E.L.; Bang, Y.J.; Camidge, D.R.; Shaw, A.T.; Solomon, B.; Maki, R.G.; Ou, S.H.; Dezube, B.J.; Jänne, P.A.; Costa, D.B.; et al. Anaplastic lymphoma kinase inhibition in non-small-cell lung cancer. *N. Engl. J. Med.* **2010**, *363*, 1693–1703. [CrossRef]
10. Lim, T.K.H.; Skoulidis, F.; Kerr, K.M.; Ahn, M.-J.; Kapp, J.R.; Soares, F.A.; Yatabe, Y. KRAS G12C in advanced NSCLC: Prevalence, co-mutations, and testing. *Lung Cancer* **2023**, *184*, 107293. [CrossRef]

11. Barlesi, F.; Mazieres, J.; Merlio, J.-P.; Debieuvre, D.; Mosser, J.; Lena, H.; Ouafik, L.H.; Besse, B.; Rouquette, I.; Westeel, V.; et al. Routine molecular profiling of patients with advanced non-small-cell lung cancer: Results of a 1-year nationwide programme of the French Cooperative Thoracic Intergroup (IFCT). *Lancet* 2016, *387*, 1415–1426. [CrossRef] [PubMed]
12. Pillai, R.N.; Behera, M.; Berry, L.D.; Rossi, M.R.; Kris, M.G.; Johnson, B.E.; Bunn, P.A.; Ramalingam, S.S.; Khuri, F.R. HER2 mutations in lung adenocarcinomas: A report from the Lung Cancer Mutation Consortium. *Cancer* 2017, *123*, 4099–4105. [CrossRef] [PubMed]
13. Michels, S.; Scheel, A.H.; Scheffler, M.; Schultheis, A.M.; Gautschi, O.; Aebersold, F.; Diebold, J.; Pall, G.; Rothschild, S.; Bubendorf, L.; et al. Clinicopathological Characteristics of RET Rearranged Lung Cancer in European Patients. *J. Thorac. Oncol.* 2016, *11*, 122–127. [CrossRef] [PubMed]
14. Westphalen, C.B.; Krebs, M.G.; Le Tourneau, C.; Sokol, E.S.; Maund, S.L.; Wilson, T.R.; Jin, D.X.; Newberg, J.Y.; Fabrizio, D.; Veronese, L.; et al. Genomic context of NTRK1/2/3 fusion-positive tumours from a large real-world population. *NPJ Precis. Oncol.* 2021, *5*, 69. [CrossRef] [PubMed]
15. Hendriks, L.E.; Kerr, K.M.; Menis, J.; Mok, T.S.; Nestle, U.; Passaro, A.; Peters, S.; Planchard, D.; Smit, E.F.; Solomon, B.J.; et al. Oncogene-addicted metastatic non-small-cell lung cancer: ESMO Clinical Practice Guideline for diagnosis, treatment and follow-up. *Ann. Oncol.* 2023, *34*, 339–357. [CrossRef] [PubMed]
16. Zehir, A.; Benayed, R.; Shah, R.H.; Syed, A.; Middha, S.; Kim, H.R.; Srinivasan, P.; Gao, J.; Chakravarty, D.; Devlin, S.M.; et al. Mutational landscape of metastatic cancer revealed from prospective clinical sequencing of 10,000 patients. *Nat. Med.* 2017, *23*, 703–713. [CrossRef] [PubMed]
17. Imielinski, M.; Berger, A.H.; Hammerman, P.S.; Hernandez, B.; Pugh, T.J.; Hodis, E.; Cho, J.; Suh, J.; Capelletti, M.; Sivachenko, A.; et al. Mapping the hallmarks of lung adenocarcinoma with massively parallel sequencing. *Cell* 2012, *150*, 1107–1120. [CrossRef]
18. Provencio-Pulla, M.; Pérez-Parente, D.; Olson, S.; Hasan, H.; Balea, B.C.; Rodríguez-Abreu, D.; Piqueras, M.L.-B.; Pal, N.; Wilkinson, S.; Vilas, E.; et al. Identification of non-actionable mutations with prognostic and predictive value in patients with advanced or metastatic non-small cell lung cancer. *Clin. Transl. Oncol.* 2024, *26*, 1384–1394. [CrossRef] [PubMed]
19. Passaro, A.; Attili, I.; Rappa, A.; Vacirca, D.; Ranghiero, A.; Fumagalli, C.; Guarize, J.; Spaggiari, L.; de Marinis, F.; Barberis, M.; et al. Genomic Characterization of Concurrent Alterations in Non-Small Cell Lung Cancer (NSCLC) Harboring Actionable Mutations. *Cancers* 2021, *13*, 2172. [CrossRef]
20. Attili, I.; Del Re, M.; Guerini-Rocco, E.; Crucitta, S.; Pisapia, P.; Pepe, F.; Barberis, M.; Troncone, G.; Danesi, R.; de Marinis, F.; et al. The role of molecular heterogeneity targeting resistance mechanisms to lung cancer therapies. *Expert Rev. Mol. Diagn.* 2021, *21*, 757–766. [CrossRef]
21. Passaro, A.; Malapelle, U.; Del Re, M.; Attili, I.; Russo, A.; Guerini-Rocco, E.; Fumagalli, C.; Pisapia, P.; Pepe, F.; De Luca, C.; et al. Understanding EGFR heterogeneity in lung cancer. *ESMO Open* 2020, *5*, e000919. [CrossRef] [PubMed]
22. Al Bakir, M.; Huebner, A.; Martínez-Ruiz, C.; Grigoriadis, K.; Watkins, T.B.K.; Pich, O.; Moore, D.A.; Veeriah, S.; Ward, S.; Laycock, J.; et al. The evolution of non-small cell lung cancer metastases in TRACERx. *Nature* 2023, *616*, 534–542. [CrossRef] [PubMed]
23. Karachaliou, N.; Chaib, I.; Cardona, A.F.; Berenguer, J.; Bracht, J.W.P.; Yang, J.; Cai, X.; Wang, Z.; Hu, C.; Drozdowskyj, A.; et al. Common Co-activation of AXL and CDCP1 in EGFR-mutation-positive Non-smallcell Lung Cancer Associated with Poor Prognosis. *EBioMedicine* 2018, *29*, 112–127. [CrossRef] [PubMed]
24. VanderLaan, P.A.; Rangachari, D.; Mockus, S.M.; Spotlow, V.; Reddi, H.V.; Malcolm, J.; Huberman, M.S.; Joseph, L.J.; Kobayashi, S.S.; Costa, D.B. Mutations in TP53, PIK3CA, PTEN and other genes in EGFR mutated lung cancers: Correlation with clinical outcomes. *Lung Cancer* 2017, *106*, 17–21. [CrossRef] [PubMed]
25. Kim, Y.; Lee, B.; Shim, J.H.; Lee, S.H.; Park, W.Y.; Choi, Y.L.; Sun, J.M.; Ahn, J.S.; Ahn, M.J.; Park, K. Concurrent Genetic Alterations Predict the Progression to Target Therapy in EGFR-Mutated Advanced NSCLC. *J. Thorac. Oncol.* 2019, *14*, 193–202. [CrossRef] [PubMed]
26. Skoulidis, F.; Goldberg, M.E.; Greenawalt, D.M.; Hellmann, M.D.; Awad, M.M.; Gainor, J.F.; Schrock, A.B.; Hartmaier, R.J.; Trabucco, S.E.; Gay, L.; et al. STK11/LKB1 Mutations and PD-1 Inhibitor Resistance in KRAS-Mutant Lung Adenocarcinoma. *Cancer Discov.* 2018, *8*, 822–835. [CrossRef] [PubMed]
27. Attili, I.; Passaro, A.; Pisapia, P.; Malapelle, U.; de Marinis, F. Uncommon EGFR Compound Mutations in Non-Small Cell Lung Cancer (NSCLC): A Systematic Review of Available Evidence. *Curr. Oncol.* 2022, *29*, 255–266. [CrossRef] [PubMed]
28. Zhao, Y.; Wang, S.; Yang, Z.; Dong, Y.; Wang, Y.; Zhang, L.; Hu, H.; Han, B. Co-Occurring Potentially Actionable Oncogenic Drivers in Non-Small Cell Lung Cancer. *Front. Oncol.* 2021, *11*, 665484. [CrossRef]
29. Skoulidis, F.; Heymach, J.V. Co-occurring genomic alterations in non-small-cell lung cancer biology and therapy. *Nat. Rev. Cancer* 2019, *19*, 495–509. [CrossRef]
30. Yu, H.A.; Goldberg, S.B.; Le, X.; Piotrowska, Z.; Goldman, J.W.; De Langen, A.J.; Okamoto, I.; Cho, B.C.; Smith, P.; Mensi, I.; et al. Biomarker-Directed Phase II Platform Study in Patients with EGFR Sensitizing Mutation-Positive Advanced/Metastatic Non-Small Cell Lung Cancer Whose Disease Has Progressed on First-Line Osimertinib Therapy (ORCHARD). *Clin. Lung Cancer* 2021, *22*, 601–606. [CrossRef]

Disclaimer/Publisher's Note: The statements, opinions and data contained in all publications are solely those of the individual author(s) and contributor(s) and not of MDPI and/or the editor(s). MDPI and/or the editor(s) disclaim responsibility for any injury to people or property resulting from any ideas, methods, instructions or products referred to in the content.

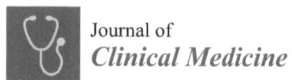

Article

Mini-Invasive Thoracic Surgery for Early-Stage Lung Cancer: Which Is the Surgeon's Best Approach for Video-Assisted Thoracic Surgery?

Beatrice Trabalza Marinucci *, Alessandra Siciliani, Claudio Andreetti, Matteo Tiracorrendo, Fabiana Messa, Giorgia Piccioni, Giulio Maurizi, Antonio D'Andrilli, Cecilia Menna, Anna Maria Ciccone, Camilla Vanni, Giacomo Argento, Erino Angelo Rendina and Mohsen Ibrahim

Department of Thoracic Surgery, Sant'Andrea Hospital, Sapienza University, 00189 Rome, Italy; alessandrasiciliani@gmail.com (A.S.); claudio.andreetti@uniroma1.it (C.A.); tiracorrendomatteo@gmail.com (M.T.); fabiana.messa@uniroma1.it (F.M.); giorgia.piccioni@uniroma1.it (G.P.); giulio.maurizi@uniroma1.it (G.M.); adandrilli@hotmail.com (A.D.); cmrossi.85@gmail.com (C.M.); cicconeam@gmail.com (A.M.C.); camillavanni.1@gmail.com (C.V.); giacomo.argento@uniroma1.it (G.A.); erinoangelo.rendina@uniroma1.it (E.A.R.); mohsen.ibrahim@uniroma1.it (M.I.)
* Correspondence: beatrice.trabalzamarinucci@uniroma1.it

Abstract: Objectives: The choice of the best Video-Assisted Thoracic Surgery (VATS) surgical approach is still debated. Surgeons are often faced with the choice between innovation and self-confidence. The present study reports the experience of a high-volume single institute, comparing data of uni-portal, bi-portal and tri-portal VATS, to find out the safest and most effective mini-invasive approach, leading surgeon's choice. **Methods:** Between 2015 and 2022, a total of 210 matched patients underwent VATS lobectomy for early-stage cancer, using uni-portal (fifth intercostal space), bi-portal (seventh space for optic and the fifth), and tri-portal (seventh and the fifth/four) access. Patients were matched for age, BPCO, smoke, comorbidities, lesions (size and staging) to obtain three homogenous groups (A: uni-portal; B: bi-portal; C: tri-portal). The surgeons had comparable expertise. Data were retrospectively collected from institutional database and analyzed. **Results:** No differences were detected considering time of surgery, length of hospital stay, complications, conversion rate, specific survival, and days of chest tube length of stay. Better results on chest tube removal were described in group A (mean 1.1 days) compared to B (mean 2.6 days) and C (mean 4.7 days); nevertheless, they not statistically significant ($p = 0.106$). **Conclusions:** No significant differences among the groups were described, except for the reduction in chest tube permanence in group A. This allows to hypothesize an enhanced recovery after surgery in this group but the different approaches in this series seem to guarantee comparable safety and effectiveness. Considering no superiority of one method above the others, the best suggested approach should be the one for which the surgeon feels more confident.

Keywords: video-assisted thoracic surgery; lung cancer; minimally invasive

Citation: Trabalza Marinucci, B.; Siciliani, A.; Andreetti, C.; Tiracorrendo, M.; Messa, F.; Piccioni, G.; Maurizi, G.; D'Andrilli, A.; Menna, C.; Ciccone, A.M.; et al. Mini-Invasive Thoracic Surgery for Early-Stage Lung Cancer: Which Is the Surgeon's Best Approach for Video-Assisted Thoracic Surgery? *J. Clin. Med.* **2024**, *13*, 6447. https://doi.org/10.3390/jcm13216447

Academic Editors: Shun Lu and Tawee Tanvetyanon

Received: 6 September 2024
Revised: 6 October 2024
Accepted: 22 October 2024
Published: 28 October 2024

Copyright: © 2024 by the authors. Licensee MDPI, Basel, Switzerland. This article is an open access article distributed under the terms and conditions of the Creative Commons Attribution (CC BY) license (https://creativecommons.org/licenses/by/4.0/).

1. Introduction

The advantages of Video-assisted Thoracic Surgery (VATS) for an enhanced recovery after surgery are well known. In fact, as a novel mini- and minimally invasive thoracic surgery technique, VATS enables surgeons to perform surgery through smaller incisions, guaranteeing less morbidity and a faster recovery compared to open thoracotomy, reducing postoperative pain, hospital stay, and improving patient quality of life and satisfaction [1]. VATS represent one of the major progresses in the history of thoracic surgery: the development of VATS and its learning curve from multi-portal to bi-portal, to uni-portal access, has been a great advance in thoracic surgery in the last 30 years. VATS is being constantly rejuvenated by the development of the techniques, with the aim to reduce the size and/or number of accesses to reduce surgical access trauma. In fact, over the past decade, VATS with three or four ports (including a 2–4 cm utility incision for delivery of the resected lobe) has been evolved to produce bi-portal (utility mini-thoracotomy with another additional thoracoscopic port), for which the locations of incision varied according to the preference of the surgeon, and finally to uni-portal (only 1-utility mini-thoracotomy) [2]. Uni-portal minimally invasive surgery has developed rapidly since Dr. Rocco first reported it in 2013, expanding from the minor thoracic procedures, such as wedge resection, to complex operations, such as lobectomy, segmentectomy, and even bronchial or pulmonary angioplasty [3].

Bi-portal VATS imply two radical changes in perspectives from the traditional three-portal technique. For double port VATS lower lobectomies, all the instrumentation and stapler insertions are performed through the utility incision. To introduce staplers without the third conventional posterior port, the location of the endostapler and the thoracoscope have to be interchanged between the two incisions. There is another important aspect, related to the instrumentation interference. In fact, instrumentation with both proximal and distal articulation, modern articulated staplers, high definition 30° cameras and energy devices seem to be more fitted for successful biportal VATS lobectomy. Moreover, bi-manual instrumentation using a cross-hand technique is often used [4]

In recent years, uni-portal VATS (U-VATS) has become a new safe and effective technique in the surgical treatment for non-small cell lung cancer (NSCLC) [5].

The single, uni-portal VATS is an approach meant to reproduce the open technique transferring the operative fulcrum inside the chest secondary to the introduction of articulating instruments. The approach is different than conventional, three- VATS because it develops along a sagittal plane, rather than a latero-lateral one. The advantage of using the camera in coordination with the instruments is that the vision is directed to the target tissue, bringing the instruments to address the target lesion from a straight perspective and, thus, it is possible to obtain similar angle of view as for open surgery. This evolution in the approach from three ports to the single port technique required a new learning curve related to different lung exposures and learning how to coordinate the instruments and the camera with no interference during surgery. So, the innovation leading to bi-VATS consisted mainly of: removing the posterior port; placing the camera at the posterior part of utility incision for lower lobectomies; using bimanual instrumentation with curved instruments; placing the camera through utility incision and use inferior port only for stapler insertion or for instrumentation for upper lobectomies; using the inferior port only to expose the lung (camera, staplers, and instrumentation through the incision) [3]. The evolution through U-Vats consists of removing the inferior port; using vascular clips when no angle for staplers; always inserting the staplers with angulation for vascular division; adopting the Anterior small thoracotomy approach (10–12 cm incision); removing the rib spreader and moving the instruments and camera along the 10 cm incision; and finally reducing, progressively, the size of the incision after gained experience [6].

Many studies in the literature have already been focused on the feasibility and on the differences in the various VATS approaches, and several studies showed no difference between them, in terms of intra- and postoperative outcomes [7]. So, the comparative clinical outcomes of U-VATS versus multiportal VATS (M-VATS) remain uncertain, and the choice of the best mini-invasive surgical approach is still being debated, considering the pro and contra of every single approach. VATS is established today as the preferred approach for early-stage lung cancer, according to the American College of Chest Physicians (ACCP) and the European Society of Medical oncology (ESMO). Although VATS has greatly reduced surgical morbidity compared to open thoracotomy, it has not eliminated it. Studies have shown that after VATS, up to 32% of patients still experience some residual discomfort. Moreover, with the increasing spread of Robot systems, VATS is now considered one of the possible minimally invasive techniques for early-stage lung cancer. In consequence, VATS is being constantly rejuvenated by the development of the technique, aimed to reduce the size and/or number of access (three-porta, two-port, and uni-portal VATS), and there is no evidence of the superiority of one over the others. Therefore, among the different VATS approaches for NSCLC treatment, the best one has not been standardized, and the surgeon is often faced with the choice between the most innovative technique and the one that gives him the most confidence.

The objective of the present study is to report the experience of a high-volume single institute, comparing data of uni-portal, bi-portal, and tri-portal VATS, to discuss the safest and most effective mini-invasive approach, helping to lead the surgeon's choice.

2. Materials and Methods

Between 2015 and 2022, a total of 240 patients underwent VATS lobectomy for early-stage lung cancer in a single center.

Inclusion criteria consisted of patients >18 years old affected by early lung cancer (stage I–IIB, excluded T3), so none underwent neoadjuvant therapy, and patients eligible for surgery using mini-invasive approach were included for upfront surgery.

Exclusion criteria included: locally advanced stages, metastatic disease, patients with low performance status not eligible for surgery, and previous thoracic and/or cardiac surgery.

To minimize selection bias, a 1:1:1 propensity score matching was performed based on predetermined confounders and baseline characteristics (age, BPCO, smoking habits, comorbidities, lesion characteristics in terms of size and staging) to identify three homogenous groups of patients. A total of 210 patients were included and divided into group A (70) that underwent uni-portal VATS; group B (70) that underwent bi-portal VATS and group C (70) that underwent tri-portal VATS. Based on the propensity score matching, 30 patients were excluded because they did not match the variables.

All patients received pre-operative assessment, including physical examination, routine blood tests, pulmonary functional tests (spirometry and blood gas analysis) and pre-operative cardiovascular tests. Imaging included Total Body Computed Tomography (CT) and Positron Emission Tomography (PET). Central tumors required bronchoscopy for endobronchial assessment and eventual diagnosis.

Included patients underwent lung resection by a mini-invasive approach: uni-portal VATS (U-VATS) consisted of a single 3–4 cm instrument port [8] at either the fourth or fifth intercostal space at the anterior axillary line (Figure 1), and eventually an XS-sized Alexis wound protector (Applied Medical, Rancho Santa Margarita, CA/USA) was applied at the utility port; bi-portal VATS (BI-VATS) consisted of 1 cm camera access at the seventh–eight intercostal space, along the medium axillary line and the second 3 cm surgical access site at the fourth–fifth space at the anterior axillary line [4]; tri-portal (TRI-VATS) consisted of access of the 1 cm camera at the seventh–eight space on the mid-axillary line and the other 1 cm port instrument at the fourth–fifth intercostal space on the anterior and the posterior axillary lines (Figure 2) [9]. A 30° 10 mm thoracoscope was used for vision.

Patients received lobectomy performed in the usual manner with lymph nodes sampling. Broncho-vascular structures were sutured and divided using Endo-GIA (Covidien, Mansfield, MA, USA) or Echelon Flex (Ethicon Endo-Surgery Inc., Blue Ash, OH, USA). The resected lobe is placed inside a specimen bag before being delivered out.

As usually performed in our clinical practice, all patients received local analgesia (Ropivacaine injection in the intercostal spaces) and systemic endo-venous analgesia (Acetaminophen 1 g, three times in a day and Ketorolac 30 mg, three times in a day). Tramadol was used in case of pain persistence with the previous medicaments. Ropivacaine can have cardiotoxic side effects, and an alternative for local analgesia could be Bupivacaine. However, Ropivacaine is believed to have a lower incidence of clinical cardiac side effects than bupivacaine. The replacement of the butyl group in bupivacaine by a propyl group in ropivacaine alters its physicochemical properties. After molecular weight, the principal difference is the lower lipid solubility of ropivacaine. Physicochemical characteristics, such as lipophilicity and molecular weight, are different between ropivacaine and bupivacaine and are caused by the replacement of the butyl group by a propyl group. These appear to be significant factors that modulate potential cardiotoxic effects. Higher concentrations of bupivacaine and ropivacaine can block voltage-gated ion channels and intracellular enzyme systems, leading to reduced cardiac membrane potential and intracellular metabolism. Cardiac output may decrease because of ventricular dysrhythmias, contractile failure, or veno-vasodilation. Supraclinical concentrations of bupivacaine can result in death because of cardiovascular collapse. In fact, differences between the isomers and their physicochemical characteristics cause different binding of the isomers to the target site. This results in modulated potential cardiotoxic effects for Ropivacaine compared to Bupivacaine [10].

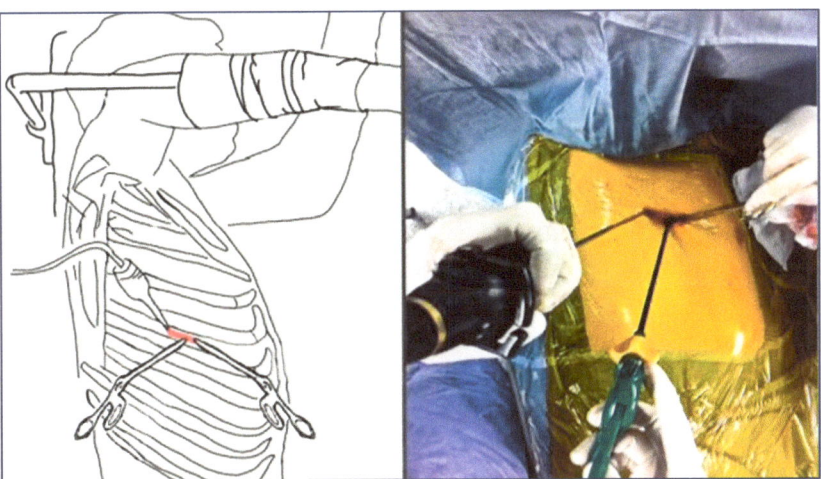

Figure 1. Uni-portal VATS approach.

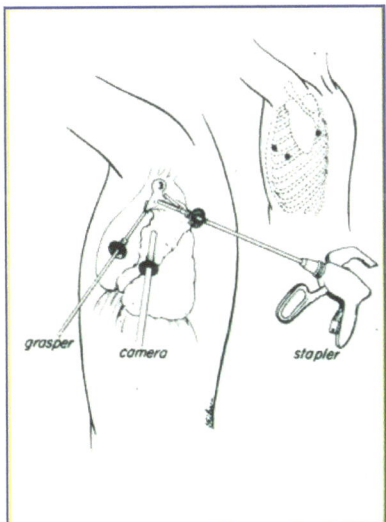

Figure 2. Tri-portal VATS approach.

Chest tubes were connected to a pleur-evac device and Chest X-Rays were performed on post-operative day 1. Pulmonary re-expansion was defined complete if the lung achieved >90% of the pleural surface at chest XR; otherwise, it was defined incomplete; the rate of lung surface was calculated evaluating the "mean interpleural distance", estimated according to the average distances between the lung and chest wall calculated at three points (apex, costophrenic sinus, midpoint) at chest XR [11].

Intra- and post-operative complications were registered. Cardiovascular post-operative complications included: atrial fibrillation (AF), hypertension, and coronary heart disease (CAD). Respiratory post-operative complications included: acute and/or chronic respiratory failure and pulmonary edema. Other complications explored in the study refer to: prolonged air leaks, intra-operative bleeding, and chronic pain.

Pain control was assessed using a Numeral Rating Scale (NRS), from 0 (no pain) to 10 (maximum level of pain) at 24 h and 72 h from surgery.

All patients started pulmonary rehabilitation programs (mobilization and respiratory exercises) on day 1. Chest tube drainage was removed after the radiological evidence of complete or near complete pulmonary expansion, absence of air leak in the pleur-evac system, and a median drain amount 5 mL/kg [12]. Pre-operative and intra-operative characteristics, post-operative minor complications (cardiovascular: atrial fibrillation; pulmonary embolism; respiratory: acute respiratory failure, pulmonary edema), pain, and specific survival were compared among the three groups.

This original retrospective observational study received institutional review board approval (Prot. n. 7 SA_2023 RIF. CE 7031/2022), and it was conducted in accordance with the Declaration of Helsinki. Written informed consent was obtained from all patients. Data are available in the text (Figure 3).

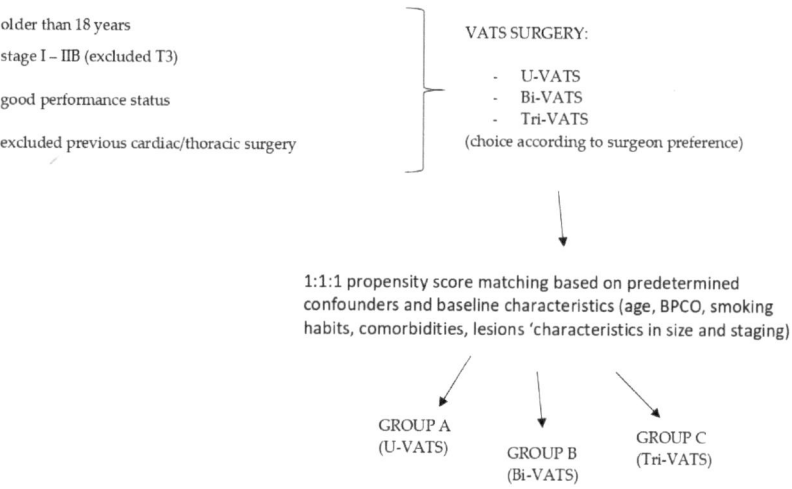

Figure 3. Diagram of patient recruitment.

Statistical Analysis

Data were collected and stored in an Excel database (Microsoft Corp, Redmond, WA, USA) and were analyzed using statistical package SPSS, version 25.0 (SPSS Software, IBM Corp., Armonk, NY, USA). The data collected were analyzed and compared between the three groups. Continuous variables were expressed as mean ± standard deviation (SD) and categorical variables were expressed as absolute number and percentage. The comparison of categorical variables was performed by the $c2$ test using Fisher's exact test between the three groups. Comparison of continuous variables was performed by the one-way ANOVA test and post hoc Bonferroni test. Significance was defined as a p value of less than 0.05.

3. Results

General characteristics of the population are described in Table 1.

Table 1. General characteristics of the population.

	UVATS	BIVATS	TRIVATS	p
Smoke, n (%)	50 (71.4%)	20 (28.6%)	40 (57%)	0.263
Cardiovascular comorbidity, n (%)	30 (42.8%)	10 (14.3%)	40 (57%)	0.243
BPCO, n (%)	40 (57%)	30 (42.8%)	20 (28.6%)	0.558
Conversion rate, n (%)	0	0	0	1.000
Intra-operative massive bleeding, n (%)	0	0	0	1.000
Post-op. Cardiovascular Complications, n (%)	10 (14.3%)	0	20 (28.6%)	0.311
Post-op Respiratory Complications, n (%)	10 (14.3%)	10 (14.3%)	10 (14.3%)	1.000
Prolonged Air Leak, n (%)	0	0	0	1.000
Incomplete pulmonary expansion in post-op day 1, n (%)	20 (28.6%)	10 (14.3%)	30 (42.8%)	0.497
Subcutaneous enphisema, n (%)	30 (42.8%)	20 (28.6%)	20 (28.6%)	0.807
Pain at 24 h, n (%)	3 (4.3%)	4 (5.7%)	4 (5.7%)	1.000

The mean age of the general population was 60.55 ± 7.1. In total, 100 patients were male (30 in group A, 30 in group B and 40 in group C, $p = 0.826$).

In total, 110 patients were smokers (50 in group A, 20 in group B, 40 in group C) without a statistically significant difference between groups ($p = 0.263$).

Cardiovascular comorbidities were referred by 30 patients in group A (42.8%), 10 in group B (14.3%), and 40 in group C (57%) ($p = 0.243$).

BPCO was detected in 40 (57%) patients in group A, 30 (42.8%) patients in group B, and 20 (28.6%) in group C ($p = 0.558$).

Stage IA3 was the most frequent, detected in 50 (71.4%) in group A, 20 (28.6%) in group B, and 40 (57%) in group C without a statistically significant difference between groups ($p = 0.263$).

The mean size of the tumor was 2.5 ± 1.2, without significant difference among the groups.

Left side lesions were described in 40 (57%) patients in group A, 40 (57%) patients in group B, and 50 (71.4%) patients in group C, without a statistically significant difference among the groups ($p = 0.817$).

LLL was performed in 20 (28.6%) patients in group A, 20 (28.6%) in group B, and 20 (28.6%) in group C, ($p = 1.000$).

LUL was performed in 20 (28.6%) patients in group A, 20 (28.6%) in group B, and 30 (42.8%) in group C, ($p = 0.807$).

RLL was performed in 20 (28.6%) in group A, 20 (28.6%) in group B, and 10 (14.3%) in group C, ($p = 0.769$).

RUL was performed in 10 (14.3%) in group A, 10 (14.3%) in group B, and 10 (14.3%) in group C ($p = 1.000$).

Surgery time was a mean of 103.20 ± 20.21, without a significant difference among the groups in the ANOVA analysis ($p = 0.870$) and in the post hoc Bonferroni test ($p = 1.000$).

The conversion rate and intra-operative massive bleeding were 0 in all the groups ($p = 1.000$).

Cardiovascular complications (atrial fibrillation-AF, hypertension, coronary heart disease-CAD) occurred in 10 patients in group A (6 AF, 3 hypertensions, 1 CAD), 0 patients in group B, and 20 patients in group C (7 AF, 12 hypertensions, 1 CAD, ($p = 0.311$).

Respiratory complications occurred in 10 (14.3%) patients in group A, 10 (14.3%) in group B, and 10 (14.3%) in group C ($p = 1.000$).

The pain score was a mean of 4.3 ± 0.5 at 24 h and 3.2 ± 1.7 at 72 h, without a significant difference among the groups.

PAL was detected in 0 patients in all groups ($p = 1.000$). Subcutaneous emphysema was described in 30 (42.8%) patients in group A, 30 (42.8%) in group B, and 20 (28.6%) in group C, ($p = 0.807$).

Incomplete pulmonary expansion in the first post-operative day was detected in 20 (28.6%) patients in group A, 10 (14.3%) in group B, and 30 (42.8%) in group C, without a statistically significant difference among the groups ($p = 0.497$).

The days of chest tube permanence were 1.14 ± 2.5 in group A, 2.6 ± 2.1 in group B, and 4.72 ± 1.5 in group C, which were not statistically significantly different according to the ANOVA test ($p = 0.106$) (Table 2) and the Bonferroni test (Table 3), considering the difference between group A and C ($p = 0.114$).

Table 2. ANOVA test.

	Sum of Squares	gl	Mean Square	F	p
Time of surgery	402.381	2	201.190	0.141	0.870
Days of chest tube	45.238	2	22.619	2.545	0.106
Length of stay	20.095	2	10.048	1.942	0.172

Table 3. Bonferroni test.

Variable	Surgical Type (i)	Surgical Type (ii)	Mean Difference	SD	p
Time of surgery (mean 103.20)	UVATS	BIVATS TRIVATS	5.714 −5.000	20.206	1.000
	BIVATS	UVATS TRIVATS	−5.714 −10.714	20.206	1.000
	TRIVATS	UVATS BIVATS	5.000 −1.429	20.206	1.000
Days of chest tube	UVATS	BIVATS TRIVATS	−1.429 −3.571	1.594	1.000 0.114
	BIVATS	UVATS TRIVATS	−1.429 −2.143	1.594	1.000 0.586
	TRIVATS	UVATS BIVATS	3.571 2.143	1.594	0.114 0.586
Length of stay	UVATS	BIVATS TRIVATS	2.000 −0.143	1.216	0.352 1.000
	BIVATS	UVATS TRIVATS	−2.000 −2.143	1.216	0.352 0.285
	TRIVATS	UVATS BIVATS	0.143 2.143	1.216	1.000 0.285

The mean total hospital stay was 4.5 ± 3.8, without a statistically significant difference among the groups according to the ANOVA test ($p = 0.172$), shown in Table 2, and the Bonferroni test (Table 3).

Peri-operative mortality was 0 in all groups.

At 1 year of follow-up, we registered no mortality nor recurrence in all the groups.

4. Discussion

Vats first appeared in 1990 [13], and in 1993 a VATS study group was formed from multiple institutions, analyzing more than 1700 cases [14].

Many studies have already reported the advantages of VATS compared to thoracotomy, such as lower morbidity, reduced postoperative pain, better cosmetic results, and better quality of life [15]. Conventionally, the traditional VATS, known as multiportal VATS (M-VATS), was performed through 3 or 4 small accesses. M-VATS has proven to offer reliable safety and feasibility, and it was introduced as a standard procedure for surgical treatment of early-staged NSCLC [16].

With the increasing technological advances relating to thoracic surgery, VATS lobectomy has evolved from tri-portal VATS (TRI-VATS) to bi-portal (BI-PORTAL) and finally to uni-portal (U-VATS) approach.

McKenna et al. published in 2006 the largest tri-portal VATS lobectomies series [17]. A few years later, the procedure was refined to bi-portal, with only one working port for thoracoscopy and a second for utility minithoracotomy access. D'Amico et al. described one of the largest bi-portal VATS series, including more than 600 cases of VATS lobectomy and segmentectomies [18]. Yamamoto et al. [19] and Rocco et al. in 2013 [3] were the first to introduce uni-portal VATS for pleural biopsy or minor lung resections, such as wedge resections. Finally, Gonzalez-Rivas et al. [20] described a series of major lung resection (including lobectomy, segmentary resections, and even complex surgical procedures) using the uni-portal VATS approach.

In the beginning, evolution from multi-portal to bi-portal, then to uni-portal VATS seemed to reduce unnecessary working ports; however, there are several major differences such as operation field perspective (U-VATS simulating the vision of open approach as the one of the most positive aspects of this procedure, facilitating even the operative approach for more technically-demanding procedures). However, the main limitation of U-VATS is reported to be the limited flexibility of instrument circulation; in fact, for M-VATS and BI-VATS, the camera and instruments can be placed among the utility thoracotomy and ports, while in U-VATS the intense jamming and interference of instruments is inevitable [21].

Recently, several meta-analyses have compared the peri-operative outcomes of U-VATS and M-VATS [22,23]. Some Authors have demonstrated several potential advantages of U-VATS over the others approaches, such as less intraoperative blood loss, shorter hospital stay, and reduced postoperative pain [3,24], but the results of these studies were highly heterogeneous. In fact, Lin et al. indicated that U-VATS significantly increased operation time compared to M-VATS [25]. A study by Mu et al. reported a shorter average hospital stay with U-VATS [26], while in the study of Al-Ameri et al. it was longer [27].

Some studies (Yang X.Y. et al.; Yang Z. et al.) reported that patients in U-VATS group had a significant reduction regarding blood loss, length of stay, and pain [28,29], but other studies [30] demonstrated that there was no significant difference between the U-VATS and M-VATS approach in terms of length of postoperative stay.

However, many of these meta-analyses presented some limitations. In fact, most of them were focused on benign disease, including patients who underwent wedge resections but not the surgery for NSCLC, requiring radical resection of the primary lesion and lymph node dissection, which requires anatomical pulmonary resection (segmentectomy or lobectomy).

Han et al. demonstrated that there was no significant difference between a single-incision group, two-incision group, and three-incision group in both recurrence-free survival and overall survival [30]. U-VATS might have some potential advantages over M-VATS in reducing postoperative pain and drainage duration, even though these advantages are not significant.

At the end, the previous results reported in the literature showed that U-VATS is as safe, feasible, and effective method as BI- and TRI-VATS in major lung resection, indicating that there is no significant difference in peri-operative outcomes among the different approaches [31].

The absence of cardiovascular complications in Group B is just an occasional finding, probably due to the selection of patients obtained by the matching analysis, and the result is not related to the specific type of approach. The absence of cardiovascular complications in this set of patients is probably because such complications did not occur in those patients selected by the matching analysis, so it is just an occasional finding. Moreover, the comparative analysis showed no statistical difference among the groups.

The higher incomplete expansion in the TRI-VATS group could be related to air accumulation in the subcutis, which could leak into the pleural cavity more easily with triportal access than bi-portal access. However, the difference is not diriment and not statistically significant, and finally, prolonged air leak (air leak lasting after the first 5 post-operative days) was null in all the groups.

Even in the present study, with the limit of a single institution retrospective analysis, no differences were detected regarding the time of surgery, length of hospital stay, complications, conversion rate, specific survival, and days of chest tube length of stay. Better results regarding chest tube removal were described in group A (mean 1.1 days) compared to group B (mean 2.6 days) and C (mean 4.7 days); nevertheless, this was not statistically significant ($p = 0.106$). This result allows us to hypothesize an enhanced recovery after surgery in this set of patients but, with the limits of results confined to peri-operative outcomes and a brief long-term follow-up. The three surgical approaches in this series seem to guarantee comparable results in terms of safety, effectiveness, oncological results, and patient satisfaction. Many studies in the literature have already been focused on the feasibility and on the differences in the various VATS approaches, and several studies showed no difference between them in terms of intra- and post-operative outcomes. So, the comparative clinical outcomes of U-VATS versus multi-port VATS (M-VATS) remain uncertain, and the choice of the best mini-invasive surgical approach is still being debated, considering the pro and contra of every single approach. The majority of constituent papers included in the meta-analysis were retrospective series or simpler case–control studies. The heterogeneity of the studies on this topic makes it difficult to achieve a standardized technique. Another effect of heterogeneity of these studies is the different surgeon experience and skills in the different centers. However, all these studies deal with safety and effectiveness of the different approaches. Considering the morbidity, mortality, and QoL, with particular attention towards the safety of VATS hilar dissection, the adequacy of oncological clearance, the long-term advantages over open surgery, and the relatively high costs of instruments and consumables, the efficacy regarding the treatment of the lung cancer was measured according to completeness of resection and survival.

The originality of our study is the comparison of the techniques with the specific aim of helping the surgeon in their choice of the correct approach for the patient, highlighting the importance of a personalized medicine based not only on the technical innovation but above all, on the operator's best confidence to achieve the best result for the patient. Thus, a single-institution experience reinforces the comparability of the techniques, taking into consideration the equivalent expertise of the whole surgical équipe. Thus, there are no differences subjected to bias related to different operator skills. In conclusion, considering the equivalence of the team and procedures, our original work aims to support the surgeon's choice in the approach to VATS.

5. Conclusions

In conclusion, considering no superiority of one method above the others, the best suggested approach should be the one for which the surgeon feels more confident. Less accesses are not synonymous with less complications, and self-confidence and personal safety for surgeons give the most effective result for patients.

In fact, innovation of surgical approaches is of great importance, but minimizing the size and number of incisions is only one part of minimally invasive surgery, which should always aim to preserve function, prolonging survival, and improving quality of life [27].

In conclusion, self-confidence and personal safety for the surgeon guarantee the best result for the patient, and less incisions should not to always be considered synonymous with less complications.

Author Contributions: Conceptualization, B.T.M., A.S. and M.I.; methodology, B.T.M., A.S. and M.I.; software, B.T.M., M.T., G.A. and F.M.; validation, E.A.R. and M.I.; formal analysis, B.T.M., A.S. and C.M.; investigation, B.T.M., G.M., A.D. and C.A.; resources, B.T.M. and M.T.; data curation, B.T.M., G.P., F.M., C.V. and M.T.; writing—review and editing, B.T.M. and A.S.; visualization and supervision, E.A.R., A.M.C. and M.I. All authors have read and agreed to the published version of the manuscript.

Funding: This research received no external funding.

Institutional Review Board Statement: The study was conducted according to the guidelines of the Declaration of Helsinki and approved by the Institutional Review Board: Prot. n. 7 SA_2023 RIF. CE 7031/2022, 1 February 2023.

Informed Consent Statement: Informed consent was obtained from all subjects involved in the study.

Data Availability Statement: The original contributions presented in this study are included in this article; further inquiries can be directed to the corresponding author.

Conflicts of Interest: The authors declare no conflicts of interest.

References

1. Bendixen, M.; Jorgensen, O.D.; Kronborg, C.; Andersen, C.; Licht, P.B. Postoperative pain and quality of life after lobectomy via video-assisted thoracoscopic surgery or anterolateral thoracotomy for early stage lung cancer: A randomised controlled trial. *Lancet Oncol.* **2016**, *17*, 836–844. [CrossRef] [PubMed]
2. Sihoe, A.D.L. Video-assisted thoracoscopic surgery as the gold standard for lung cancer surgery. *Respirology* **2020**, *25* (Suppl. 2), 49–60. [CrossRef] [PubMed]
3. Rocco, G.; Martucci, N.; La Manna, C.; Jones, D.R.; De Luca, G.; La Rocca, A.; Cuomo, A.; Accardo, R. Ten-year experience on 644 patients undergoing single-port (uni-portal) video-assisted thoracoscopic surgery. *Ann. Thorac. Surg.* **2013**, *96*, 434–438. [CrossRef] [PubMed]
4. Wang, G.S.; Wang, Z.; Wang, J.; Rao, Z.P. Biportal complete video-assisted thoracoscopic lobectomy and systematic lymphadenectomy. *J. Thorac. Dis.* **2013**, *5*, 875–881. [CrossRef] [PubMed] [PubMed Central]
5. Sihoe, A.D. The evolution of minimally invasive thoracic surgery: Implications for the practice of uni-portal thoracoscopic surgery. *J. Thorac. Dis.* **2014**, *6*, S604–S617.
6. Gonzalez-Rivas, D.; Fieira, E.; Delgado, M.; Mendez, L.; Fernandez, R.; de la Torre, M. Evolving from conventional video-assisted thoracoscopic lobectomy to uni-portal: The story behind the evolution. *J. Thorac. Dis.* **2014**, *6*, S599–S603. [CrossRef]
7. Yan, Y.; Huang, Q.; Han, H.; Zhang, Y.; Chen, H. Uni-portal versus multiportal video-assisted thoracoscopic anatomical resection for NSCLC: A meta-analysis. *J. Cardiothorac. Surg.* **2020**, *15*, 238. [CrossRef] [PubMed] [PubMed Central]
8. Sihoe, A.D. Uni-portal video-assisted thoracic (VATS) lobectomy. *Ann. Cardiothorac. Surg.* **2016**, *5*, 133–144. [CrossRef] [PubMed] [PubMed Central]
9. Sihoe, A.D.; Yim, A.P. Video-assisted pulmonary resections. In *Pearson's Thoracic and Esophageal Surgery*, 3rd ed.; Patterson, G.A., Cooper, J.D., Deslauriers, J., Meyerson, S.L., Patterson, A., Eds.; Elsevier: Philadelphia, PA, USA, 2008; pp. 970–988.
10. Graf, B.M.; Abraham, I.; Eberbach, N.; Kunst, G.; Stowe, D.F.; Martin, E. Differences in cardiotoxicity of bupivacaine and ropivacaine are the result of physicochemical and stereoselective properties. *Anesthesiology* **2002**, *96*, 1427–1434. [CrossRef] [PubMed]
11. Ruffini, E.; Albera, C.; Carpagnano, G.E.; De Rose, V.; Foschino Barbaro, M.P.; Leo, F.; Novello, S.; Resta, O.; Scagliotti, G.V.; Sollitto, F. Malattie dell'apparato Respiratorio. Pneumologia e Chirurgia Toracica. In *Capitolo: Patologia della pleura—Pneumotorace*; Vanni, C., Andreetti, C., Marinucci, B.T., Rendina, E.A., Eds.; Edizioni Minerva Medica: Torino, Italy, 2021; ISBN 978-88-5532-054-2.
12. Stamenovic, D.; Dusmet, M.; Schneider, T.; Roessner, E.; Messerschmidt, A. A simple size-tailored algorithm for the removal of chest drain following minimally invasive lobectomy: A prospective randomized study. *Surg. Endosc.* **2022**, *36*, 5275–5281. [CrossRef] [PubMed] [PubMed Central]
13. Marchetti, G.P.; Pinelli, V.; Tassi, G.F. 100 years of thoracoscopy: Historical notes. *Respiration* **2011**, *82*, 187–192. [CrossRef] [PubMed]
14. Yan, T.D.; Cao, C.; D'Amico, T.A.; Demmy, T.L.; He, J.; Hansen, H.; Swanson, S.J.; Walker, W.S.; Casali, G.; Donning, J.; et al. Video-assisted thoracoscopic surgery lobectomy at 20 years: A consensus statement. *Eur. J. Cardio-Thorac. Surg. Off. J. Eur. Assoc. Cardio-Thorac. Surg.* **2013**, *45*, 633–639. [CrossRef] [PubMed]
15. Palade, E.; Guenter, J.; Kirschbaum, A.; Wiesemann, S.; Passlick, B. [Postoperative pain in the acute phase after surgery: VATS lobectomy vs. open lung resection: Results of a prospective randomised trial]. *Zentralblatt Chir.* **2014**, *139* (Suppl. 1), S59–S66.
16. Long, H.; Tan, Q.; Luo, Q.; Wang, Z.; Jiang, G.; Situ, D.; Lin, Y.; Su, X.; Liu, Q.; Rong, T. Thoracoscopic surgery versus thoracotomy for lung Cancer: Short-term outcomes of a randomized trial. *Ann. Thorac. Surg.* **2018**, *105*, 386–392. [CrossRef] [PubMed]
17. McKenna, R.J., Jr.; Houck, W.; Fuller, C.B. Video-assisted thoracic surgery lobectomy: Experience with 1100 cases. *Ann. Thorac. Surg.* **2006**, *81*, 421–425, discussion 425–426. [CrossRef]

18. Berry, M.F.; D'Amico, T.A.; Onaitis, M.W.; Kelsey, C.R. Thoracoscopic approach to lobectomy for lung cancer does not compromise oncologic efficacy. *Ann. Thorac. Surg.* **2014**, *98*, 197–202. [CrossRef]
19. Yamamoto, H.; Okada, M.; Takada, M.; Mastuoka, H.; Sakata, K.; Kawamura, M. Video-assisted thoracic surgery through a single skin incision. *Arch. Surg.* **1998**, *133*, 145–147. [CrossRef]
20. Gonzalez-Rivas, D.; Yang, Y.; Stupnik, T.; Sekhniaidze, D.; Fernandez, R.; Velasco, C.; Zhu, Y.; Jiang, G. Uni-portal video-assisted thoracoscopic bronchovascular, tracheal and carinal sleeve resections dagger. *Eur. J. Cardiothorac. Surg.* **2016**, *49* (Suppl. 1), i6–i16.
21. Gonzalez-Rivas, D.; Paradela, M.; Fernandez, R.; Delgado, M.; Fieira, E.; Mendez, L.; Velasco, C.; de la Torre, M. Uni-portal video-assisted thoracoscopic lobectomy: Two years of experience. *Ann. Thorac. Surg.* **2013**, *95*, 426–432. [CrossRef]
22. Abouarab, A.A.; Rahouma, M.; Kamel, M.; Ghaly, G.; Mohamed, A. Single versus multi-incisional video-assisted thoracic surgery: A systematic review and Meta-analysis. *J. Laparoendosc. Adv. Surg. Tech. Part A* **2018**, *28*, 174–185. [CrossRef]
23. Ng, C.S.H.; MacDonald, J.K.; Gilbert, S.; Khan, A.Z.; Kim, Y.T.; Louie, B.E.; Blair Marshall, M.; Santos, R.S.; Scarci, M.; Shargal, Y.; et al. Optimal Approach to Lobectomy for Non-Small Cell Lung Cancer: Systemic Review and Meta-Analysis. *Innovations* **2019**, *14*, 90–116. [CrossRef] [PubMed]
24. Ng, C.S.; Kim, H.K.; Wong, R.H.; Yim, A.P.; Mok, T.S.; Choi, Y.H. Single-port video-assisted thoracoscopic major lung resections: Experience with 150 consecutive cases. *Thorac. Cardiovasc. Surg.* **2016**, *64*, 348–353. [CrossRef] [PubMed]
25. Lin, F.; Zhang, C.; Zhang, Q.; Cheng, K.; Zhao, Y. Uni-portal video-assisted thoracoscopic lobectomy: An alternative surgical method for pulmonary carcinoma. *Pak. J. Med. Sci.* **2016**, *32*, 1283–1285. [PubMed]
26. Mu, J.W.; Gao, S.G.; Xue, Q.; Mao, Y.S.; Wang, D.L.; Zhao, J.; Gao, Y.S.; Huang, J.F.; He, J. A propensity matched comparison of effects between video assisted thoracoscopic single-port, two-port and three-port pulmonary resection on lung cancer. *J. Thorac. Dis.* **2016**, *8*, 1469–1476. [CrossRef] [PubMed]
27. Al-Ameri, M.; Sachs, E.; Sartipy, U.; Jackson, V. Uni-portal versus multiportal video-assisted thoracic surgery for lung cancer. *J. Thorac. Dis.* **2019**, *11*, 5152–5161. [CrossRef]
28. Yang, X.; Li, M.; Yang, X.; Zhao, M.; Huang, Y.; Dai, X.; Jiang, T.; Feng, M.; Zhan, C.; Wang, Q. Uniport versus multiport video-assisted thoracoscopic surgery in the perioperative treatment of patients with T1-3N0M0 non-small cell lung cancer: A systematic review and meta-analysis. *J. Thorac. Dis.* **2018**, *10*, 2186–2195. [CrossRef]
29. Yang, Z.; Shen, Z.; Zhou, Q.; Huang, Y. Single-incision versus multiport video-assisted thoracoscopic surgery in the treatment of lung cancer: A systematic review and meta-analysis. *Acta Chir. Belg.* **2018**, *118*, 85–93. [CrossRef]
30. Han, K.N.; Kim, H.K.; Choi, Y.H. Midterm outcomes of single port thoracoscopic surgery for major pulmonary resection. *PLoS ONE* **2017**, *12*, e0186857. [CrossRef]
31. Cheng, X.; Onaitis, M.W.; D'Amico, T.A.; Chen, H. Minimally invasive thoracic surgery 3.0: Lessons learned from the history of lung Cancer surgery. *Ann. Surg.* **2018**, *267*, 37–38. [CrossRef]

Disclaimer/Publisher's Note: The statements, opinions and data contained in all publications are solely those of the individual author(s) and contributor(s) and not of MDPI and/or the editor(s). MDPI and/or the editor(s) disclaim responsibility for any injury to people or property resulting from any ideas, methods, instructions or products referred to in the content.

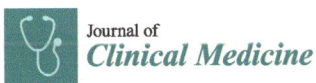

Article

Two-Year Experience of a Center of Excellence for the Comprehensive Management of Non-Small Cell Lung Cancer at a Fourth-Level Hospital in Bogota, Colombia: Observational Case Series Study and Retrospective Analysis

Luis Gerardo García-Herreros *, Enid Ximena Rico-Rivera and Olga Milena García Morales

Fundación Santa Fe de Bogotá Centro de Cuidado Clínico de Cáncer de Pulmón, Bogotá 110111, Colombia
* Correspondence: luis.garciah@fsfb.org.co

Abstract: Background: This study aimed to provide a comprehensive analysis of 56 patients admitted to the Lung Cancer Clinical Care Center (C3) at Fundación Santa Fe de Bogotá (FSFB) between 2 May 2022 and 22 April 2024. The focus was on demographic characteristics, smoking history, comorbidities, lung cancer types, TNM classification, treatment modalities, and outcomes. **Methods:** This observational case series study reviewed medical records and included patients over 18 years with a confirmed diagnosis of non-small cell lung cancer (NSCLC). Data were collected and analyzed for demographics, comorbidities, treatment types, biomolecular profiling, and survival rates. Ethical approval was obtained, and data were anonymized. **Results:** The mean age was 71.8 years with a female predominance (53.6%). A history of smoking was present in 71.4% of patients. Adenocarcinoma was the most common type (75.0%), followed by squamous cell carcinoma (19.6%). At admission, the most frequent TNM stages were IA2 (17.9%) and IVA (16.1%). One-year survival was 68.8%, and 94.3% of stage I–IIIA patients underwent PET scans. Biomolecular profiling revealed 69.2% non-mutated EGFR, 90.4% ALK-negative, and various PDL-1 expression levels. Immunotherapy was received by 91.4% of patients, with Alectinib and Osimertinib being common. Grade III–IV pneumonitis occurred in 5.4% of patients. **Conclusions:** The study's findings align with existing literature, highlighting significant smoking history, common adenocarcinoma, and substantial use of immunotherapy. Limitations include the observational design, small sample size, and short follow-up period, impacting the generalizability and long-term outcome assessment. Future research should address these limitations and explore longitudinal outcomes and emerging therapies.

Keywords: lung neoplasms; carcinoma; non-small-cell lung; immunotherapy; radiotherapy; survival; drug-related side effects and adverse reactions

Citation: García-Herreros, L.G.; Rico-Rivera, E.X.; García Morales, O.M. Two-Year Experience of a Center of Excellence for the Comprehensive Management of Non-Small Cell Lung Cancer at a Fourth-Level Hospital in Bogota, Colombia: Observational Case Series Study and Retrospective Analysis. J. Clin. Med. **2024**, 13, 6820. https://doi.org/10.3390/jcm13226820

Academic Editor: Kazuyoshi Imaizumi

Received: 23 September 2024
Revised: 29 October 2024
Accepted: 7 November 2024
Published: 13 November 2024

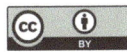

Copyright: © 2024 by the authors. Licensee MDPI, Basel, Switzerland. This article is an open access article distributed under the terms and conditions of the Creative Commons Attribution (CC BY) license (https://creativecommons.org/licenses/by/4.0/).

1. Introduction

Lung cancer, or bronchogenic carcinoma, arises in the lung parenchyma or bronchi and stands as one of the principal causes of cancer-related mortality both globally and in the United States. Since 1987, it has surpassed breast cancer as the leading cause of cancer death in women, with an estimated 225,000 new cases and 160,000 deaths occurring annually in the U.S. alone [1,2]. In 2021, projections from the International Association for the Study of Lung Cancer (IASLC) indicated 235,760 new cases and 131,880 deaths within the U.S. [3]. In Colombia, approximately 4000 new cases are diagnosed each year, with a high proportion (72%) presenting at advanced or metastatic stages, contributing to a low 5-year survival rate of 8.7% [4]. Lung cancer incidence has increased sharply over the 20th century, largely attributable to the rise in tobacco use [1,2]. Globally, lung cancer is the leading cause of cancer death and the second most common cancer after breast cancer, comprising around 12.4% of all cancer diagnoses and responsible for approximately 1.8 million deaths annually [5–9]. In developing regions, incidence rates have grown significantly, with nearly half (49.9%) of new cases now occurring in these areas [10]. In the U.S., lung cancer mortality is generally higher in men, with African American men experiencing higher age-adjusted mortality rates compared to Caucasian men, though no significant racial differences are noted among women [11]. Tobacco smoking remains the primary cause of lung cancer, linked to roughly 90% of cases [11]. Additional risk factors include asbestos exposure, radon, passive smoking (which increases risk by 20–30%), previous radiation therapy (particularly for cancers like non-Hodgkin lymphoma and breast cancer), and specific occupational exposures to metals and hydrocarbons [11–14]. Radon, especially in mining settings, and residential radon exposure have both been associated with increased lung cancer mortality, particularly among smokers [6,7].

In Colombia, fragmented healthcare access for lung cancer patients often results in delayed diagnosis, suboptimal treatment, and insufficient follow-up, leading to worse patient outcomes and heightened mortality. These barriers, coupled with frequent hospitalizations and prolonged treatments, contribute to a significant economic burden on the healthcare system [4]. In response to these challenges, Fundación Santa Fe de Bogotá (FSFB) established the Lung Cancer Clinical Care Center (C3) in 2020. This center aims to improve lung cancer outcomes through a model of high-quality care based on four pillars: advanced clinical management, high-impact metrics, patient-centered care, and research. This case series describes C3's lung cancer management experience and presents the institutional registry of non-small-cell lung cancer (NSCLC) patients. The registry is designed to systematize case records, elevate care standards, and provide a foundation for ongoing research in lung cancer [4].

2. Materials and Methods

This is a descriptive observational study of a case series. The study population consisted of patients enrolled in the Lung Cancer Clinical Care Center (C3) at Fundación Santa Fe de Bogotá (FSFB) from the start of systematic data collection on 2 May 2022, until the last patient enrollment on 22 April 2024.

2.1. Selection Criteria

2.1.1. Inclusion Criteria

The inclusion criteria for this study are the same as those of the C3 Lung Cancer Center at FSFB and included:

- Patients over 18 years old.
- Patients with a confirmed diagnosis of primary lung cancer, including non-small cell lung cancer (NSCLC), of all histological subtypes and stages according to the most recent version of the TNM classification.
- Patients initially diagnosed at FSFB or referred from other institutions with confirmed pathology for continued therapy at C3.
- Patients for whom protocol continuity can be ensured at the institution.

2.1.2. Exclusion Criteria

The exclusion criteria for this study are the same as those of the C3 Lung Cancer Center at FSFB and included:

- Patients with lung metastases from a primary tumor located elsewhere.
- Patients with lung cancer and a life expectancy of less than 6 months (e.g., those with high tumor burden, refractory to multiple treatment lines, or in irreversible functional decline treated outside the C3 protocol).
- Patients who refused to receive comprehensive care at FSFB.

2.2. Patient Evaluation and Management Definition

After confirming the histopathological diagnosis of non-small-cell lung cancer (NSCLC) with the appropriate biomarkers, either through biopsy or surgical resection (pTNM), the C3 proceeded with disease staging. This was carried out using the 8th edition of the TNM classification to define the stage and guide the appropriate treatment. This record was used for the purpose of this research. Staging was performed non-invasively with a chest CT scan and, in all cases, a PET scan, along with an MRI of the brain in special cases to assess the probability of metastasis. Invasive staging was performed using procedures such as mediastinoscopy or endobronchial ultrasound (EBUS) if the chest CT or PET scan revealed mediastinal involvement or probable involvement of N1 lymph nodes.

Tumor size alone was not a criterion for invasive staging, as this had a level C evidence grade, and each case was individually evaluated [15]. According to the experience of the C3, central tumors dependent on lobar bronchi always required invasive staging. Initial pathological samples used for histopathological diagnosis underwent at least biomarker testing for ALK, PD-L1, and EGFR. Depending on the specific characteristics of each patient, additional biomarkers were tested. In surgical specimens, criteria for pathological staging were evaluated, and if necessary, the pathology team reclassified the tumor. New biomarker tests could be performed based on available treatments and the multidisciplinary team's decisions. Upon confirming the NSCLC diagnosis histologically, the treating physician determined the most beneficial treatment for the patient, which could include oncological management, surgical management, or a combination of both.

2.2.1. Tumor Classification by Histological Subtype

The histopathological classification of lung cancers was based on cellular and molecular subtypes, which is essential for diagnosis and management. The World Health Organization (WHO) 2021 lung tumor classification system divides lung cancers as follows [16]:

- Adenocarcinomas;
- Squamous cell carcinomas;
- Precursor glandular lesions;
- Adenosquamous carcinomas;
- Precursor squamous lesions;
- Large-cell carcinomas;
- Sarcomatoid carcinomas;
- Pulmonary neuroendocrine neoplasms;
- Salivary gland-type tumors;
- Neuroendocrine tumors;
- Neuroendocrine carcinomas;
- Other epithelial tumors.

According to the WHO, identifying histological characteristics, measuring the depth of invasion, and the mode of spread have prognostic value [16]. For example, tumor spread through airways is associated with a higher recurrence rate after limited resections and should be reported in pathology evaluations [16]. The WHO has removed previously described subtypes such as clear cell, rhabdoid, and signet ring from its latest classification, as these appear to be cytological features that can occur in any adenocarcinoma [16]. The WHO classification emphasizes immunohistochemical staining to classify cancers that may not have typical cytological features under optical microscopy [16]. In the WHO 2015 classification system, poorly differentiated carcinomas were reclassified as squamous cell carcinomas if they expressed p40; as solid adenocarcinomas if they expressed thyroid transcription factor 1; and as neuroendocrine carcinomas if positive for chromogranin and synaptophysin [17].

Given that C3 only includes patients with NSCLC within the inclusion criteria, only histological subtypes corresponding to this type of cancer were considered for this study.

2.2.2. Lung Cancer Staging (TNM System) in the Studied Population

Staging was conducted using the TNM classification system in its last version [15] to plan treatment and guide prognosis for each patient. This classification was used to evaluate the anatomical extent of the disease both clinically and from a histopathological point of view.

2.2.3. Evaluation of Biomarkers in the Studied Population

The pathophysiology of lung cancer is highly complex and not fully understood. It is believed that repeated exposure to carcinogens such as cigarette smoke leads to pulmonary epithelial dysplasia. Continued exposure can induce genetic mutations, thereby affecting protein synthesis [18]. This disruption causes cell cycle dysregulation and fosters carcinogenesis. The most common genetic mutations involved in lung cancer include MYC, BCL2, and p53 for small-cell lung cancer (SCLC), and EGFR, KRAS, and p16 for non-small-cell lung cancer (NSCLC) [19,20].

These biomarkers are crucial because the primary treatment for metastatic NSCLC relies on identifying specific driver genetic mutations. These include alterations in the epidermal growth factor receptor (EGFR) and rearrangements in the anaplastic lymphoma kinase (ALK) gene [19–21]. Additionally, PD-L1 expressions have been associated with increased tumor proliferation, cancer aggressiveness, and reduced survival in NSCLC patients, particularly those diagnosed with adenocarcinoma [22].

Therefore, during the histopathological diagnosis of lung cancer at C3, it was crucial to conduct a minimum biomarker analysis including ALK, PD-L1, and EGFR using the initial pathological sample, especially for patients in stages III and IV of the disease, to ensure targeted therapy [21,22]. The assessment of these biomarkers was considered for research purposes. This initial evaluation could be expanded to include other biomarkers based on each patient's specific characteristics. Thus, whenever the treating physician requested evaluation of biomarkers other than those mentioned, these were documented in the study's results section.

2.2.4. Functional Impact of Oncologic Disease (ECOG Performance Status) and Its Evaluation in the Study Population

Clinical research involving cancer patients necessitates the use of standardized criteria to measure the disease's impact on patients' ability to perform daily activities, known as the patient's functional status. The Eastern Cooperative Oncology Group (ECOG) Performance Status Scale corresponds to a well-established system widely referenced in the literature for such measurements [23].

This scale describes a patient's level of functioning in terms of their ability to self-care, perform daily activities, and engage in physical activities (e.g., walking, working, etc.) [23]. Researchers worldwide consider the ECOG Performance Status Scale when planning oncologic clinical trials to study new treatments. This numerical rating system helps define the patient population for the trial and guides physicians enrolling patients in these studies. It also allows physicians to monitor changes in a patient's functional level resulting from treatment during a clinical trial [23]. The updated ECOG Scale was used in this study to evaluate the impact of the disease on the quality of life of the participants.

For study purposes, the ECOG Performance Status scores were recorded and analyzed at the initial assessments of the patients to ascertain the presence and potential magnitude of differences in patient functionality between the time of admission to C3 and their current status.

2.3. Study Procedures

2.3.1. Data Collection, Tabulation, and Data Cleaning

As part of the routine clinical practice at C3, all necessary information to meet the study objectives was collected from each patient's medical records. At FSFB, a university hospital, all patients must sign an informed consent allowing the use of their data for research, in accordance with approval from the Institutional Research Ethics Committee.

Subsequently, an epidemiologist and hospital physician from FSFB with research experience reviewed all C3 medical records starting from 2 May 2022. She tabulated all the information into a Microsoft Excel® database specifically designed for this study, which was further analyzed for the final report. This database incorporates all variables outlined in the study protocol.

2.3.2. Description of Potential Biases and Measures to Control Them

As an observational case series study, the primary bias that could arise is information bias, which occurs when collected information about cases is inaccurate or incomplete. This may result from errors in data collection, interpretation, or inadequate record-keeping. To mitigate and minimize the likelihood of this bias, the following strategies were implemented:

- Double review of medical records: Information from medical records was reviewed in duplicate to minimize errors in interpretation and recording.
- Training and expertise of personnel: The data collection process was overseen by a hospital physician from C3, an epidemiologist experienced in research, data collection, and conducting observational studies.

2.3.3. Statistical Analysis

For this study, data description included qualitative and quantitative variables, with corresponding frequency and percentage analysis for each category, as well as frequency distribution for variables of interest in qualitative data. Summary measures such as mean, range, and standard deviation were used for quantitative variables.

All statistical analyses were conducted using the latest versions of Microsoft Excel® and SPSS.

2.3.4. Ethical Aspects of This Study

This study was classified as minimal-risk research, according to definitions outlined in Resolution 8430 of 1993 by the Colombian Ministry of Health [24], which regulates clinical research in Colombia. Approval from the FSFB Research Ethics Committee was obtained to conduct this study (CCEI-16751-2024).

As an observational descriptive study, this research did not involve administering or modifying treatment regimens for participating patients. This study adhered to and respected established norms for research involving humans, as defined by national and international regulations, including the Declaration of Helsinki and its subsequent revisions [25].

Furthermore, all patients at FSFB, being a university hospital, provided informed consent upon admission to C3, voluntarily agreeing to the use of their data for research purposes. All information was handled confidentially. Results were presented in aggregate form to ensure anonymity and protect the identity of each participant.

3. Results

3.1. Baseline Characteristics and Smoking History

Fifty-six patients were admitted to C3 between 2 May 2022 and 22 April 2024. The age range was between 49 and 90 years, with a mean age of 71.8 years. Regarding gender distribution, 30 (53.6%) patients were female, while the remaining 26 (46.4%) patients were male.

In the analysis of the 56 patients, it was found that 71.4% (n = 40) were smokers at some point in their lives, while 28.6% (n = 16) never smoked. Additionally, none of the patients currently smoke, indicating a significant prevalence of smoking history, though without the presence of active smokers in the studied population (Table 1).

In the initial analysis of the patients' functional condition, evaluated using the ECOG Scale, it was found that most patients had an ECOG level of 0 and 1, with 18 and 23 cases, respectively. Only one patient was classified as ECOG 2 at the time of admission. This result suggests that most patients maintained an adequate level of activity and could carry out light work.

Table 1. Baseline characteristics and smoking history.

Characteristic	Value
Number of patients	56
Age range (years)	49–90
Mean age (years)	71.8
Female, n (%)	30 (53.6%)
Male, n (%)	26 (46.4%)
Ever smoked, n (%)	40 (71.4%)
Never smoked, n (%)	16 (28.6%)
Currently smoking, n (%)	0 (0%)

3.2. Baseline Pathologies and Medications

In the analysis of the 56 patients, the most frequent pathologies were hypertension (21.4%), diabetes mellitus (14.3%), chronic obstructive pulmonary disease (COPD) (10.7%), ischemic heart disease (8.9%), dyslipidemia (7.1%), hypothyroidism (5.4%), previous cancer (3.6%), and chronic renal failure (3.6%), with various other pathologies representing 25.0%. The most frequently used medications were atorvastatin (21.4%), omeprazole (14.3%), metformin (10.7%), enalapril (8.9%), levothyroxine (7.1%), metoprolol (5.4%), insulin (3.6%), and aspirin (3.6%), with various other medications representing 25.0%. These results highlight the prevalence of chronic diseases such as hypertension and diabetes and the common use of medications for their control (Table 2).

Table 2. Pathologies and medications.

Pathologies	n (%) Pathologies	Medications	n (%) Medications
Hypertension	12 (21.4%)	Atorvastatin	12 (21.4%)
Diabetes mellitus	8 (14.3%)	Omeprazole	8 (14.3%)
Chronic obstructive pulmonary disease (COPD)	6 (10.7%)	Metformin	6 (10.7%)
Ischemic heart disease	5 (8.9%)	Enalapril	5 (8.9%)
Dyslipidemia	4 (7.1%)	Levothyroxine	3 (5.4%)
Hypothyroidism	3 (5.4%)	Metoprolol	3 (5.4%)
Previous cancer	2 (3.6%)	Insulin	2 (3.6%)
Chronic renal failure	2 (3.6%)	Aspirin	2 (3.6%)
Other pathologies	14 (25.0%)	Other medications	15 (26.7%)

3.3. Lung Cancer Type and TNM Stage

Regarding the type of lung cancer, 42 (75.0%) patients were diagnosed with adenocarcinoma, 11 (19.6%) patients with squamous cell carcinoma, 2 (3.6%) patients with poorly differentiated carcinoma, and 1 (1.8%) patient with infiltrating carcinoma with neuroendocrine differentiation (Table 3).

Regarding the TNM classification at the time of admission to C3, one patient was classified as stage IA1 (1.8%), ten patients as IA2 (17.9%), three patients as IA3 (5.4%), eight patients as IB (14.3%), one patient as IIA (1.8%), six patients as IIB (10.7%), six patients as IIIA (10.7%), four patients as IIIB (7.1%), two patients as IIIC (3.6%), nine patients as IVA (16.1%), and six patients as IVB (10.7%) (Table 3).

Table 3. Lung cancer types and the TNM classification.

Lung Cancer Type	n (%) Lung Cancer Type	Initial TNM Stage	n (%) Initial TNM	Current TNM Stage	n (%) Current TNM
Adenocarcinoma	42 (75.0%)	IA1	1 (1.8%)	IA1	1 (1.8%)
Squamous cell carcinoma	11 (19.6%)	IA2	10 (17.9%)	IA2	9 (16.1%)
Poorly differentiated carcinoma	2 (3.6%)	IA3	3 (5.4%)	IA3	3 (5.4%)
Infiltrating carcinoma with neuroendocrine differentiation	1 (1.8%)	IB	8 (14.3%)	IB	8 (14.3%)
		IIA	1 (1.8%)	IIA	1 (1.8%)
		IIB	6 (10.7%)	IIB	4 (7.1%)
		IIIA	6 (10.7%)	IIIA	6 (10.7%)
		IIIB	4 (7.1%)	IIIB	4 (7.1%)
		IIIC	2 (3.6%)	IIIC	2 (3.6%)
		IVA	9 (16.1%)	IVA	9 (16.1%)
		IVB	6 (10.7%)	IVB	9 (16.1%)

On the other hand, the current TNM stage at the time of the last visit to C3 was as follows: one patient was classified as stage IA1 (1.8%), nine patients as IA2 (16.1%), three patients as IA3 (5.4%), eight patients as IB (14.3%), one patient as IIA (1.8%), four patients as IIB (7.1%), six patients as IIIA (10.7%), four patients as IIIB (7.1%), two patients as IIIC (3.6%), nine patients as IVA (16.1%), and nine patients as IVB (16.1%). Disease progression was documented in only three of the 56 patients (Table 3).

3.4. One-Year Survival and PET Scan Results

The one-year survival analysis from diagnosis was conducted in 16 patients who completed one year of follow-up. The results indicate that 11 of these patients, representing 68.8% of the analyzed group, survived at least one year after the initial diagnosis. In contrast, five patients, equivalent to 31.2% of the group, died within the first year.

In the evaluation of PET scan use in patients diagnosed with stage I–IIIA cancer (35 patients), it was observed that a high percentage of these patients, specifically 94.3%, received a PET scan as part of their initial diagnostic evaluation. Two patients, representing 5.7%, did not undergo this diagnostic procedure.

In the combined analysis of patients diagnosed with stage I–IIIA cancer who received a PET scan, it was observed that of those who underwent the procedure, 24 patients, equivalent to 72.7%, obtained a negative result, indicating the possible absence of significant tumor activity or the effectiveness of previous treatments. On the other hand, nine patients, representing 27.3% of the evaluated group, showed positive results in the PET scan, suggesting the presence of active tumor activity or recurrence.

3.5. Surgical Procedures

Out of a total of 56 patients in the database, 39 patients, corresponding to 69.6%, underwent surgical procedures for lung cancer treatment. Of these 39 patients, 8 of them, representing 20.5%, had to undergo more than one surgical intervention at different times.

The analysis of surgical treatments in the database indicates that various surgical interventions were performed, each specifically tailored to the individual patient's needs, including segmental lobectomies, wedge resections, mediastinoscopies with biopsies, and combinations of thoracoscopies with pleurodesis, among others. Each type of surgery was documented in a single instance, highlighting the personalization of surgical treatment. Most of these interventions (84.6%) resulted in an R0 resection, indicating no cancer cells were found in the resected tissue margins. Regarding postoperative recovery, 76.9% of patients did not require hospital readmission within 30 days post-operation, while 23.1% of patients were readmitted for various reasons such as infection, medication adjustments, and gastrointestinal problems, among others. This analysis shows effective surgical management, with a minority of cases experiencing significant postoperative complications.

3.6. Biomolecular Profiles and Biomarker Analysis

Fifty-two of the fifty-six patients included in this study underwent biomolecular analysis for the biomarkers EGFR, ALK, and PDL-1. This analysis was primarily conducted in patients with stage III to IV cancer, indicating that most of the evaluated sample received detailed biomolecular assessments to guide more personalized and targeted treatment decisions.

In the analysis conducted with 52 patients who underwent EGFR biomarker analysis, it was found that the majority, 69.2%, had non-mutated EGFR. Specific mutations were also identified, with 15.4% of patients showing the EX19DEL mutation, while the EX20INS and L858R mutations were present in 7.7% each.

In the ALK biomarker analysis conducted on 52 patients, it was observed that the majority, 90.4%, were ALK negative, indicating the absence of the ALK mutation in most of the evaluated patients. Additionally, 7.7% of patients were ALK positive, while 1.9% showed a weak positive ALK result.

Regarding the PDL-1 analysis conducted in 52 patients, it was found that 11.5% of patients showed 0% expression, while 34.6% exhibited less than 1% expression. Expressions of 1% and 3% were observed in 3.8% and 5.8% of patients, respectively. The expression of 5% was reported by 11.5% of patients. Other expressions, such as 10%, 20%, and 30%, were present in 5.8%, 7.7%, and 5.8%, respectively. Expressions of 35%, 40%, 70%, 80%, and 90% were less common, recorded in 1.9% of patients each.

3.7. Oncological Management, Therapies, and Adverse Events

Thirty-seven patients, equivalent to 66.1% of the evaluated sample, received oncological management. Of these patients, 91.4% received immunotherapy, with the most frequently used treatments being Alectinib in 11.11% of cases, followed by Osimertinib with 8.3%. Other medications had a more dispersed distribution, each representing 2.8% of the total. The treatment intention was mainly distributed between adjuvant (43.2%) and palliative (40.6%), with a smaller proportion of neoadjuvant (16.2%). Of the 37 patients evaluated, 19 (51.4%) received second-line therapies, and only 3 (8.1%) received third-line therapies for lung cancer. These results indicate a significant proportion of patients progressing to second-line treatments, while a smaller fraction required third-line treatments. Regarding pulmonary adverse events, only two patients (5.4%) developed grade III and IV adverse events consistent with pneumonitis.

Regarding radiotherapy, it was initiated in 19 of the 56 patients (33.9%), with the most used modality being SBRT (Stereotactic Body Radiation Therapy) in 10 cases (52.6%), followed by IMRT (Intensity-Modulated Radiation Therapy) in 9 patients (47.4%). The number of radiotherapy cycles varied from 3 to 30 depending on the patient, with a mean of 12 cycles. No radiotherapy toxicity events were documented according to the RTOG (Radiation Therapy Oncology Group) and EORTC (European Organisation for Research and Treatment of Cancer) criteria.

3.8. Mortality and Causes of Death

Eight of the patients in this study died during the follow-up period (14.3%). The most common causes of death were tumor progression in five patients and septic shock, stroke, and decompensated heart failure in each of the remaining three patients.

4. Discussion

The present study provides a comprehensive analysis of 56 patients admitted to C3 between 2 May 2022 and 22 April 2024, focusing on demographic characteristics, smoking history, comorbidities, lung cancer types, TNM classification, treatment modalities, and outcomes. Our findings are consistent with previous research and provide valuable insights into the management and prognosis of lung cancer patients [1–4,11,12].

The demographic data revealed a predominance of elderly patients with a mean age of 71.8 years. The gender distribution showed a slightly higher proportion of females (53.6%) compared to males (46.4%). These findings align with the general epidemiological trends observed in lung cancer, where age and gender are significant risk factors [11,12].

The smoking history analysis indicated that 71.4% of patients had a history of smoking, while 28.6% had never smoked. This is significantly higher than the prevalence of tobacco use in the Colombian general population, which is approximately 33% [4]. Notably, none of the patients were current smokers at the time of this study. This is significant, as smoking is a well-established risk factor for lung cancer, and smoking cessation is known to improve prognosis and reduce recurrence rates [26].

Comorbidities were prevalent among the patient cohort, with hypertension (21.4%), diabetes mellitus (14.3%), and chronic obstructive pulmonary disease (COPD) (10.7%) being the most common. The correlation between these comorbidities and the medications prescribed highlights the importance of comprehensive management in lung cancer patients. For instance, hypertension was commonly treated with antihypertensive medications such as enalapril and losartan, while diabetes mellitus management included metformin and insulin. These findings underscore the necessity of addressing comorbid conditions to optimize overall patient outcomes.

In terms of lung cancer types, adenocarcinoma was the most prevalent, accounting for 75.0% of cases, followed by squamous cell carcinoma at 19.6%. This distribution is consistent with global patterns, where adenocarcinoma is the most common histological subtype of lung cancer [15–17]. The TNM classification at admission and the last visit showed a progression in some patients, emphasizing the aggressive nature of the disease and the need for continuous monitoring and treatment adjustments [27].

The survival analysis revealed that 68.8% of patients survived at least one year post-diagnosis, while 31.2% succumbed within the first year. This survival rate is like or even higher than what has been reported in the literature [8–10]. The utilization of PET scans was high, with 94.3% of stage I–IIIA patients undergoing this diagnostic procedure, which is crucial for accurate staging and treatment planning [28–30]. PET scan results indicated a high rate of negative findings (72.7%), suggesting effective initial treatments or low tumor activity at the time of evaluation.

Biomolecular profiling and biomarker analysis showed most of the patients included in this study underwent profiling, with non-mutated EGFR being the most common result (69.2%). This aligns with the current understanding that EGFR mutations, although less common, have significant therapeutic implications. The presence of ALK and PDL-1 biomarkers also provides opportunities for targeted therapies, which are increasingly becoming standard care in advanced lung cancer [19–22].

Oncological management predominantly involves immunotherapy, with 91.4% of patients receiving this treatment modality. Alectinib and osimertinib were the most frequently used medications, reflecting their efficacy in targeted treatment [31–38]. Adjuvant (43.2%) and palliative (40.6%) treatments were the primary intents, highlighting the diverse therapeutic approaches based on disease stage and patient condition.

The incidence of grades III and IV pneumonitis was low (5.4%), indicating that severe pulmonary adverse events were relatively rare. This is like what has been reported in the literature [39]. Radiotherapy, particularly SBRT and IMRT, was utilized in 33.9% of patients, with a mean of 12 cycles per patient. The absence of documented radiotherapy toxicity according to RTOG and EORTC criteria suggests that these modalities were well tolerated. This is notable as it has been reported that between 10 and 30% of all patients with lung or breast cancer receiving thoracic radiotherapy develop radiation-induced pneumonitis (RIP) as a subacute treatment-associated toxicity, and they are at high risk of developing radiation-induced lung fibrosis (RILF) as late toxicity, although treatment-related death is uncommon [40]. However, it is possible that the low power of the study as well as the short follow-up period did not allow for a more accurate assessment of this outcome.

Mortality analysis revealed that 14.3% of patients died during the study period. The most common causes of death were tumor progression in five patients and septic shock, stroke, and decompensated heart failure in each of the remaining three patients. These findings emphasize the need for ongoing supportive care and early intervention to manage complications.

In the context of previous studies, our findings corroborate the established risk factors, comorbidities, and treatment outcomes in lung cancer patients. The high utilization of diagnostic and therapeutic modalities aligns with current clinical guidelines, reflecting a comprehensive approach to lung cancer management.

Despite the valuable insights provided by this study, several limitations must be acknowledged. As an observational study based on a case series and the review of medical records, it is inherently subject to selection bias, recall bias, and other limitations typical of retrospective data collection. The sample size of 56 patients, while sufficient to offer preliminary insights, limits the statistical power and may not provide a comprehensive representation of the broader population of lung cancer patients. This constraint is particularly important given the heterogeneity of lung cancer in terms of histological subtypes, stages at diagnosis, and patient demographics, which could affect the generalizability of the findings.

Additionally, the relatively short follow-up period poses a significant limitation, particularly in assessing long-term outcomes and late-onset toxicities such as radiation-induced lung fibrosis (RILF), which may take years to manifest. This limited follow-up may lead to an underestimation of the incidence of these complications, and, as a result, the conclusions about long-term efficacy and safety are necessarily incomplete. Extending the follow-up period in future studies will be essential to capture a more accurate picture of survival rates, quality of life, and the incidence of delayed adverse events.

The study's low statistical power also restricts its ability to detect smaller effect sizes or subtle differences between subgroups, which could be critical in identifying specific patient characteristics that influence treatment outcomes. For example, variations in response to treatment based on genetic factors, comorbidities, or previous treatments might not have been fully captured due to the small sample size and limited subgroup analysis. This highlights the need for larger, multi-center studies that can enroll a more diverse cohort and provide more robust statistical analyses.

Future research should aim to address these limitations by not only incorporating larger and more heterogeneous patient populations but also adopting a prospective design. Prospective studies would mitigate the inherent biases of retrospective data collection and allow for a more controlled and systematic assessment of patient outcomes, particularly in evaluating long-term efficacy and safety. Randomized controlled trials (RCTs) would further help validate these findings, offering stronger evidence for optimizing therapeutic strategies and ensuring that the results can be applied to clinical practice with greater confidence. These efforts would ultimately contribute to refining treatment protocols and improving outcomes for lung cancer patients.

To improve outcomes for NSCLC patients, several strategies could be considered. First, enhancing early detection through expanded screening programs, especially for high-risk groups, would be crucial in reducing the presentation of late-stage NSCLC. Additionally, increasing access to comprehensive biomarker testing nationwide could enable more precise, targeted therapies, optimizing treatment efficacy. This aligns with a future plan to strengthen precision medicine in Colombia by promoting accessibility to biomolecular profiling and newer targeted therapies, potentially through collaborative networks and policy adjustments. Moreover, implementing multidisciplinary lung cancer teams and streamlining referral pathways could improve patient management and ensure timely treatment, particularly for patients in underserved regions. These approaches could collectively contribute to achieving more favorable NSCLC outcomes in Colombia.

Author Contributions: Conceptualization, L.G.G.-H., E.X.R.-R. and O.M.G.M.; methodology, L.G.G.-H., E.X.R.-R. and O.M.G.M.; software, E.X.R.-R.; validation, L.G.G.-H., E.X.R.-R. and O.M.G.M.; formal analysis, L.G.G.-H., E.X.R.-R. and O.M.G.M.; investigation, L.G.G.-H., E.X.R.-R. and O.M.G.M.; resources, L.G.G.-H.; data curation, L.G.G.-H., E.X.R.-R. and O.M.G.M.; writing—original draft preparation, L.G.G.-H., E.X.R.-R. and O.M.G.M.; writing—review and editing, L.G.G.-H., E.X.R.-R. and O.M.G.M.; visualization, L.G.G.-H., E.X.R.-R. and O.M.G.M.; supervision, L.G.G.-H.; project administration, L.G.G.-H.; funding acquisition, L.G.G.-H. All authors have read and agreed to the published version of the manuscript.

Funding: The medical writing process and the payment of the open access fee for the publication were carried out by AstraZeneca.

Institutional Review Board Statement: This study was conducted in accordance with the Declaration of Helsinki and approved by the Ethics Committee of FUNDACIÓN SANTA FE DE BOGOTÁ (Protocol version 002 dated 4 July 2024), with approval code: CCEI-16751-2024.

Informed Consent Statement: Informed consent was not required for participation in the present study, as patients at this university hospital voluntarily and in writing agree that their anonymized data may be used for research purposes, subject to prior approval by the research ethics committee, as was the case in this study.

Data Availability Statement: Due to institutional policies and in compliance with the Habeas Data Law and data protection regulations applicable in Colombia, it is not possible to publicly share the corresponding database for this study. However, this information will be available upon request to other researchers.

Conflicts of Interest: The authors have no conflicts of interest to declare.

References

1. Oliver, A.L. Lung Cancer: Epidemiology and Screening. *Surg. Clin. N. Am.* **2022**, *102*, 335–344. [CrossRef] [PubMed]
2. Siddiqui, F.; Vaqar, S.; Siddiqui, A.H. Lung Cancer. [Updated 2023 May 8]. In *StatPearls [Internet]*; StatPearls Publishing: Treasure Island, FL, USA, 2024. Available online: https://www.ncbi.nlm.nih.gov/books/NBK482357/ (accessed on 24 May 2024).
3. Zhang, J.; Basu, P.; Emery, J.D.; IJzerman, M.J.; Bray, F. LC statistics in the United States: A reflection on the impact of cancer control. *Ann. Cancer Epidemiol.* **2022**, *6*, 2. [CrossRef]
4. Cuenta de Alto Costo, Instituto de Evaluación Tecnológica en Salud (IETS), Asociación Colombiana de Hematología y Oncología. Herramienta Técnica Para la Gestión del Riesgo Dirigida a Profesionales de la Salud Involucrados en el Diagnóstico, Seguimiento y Monitoreo de Pacientes con Cáncer de Pulmón [Internet]. Available online: https://cuentadealtocosto.org/herramientas_tecnica/herramienta-tecnica-cancer-de-pulmon/ (accessed on 24 May 2024).
5. Klebe, S.; Leigh, J.; Henderson, D.W.; Nurminen, M. Asbestos, smoking and lung cancer: An update. *Int. J. Environ. Res. Public Health* **2019**, *17*, 258. [CrossRef] [PubMed] [PubMed Central]
6. Grosche, B.; Kreuzer, M.; Kreisheimer, M.; Schnelzer, M.; Tschense, A. Lung cancer risk among German male uranium miners: A cohort study, 1946–1998. *Br. J. Cancer* **2006**, *95*, 1280–1287. [CrossRef] [PubMed]
7. Darby, S.; Hill, D.; Auvinen, A.; Barros-Dios, J.M.; Baysson, H.; Bochicchio, F.; Deo, H.; Falk, R.; Forastiere, F.; Hakama, M.; et al. Radon in homes and risk of lung cancer: Collaborative analysis of individual data from 13 European case-control studies. *BMJ* **2005**, *330*, 223. [CrossRef]
8. Siegel, R.L.; Miller, K.D.; Jemal, A. Cancer Statistics, 2017. *CA Cancer J. Clin.* **2017**, *67*, 7–30. [CrossRef]
9. Sung, H.; Ferlay, J.; Siegel, R.L.; Laversanne, M.; Soerjomataram, I.; Jemal, A.; Bray, F. Global Cancer Statistics 2020: GLOBOCAN Estimates of Incidence and Mortality Worldwide for 36 Cancers in 185 Countries. *CA Cancer J. Clin.* **2021**, *71*, 209–249. [CrossRef]
10. Barta, J.A.; Powell, C.A.; Wisnivesky, J.P. Global Epidemiology of Lung Cancer. *Ann. Glob. Health* **2019**, *85*, 8. [CrossRef]
11. Alberg, A.J.; Samet, J.M. Epidemiology of lung cancer. *Chest* **2003**, *123* (Suppl. S1), 21S–49S. [CrossRef]
12. de Groot, P.; Munden, R.F. Lung cancer epidemiology, risk factors, and prevention. *Radiol. Clin. North Am.* **2012**, *50*, 863–876. [CrossRef] [PubMed]
13. Lorigan, P.; Radford, J.; Howell, A.; Thatcher, N. Lung cancer after treatment for Hodgkin's lymphoma: A systematic review. *Lancet Oncol.* **2005**, *6*, 773–779. [CrossRef] [PubMed]
14. Burns, D.M. Primary prevention, smoking, and smoking cessation: Implications for future trends in lung cancer prevention. *Cancer* **2000**, *89* (Suppl. S11), 2506–2509. [CrossRef] [PubMed]

15. National Comprehensive Cancer Network. NCCN Clinical Practice Guidelines in Oncology (NCCN Guidelines®) Non-Small Cell Lung Cancer [Internet]. Version 4.2023—18 October 2023. Available online: https://www.nccn.org/professionals/physician_gls/pdf/nscl.pdf (accessed on 2 July 2024).
16. Nicholson, A.G.; Tsao, M.S.; Beasley, M.B.; Borczuk, A.C.; Brambilla, E.; Cooper, W.A.; Dacic, S.; Jain, D.; Kerr, K.M.; Lantuejoul, S.; et al. The 2021 WHO Classification of Lung Tumors: Impact of Advances Since 2015. *J. Thorac. Oncol.* **2022**, *17*, 362–387. [CrossRef] [PubMed]
17. Travis, W.D.; Brambilla, E.; Nicholson, A.G.; Yatabe, Y.; Austin, J.H.M.; Beasley, M.B.; Chirieac, L.R.; Dacic, S.; Duhig, E.; Flieder, D.B.; et al. The 2015 World Health Organization Classification of Lung Tumors: Impact of Genetic, Clinical and Radiologic Advances Since the 2004 Classification. *J. Thorac. Oncol.* **2015**, *10*, 1243–1260. [CrossRef] [PubMed]
18. Cagle, P.T.; Allen, T.C.; Olsen, R.J. Lung cancer biomarkers: Present status and future developments. *Arch. Pathol. Lab. Med.* **2013**, *137*, 1191–1198. [CrossRef]
19. Lindeman, N.I.; Cagle, P.T.; Beasley, M.B.; Chitale, D.A.; Dacic, S.; Giaccone, G.; Jenkins, R.B.; Kwiatkowski, D.J.; Saldivar, J.-S.; Squire, J.; et al. Molecular testing guideline for selection of lung cancer patients for EGFR and ALK tyrosine kinase inhibitors: Guideline from the College of American Pathologists, International Association for the Study of Lung Cancer, and Association for Molecular Pathology. *J. Mol. Diagn.* **2013**, *15*, 415–453.
20. Lindeman, N.I.; Cagle, P.T.; Aisner, D.L.; Arcila, M.E.; Beasley, M.B.; Bernicker, E.H.; Colasacco, C.; Dacic, S.; Hirsch, F.R.; Kerr, K.; et al. Updated Molecular Testing Guideline for the Selection of Lung Cancer Patients for Treatment With Targeted Tyrosine Kinase Inhibitors. *J. Mol. Diagn.* **2018**, *20*, 129–159. [CrossRef]
21. Ekin, Z.; Nart, D.; Savaş, P.; Veral, A. Comparison of PD-L1, EGFR, ALK, and ROS1 Status Between Surgical Samples and Cytological Samples in Non-Small Cell Lung Carcinoma. *Balk. Med. J.* **2021**, *38*, 287–295.
22. Pawelczyk, K.; Piotrowska, A.; Ciesielska, U.; Jablonska, K.; Glatzel-Plucinska, N.; Grzegrzolka, J.; Podhorska-Okolow, M.; Dziegiel, P.; Nowinska, K. Role of PD-L1 Expression in Non-Small Cell Lung Cancer and Their Prognostic Significance According to Clinicopathological Factors and Diagnostic Markers. *Int. J. Mol. Sci.* **2019**, *20*, 824. [CrossRef]
23. ECOG-ACRIN Cancer Research Group. ECOG Performance Status Scale [Internet]. Available online: https://ecog-acrin.org/resources/ecog-performance-status/ (accessed on 21 May 2024).
24. Ministerio de Salud y Protección Social. RESOLUCION NUMERO 8430 DE 1993 [Internet]. Available online: https://www.minsalud.gov.co/sites/rid/Lists/BibliotecaDigital/RIDE/DE/DIJ/RESOLUCION-8430-DE-1993.pdf (accessed on 24 May 2024).
25. World Medical Association. WMA Declaration of Helsinki–Ethical Principles for Medical Research Involving Human Subjects [Internet]. Available online: https://www.wma.net/policies-post/wma-declaration-of-helsinki-ethical-principles-for-medical-research-involving-human-subjects/ (accessed on 24 May 2024).
26. Park, E.; Kang, H.Y.; Lim, M.K.; Kim, B.; Oh, J.K. Cancer Risk Following Smoking Cessation in Korea. *JAMA Netw. Open* **2024**, *7*, e2354958. [CrossRef] [PubMed] [PubMed Central]
27. Matilla, J.M.; Zabaleta, M.; Martínez-Téllez, E.; Abal, J.; Rodríguez-Fuster, A.; Hernández-Hernández, J. New TNM staging in lung cancer (8th edition) and future perspectives. *J. Clin. Transl. Res.* **2020**, *6*, 145–154. [PubMed] [PubMed Central]
28. Schrevens, L.; Lorent, N.; Dooms, C.; Vansteenkiste, J. The role of PET scan in diagnosis, staging, and management of non-small cell lung cancer. *Oncologist* **2004**, *9*, 633–643. [CrossRef] [PubMed]
29. Vansteenkiste, J.F.; Stroobants, S.S. PET scan in lung cancer: Current recommendations and innovation. *J. Thorac. Oncol.* **2006**, *1*, 71–73. [CrossRef] [PubMed]
30. Vansteenkiste, J.F. PET scan in the staging of non-small cell lung cancer. *Lung Cancer* **2003**, *42* (Suppl. S1), 27–37. [CrossRef] [PubMed]
31. Hutchinson, L. Targeted therapies: Defining the best-in-class in NSCLC. *Nat. Rev. Clin. Oncol.* **2017**, *14*, 457. [CrossRef] [PubMed]
32. Uemura, T.; Hida, T. Alectinib can replace crizotinib as standard first-line therapy for ALK-positive lung cancer. *Ann. Transl. Med.* **2017**, *5*, 433. [CrossRef] [PubMed] [PubMed Central]
33. Paik, J.; Dhillon, S. Alectinib: A Review in Advanced, ALK-Positive NSCLC. *Drugs* **2018**, *78*, 1247–1257. [CrossRef] [PubMed]
34. Rossi, A. Alectinib for ALK-positive non-small-cell lung cancer. *Expert Rev. Clin. Pharmacol.* **2016**, *9*, 1005–1013. [CrossRef] [PubMed]
35. Ramalingam, S.S.; Vansteenkiste, J.; Planchard, D.; Cho, B.C.; Gray, J.E.; Ohe, Y.; Zhou, C.; Reungwetwattana, T.; Cheng, Y.; Chewaskulyong, B.; et al. Overall Survival with Osimertinib in Untreated, EGFR-Mutated Advanced NSCLC. *N. Engl. J. Med.* **2020**, *382*, 41–50. [CrossRef] [PubMed]
36. Soria, J.C.; Ohe, Y.; Vansteenkiste, J.; Reungwetwattana, T.; Chewaskulyong, B.; Lee, K.H.; Dechaphunkul, A.; Imamura, F.; Nogami, N.; Kurata, T.; et al. Osimertinib in Untreated EGFR-Mutated Advanced Non-Small-Cell Lung Cancer. *N. Engl. J. Med.* **2018**, *378*, 113–125. [CrossRef] [PubMed]
37. Bollinger, M.K.; Agnew, A.S.; Mascara, G.P. Osimertinib: A third-generation tyrosine kinase inhibitor for treatment of epidermal growth factor receptor-mutated non-small cell lung cancer with the acquired Thr790Met mutation. *J. Oncol. Pharm. Pract.* **2018**, *24*, 379–388. [CrossRef] [PubMed]
38. Mok, T.S.; Wu, Y.-L.; Ahn, M.-J.; Garassino, M.C.; Kim, H.R.; Ramalingam, S.S.; Shepherd, F.A.; He, Y.; Akamatsu, H.; Theelen, W.S.M.E.; et al. Osimertinib or Platinum-Pemetrexed in EGFR T790M-Positive Lung Cancer. *N. Engl. J. Med.* **2017**, *376*, 629–640. [CrossRef] [PubMed]

39. Tiu, B.C.; Zubiri, L.; Iheke, J.; Pahalyants, V.; Theodosakis, N.; Ugwu-Dike, P.; Seo, J.; Tang, K.; Sise, M.E.; Sullivan, R.; et al. Real-world incidence and impact of pneumonitis in patients with lung cancer treated with immune checkpoint inhibitors: A multi-institutional cohort study. *J. Immunother. Cancer* **2022**, *10*, e004670. [CrossRef] [PubMed]

40. Käsmann, L.; Dietrich, A.; Staab-Weijnitz, C.A.; Manapov, F.; Behr, J.; Rimner, A.; Jeremic, B.; Senan, S.; De Ruysscher, D.; Lauber, K.; et al. Radiation-induced lung toxicity-cellular and molecular mechanisms of pathogenesis, management, and literature review. *Radiat. Oncol.* **2020**, *15*, 214. [CrossRef] [PubMed]

Disclaimer/Publisher's Note: The statements, opinions and data contained in all publications are solely those of the individual author(s) and contributor(s) and not of MDPI and/or the editor(s). MDPI and/or the editor(s) disclaim responsibility for any injury to people or property resulting from any ideas, methods, instructions or products referred to in the content.

MDPI AG
Grosspeteranlage 5
4052 Basel
Switzerland
Tel.: +41 61 683 77 34

Journal of Clinical Medicine Editorial Office
E-mail: jcm@mdpi.com
www.mdpi.com/journal/jcm

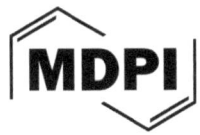

Disclaimer/Publisher's Note: The title and front matter of this reprint are at the discretion of the Guest Editor. The publisher is not responsible for their content or any associated concerns. The statements, opinions and data contained in all individual articles are solely those of the individual Editor and contributors and not of MDPI. MDPI disclaims responsibility for any injury to people or property resulting from any ideas, methods, instructions or products referred to in the content.

www.ingramcontent.com/pod-product-compliance
Lightning Source LLC
LaVergne TN
LVHW072352090526
838202LV00019B/2530